T0260254

CRC Desk Reference
for ALLERGY and ASTHMA

CRC Desk Reference Series

Series Editor
Gerald Kerkut
University of Southampton
Southampton, England

Published Titles

CRC Desk Reference for Nutrition
Carolyn Berdanier, University of Georgia, Athens, Georgia

CRC Desk Reference of Clinical Pharmacology
Manuchair Ebadi, University of Nebraska, Omaha, Nebraska

CRC Desk Reference for Hematology
N. K. Shinton, University of Warwick, Coventry, United Kingdom

CRC Desk Reference for Allergy and Asthma
Hans-Uwe Simon, University of Zurich, Davos, Switzerland

CRC Desk Reference
for ALLERGY *and* ASTHMA

Hans-Uwe Simon, M.D.
Assistant Professor of Immunology
Swiss Institute of Allergy and Asthma Research (SIAF)
University of Zurich
Davos, Switzerland

With contributions by
Cezmi A. Akdis
Laura Armetti
Thomas Bieber
Martin D. Chapman
Anthony J. Frew
Hillel S. Koren
Francesca Levi-Schaffer
Simon M. McHugh
Gerald Messer
Marie O'Neill
David Peden
Dagmar Simon
Alisa M. Smith
Elisabeth H. Weiss
Andreas Wollenberg
Donata Vercelli

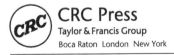

CRC Press
Taylor & Francis Group
Boca Raton London New York

CRC Press is an imprint of the
Taylor & Francis Group, an **informa** business

CRC Press
Taylor & Francis Group
6000 Broken Sound Parkway NW, Suite 300
Boca Raton, FL 33487-2742

© 2000 by Taylor & Francis Group, LLC
CRC Press is an imprint of Taylor & Francis Group, an Informa business

No claim to original U.S. Government works

ISBN-13: 9780849396847 (Hardback)

Visit the Taylor & Francis Web site at
http://www.taylorandfrancis.com

and the CRC Press Web site at
http://www.crcpress.com

Library of Congress Cataloging-in-Publication Data

CRC desk reference for allergy and asthma / [edited by] Hans-Uwe Simon ; with contributions by Cezmi A. Akdis ... [et al.].
    p.   cm. — (CRC desk reference series)
    ISBN 0-8493-9684-0
        1. Allergy—Encyclopedias. 2. Asthma—Encyclopedias. I. Simon, Hans-Uwe. II. Akdis, Cezmi A. III. Series.

RC585.C74 2000
616.97'003—dc21

99-058426
CIP

THE EDITOR

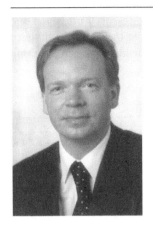

Hans-Uwe Simon, M.D., is assistant professor of immunology at the University of Zurich as well as deputy director and head of asthma research at the Swiss Institute of Allergy and Asthma Research (SIAF), located in Davos. He earned an M.Sc. in 1984 and an M.D. degree in 1986, both in pharmacology from the University of Jena, Germany. From 1986 to 1990, he was trained in clinical immunology at the same university. He completed his postdoctoral training at research units of the Mount Sinai Hospital and General Hospital in Toronto, Canada, between 1990 and 1992. He has been on the staff of SIAF since December 1992.

Dr. Simon's research has focused on the role of apoptosis in inflammatory disorders. In particular, he has investigated pathogenic mechanisms in bronchial asthma, atopic dermatitis, idiopathic eosinophilia, and cystic fibrosis. He developed the general concept of delayed apoptosis causing accumulation of effector cells in inflammatory responses. Furthermore, he defined a subgroup of patients with idiopathic eosinophilia that is characterized by abnormal clones of T cells producing interleukin-5. He continues to work in the field of inflammation and manages research programs in immunology, pharmacology, biochemistry, and molecular biology.

He has presented more than 50 invitational lectures at international meetings and has published more than 100 papers and book chapters. During his academic career, Dr. Simon has received 17 awards, including the Paul-Martini-Prize (1997) and an honorable mention from the Pharmacia Allergy Research Foundation (1998). His research has been supported by many organizations including the Swiss National Science Foundation.

Dr. Simon is a member of 14 international scientific societies, including the American Academy of Allergy, Asthma & Immunology (AAAAI) and the European Academy of Allergology and Clinical Immunology (EAACI). He serves on the editorial boards of several journals, including *Allergy, International Archives of Allergy and Immunology, Allergologie* and *Apoptosis*.

ACKNOWLEDGMENTS

The authors would like to thank and express their appreciation to Professors Kurt Blaser and Brunello Wüthrich as well as the co-workers of Hans-Uwe Simon at the Swiss Institute of Allergy and Asthma Research in Davos for critical reading and comments on the manuscript.

CONTRIBUTORS

Professor Cezmi A. Akdis
Swiss Institute of Allergy and Asthma
  Research (SIAF)
University of Zurich
Davos, Switzerland

Dr. Laura Armetti
Department of Pharmacology
Hadassah Medical School
The Hebrew University
Jerusalem, Israel

Professor Thomas Bieber
Department of Dermatology
University of Bonn
Bonn, Germany

Professor Martin D. Chapman
Asthma and Allergic Diseases Center
University of Virginia HSC
Charlottesville, Virginia

Dr. Anthony J. Frew
Southampton General Hospital
University of Southampton
Southampton, England, United Kingdom

Dr. Hillel S. Koren
National Health and Environmental Effects
  Research Laboratory
U.S. Environmental Protection Agency
Research Triangle Park,
North Carolina

Professor Francesca Levi-Schaffer
Department of Pharmacology
Hadassah Medical School
The Hebrew University
Jerusalem, Israel

Dr. Simon M. McHugh
Clinical Research Unit
Addenbrooke's Centre for Clinical
  Investigation
Addenbrooke's Hospital
Cambridge, England, United Kingdom

Dr. Gerald Messer
Department of Dermatology
University of Munich
Munich, Germany

Dr. Marie O'Neill
National Health and Environmental Effects
  Research Laboratory
U.S. Environmental Protection Agency
Research Triangle Park, North Carolina

Dr. David Peden
Center for Environmental Medicine and
  Lung Biology
University of North Carolina at Chapel Hill
Chapel Hill, North Carolina

Dr. Dagmar Simon
Clinic for Dermatology and Allergy
  (Alexanderhausklinik)
Davos, Switzerland

Dr. Hans-Uwe Simon
Swiss Institute of Allergy and Asthma
  Research (SIAF)
University of Zurich
Davos, Switzerland

Dr. Alisa M. Smith
Asthma and Allergic Diseases Center
University of Virginia HSC
Charlottesville, Virginia

Professor Elisabeth H. Weiss
Institute for Anthropology and Genetics
University of Munich
Munich, Germany

Dr. Andreas Wollenberg
Department of Dermatology
University of Munich
Munich, Germany

Dr. Donata Vercelli
Molecular Immunoregulation Unit
San Raffaele Scientific Institute
Milan, Italy

SERIES PREFACE

This series of volumes will form a set of concise medical science encyclopedias.

Very few people read a medical or science book right through from cover to cover. They tend to dip into the book, reading a few pages here and a few pages there. More often they look up subjects in the index at the back of the book and with a finger in the index page, they look up the different page references, often having difficulty in finding the reference subject on the given page. This is partly because an index usually gives the page references in numerical order (though the more important references are often printed in bold) and partly because the indexer likes to give every possible reference, major, minor, and minuscule.

The present book is in effect an annotated index. The topics are arranged in alphabetical order, so that they are easy to find. The intention is that each topic should be concise so that after having read it, the reader will be able to remember the important information in that topic. There is a "take away message." Too often in larger encyclopedias, the item has to be read several times to get the key information, i.e., such books are discursive instead of didactic. The intention in the present book is to give the time-pressed reader the necessary data quickly and concisely.

On the other hand, some subjects have to be discussed in more detail to provide the background information necessary to give a fuller understanding of the subject.

In addition the book contains "orientation" subjects that give the background and bring the reader up to date. Medicine and science advance very quickly these days and although recent graduates can be assumed to have the modern information, even those graduating 5 years ago can sometimes find themselves unsure about new facts, ideas, and terminology that are now currently mentioned in the news and have come into vogue.

It is difficult to get a correct balance between being sufficiently informative so as to be useful, being too concise so that the required information is not present, and being so long that the reader can't find the time to read the item.

It is hoped that these Desk References get near the correct balance and will be useful sources of information for the reader.

Gerald Kerkut
Series Editor

PREFACE

The prevalence of allergic diseases and asthma has increased in recent years. This has stimulated intensive research to understand the pathogenesis of these diseases. Indeed, researchers have provided key insights and new concepts that have also changed therapeutic strategies. Moreover, allergic inflammation has been something of a model that helps to further the understanding of regulatory mechanisms of inflammation in general. Here, I would like to mention just a few examples. Allergy research has contributed significantly to our current knowledge in intracellular and extracellular mechanisms of anergy, immunoglobulin class switching, and maturation of antigen-presenting cells. Moreover, the general role of delayed apoptosis to accumulate inflammatory cells as well as the biological functions of at least some cytokines (e.g., IL-4, IL-5, IL-10, IL-13) would not have been fully elucidated without studying allergic inflammation. Finally, immunotherapy represents the only utilized antigen-specific treatment in humans at the moment and, therefore, the insights obtained here are applicable to other forms of vaccination.

This book was conceived as a guide for a broad readership of medical and science students, clinicians, and researchers. It provides the latest scientific information about allergic and asthmatic diseases and considers clinical and basic science issues, both of which are presented as clearly as possible. Thus, we have tried to combine knowledge from clinical immunology and allergology with basic immunology, pharmacology, biochemistry, and molecular biology. The authors have also incorporated all newly discussed treatment strategies of allergic and asthmatic diseases. In addition, we summarized certain issues by collecting all available data and presented them in unique ways (e.g., mechanisms that limit inflammation, immunotherapy, Th1/Th2 markers, classification of urticaria, etc.). At the moment, such synthesis cannot be found in any other text.

The form of this book as an encyclopedia may have helped us to switch rapidly between basic and clinical science and demonstrate the close links between them. This could be achieved by cross-referencing, and we hope that the form we have chosen is easy to use. Very important information is highlighted in boxes, allowing rapid identification of key concepts. The organization of the book demanded a unified nomenclature throughout that will greatly assist those readers who are new in the field. Moreover, we avoided the excessive overlap and controversial presentation of issues that are usually the major problems of textbooks. Instead, information is given in a readily accessible format. Although written by many authors, special care was taken to achieve a consistent style.

There are several methods of continuing education. However, a textbook in the form of an encyclopedia, constantly present on the desk, might be indispensable. It has been my good fortune to obtain the collaboration of many well-recognized individuals in the field for this project. We hope that this work will have genuine value as a standard reference book for all individuals who are interested in allergy and asthma. Since many of the hot topics and views that we mention here were not widely published as we finished this book, we believe that it will have sustaining value in the upcoming years.

I welcome comments and criticisms from readers.

Hans-Uwe Simon, M.D.
January 2000

How to Use This Book

Entries that are of clinical or scientific importance are listed in alphabetical order. More information on a particular subject can be obtained when words are printed in *italic*. Italic indicates that there is another related entry available in this book. All *links* are given only once within one entry, although the term might be mentioned several times. We hope that this organization of *cross-referencing* will assist the reader in obtaining maximal information. "Quick" readers will find very important information in boxes. Figures and tables are included to provide concise yet comprehensive information. Because this is an alphabetical list of terms, there is no index.

LIST OF TABLES

LIST OF FIGURES

A

AAAAI

American Academy of Allergy, Asthma, and Immunology.

ABPA

(See *allergic bronchopulmonary aspergillosis.*)

ACANTHOSIS

Diffuse hyperplasia and thickening of the prickle cell layer of the *epidermis*; a common histologic finding in chronic cutaneous *inflammation*.

ACARICIDES

Acaricides are *pesticides* that kill *house-dust mites*.

ACE

(See *angiotensin-converting enzyme.*)

ACETYLCHOLINE

Acetylcholine is a neurotransmitter (see *nervous system*) of the vagus nerve that mediates its functional effects by binding to *muscarinic receptors*. Acetylcholine stimulation results in contraction of the myoepithelial cells surrounding bronchial submucosal glands and therefore in *airway obstruction.*

Acetylcholine can be used in *bronchial provocation tests* to measure *airway hyperresponsiveness.*

Besides airway *smooth muscle* cells, inflammatory cells such as *mast cells* can also be activated by acetylcholine. The effects of acetylcholine are reversed by *anticholinergic drugs*. Such drugs are useful in the treatment of *asthma* and *COPD.*

ACETYLCYSTEINE

This drug belongs to the group of sulfhydryl agents, which have a mucolytic effect (see *mucus*) due to their ability to cleave disulfide bonds.

ACETYLSALICYLIC ACID (ASA)

(See *aspirin.*)

ACID AEROSOLS

Acid *aerosols* are often the consequence of *air pollution*. They are mainly comprised of sulfuric acid (H_2SO_4) and its partial neutralization product, ammonium bisulfate, but also nitric oxide, hydrochloric acid, and hydroxymethanesulfonic acid. Most H_2SO_4 is derived from *sulfur dioxide* (SO_2) and is present in the air as droplets. The concentrations of acid in the ambient air are difficult to measure. Concentrations of sulfate or SO_2 are often used as surrogates for levels of acidity.

ACID HYDROLASES

In *phagocytes*, acid hydrolases play an important role in the lysosomal degradation of ingested material. Since *mast cell granules* are an important source of these enzymes such as *β-glucuronidase*, *β-D-galactosidase*, and *arylsulfatase*, there is some evidence that a similar mechanism may be maintained in mast cells. Acid hydrolases have an optimal activity within an acid pH range, which prevails in inflammatory processes such as *allergic inflammation*.

ACOUSTIC RHINOMETRY

This method measures cross-sectional areas of the nasal airways by sending a sound pulse, which is reflected by nose structures. The reflected signal is recorded by a microphone and then analyzed.

ACQUIRED IMMUNODEFICIENCY SYNDROME (AIDS)

AIDS was identified in a group of homosexual men in 1981. The causative agent, human immunodeficiency virus (HIV), was identified 2 years later. HIV infects *CD4+ T cells* via specific ligation to the CD4 molecule. It also infects *macrophages*, where it can replicate successfully after uptake by *phagocytosis* and successfully avoid the attentions of *CD8+* cytotoxic T cells.

CD4+ T cells undergo depletion and dysfunction during the course of an HIV infection.

T cell depletion occurs by several different mechanisms. The most evident is syncytium formation, whereby syncytia are formed between infected and uninfected CD4+ cells, thus removing a large number from the circulation. Other CD4+ cells die as a result of disruption of their *DNA* function by nonintegrated or poorly integrated HIV viral DNA. Infected CD4+ T cells, macrophages, and follicular *dendritic cells* can also be eliminated by cytotoxic T cells and *NK cells*. Inhibition of CD4+ T cell expansion, resulting in apparent depletion, may also occur by a variety of mechanisms. *Antibodies* to gp120 (a surface expressed HIV glycopeptide) can cross-react with *major histocompatibility complex* (MHC) DR and DQ molecules and "block" effective MHC class II *antigen presentation* to CD4+ T cells. Alternatively, gp120 or gp120 *immune complexes* may bind directly to CD4 and induce either *anergy* or *apoptosis*.

There is some evidence for *Th1* to *Th2 cytokine* switching within the T cell compartment as AIDS progresses. Clinically, this may be expressed as a recurrence of childhood *allergies*, an emergence of new allergic sensitivity (see *sensitization*), and *eosinophilia*.

Th1 to Th2 cytokine switching is usually transient. The evidence that this switch occurs within the CD4+ T cell compartment is not good. CD4+ T cells from AIDS patients are able to secrete both Th1 and Th2 cytokines after appropriate stimulation.

There is evidence that CD8+ T cells may be induced to switch from a predominantly *Tc1* functional phenotype to a *Tc2* cytokine-producing profile, resulting in reduced cytolytic activity and supplementation of the depleted CD4–Th2 help for *B cell immunoglobulin* production.

The mechanisms for such a switch are unclear but may be related to anergic depletion of cytotoxic CD8+ T cells by the production, expression, and release of high levels of HIV proteins. CD8+ T cells are not infected by HIV, and their relative number and activity tend to increase in early infection. They have increased cytolytic activity and have been shown to secrete high levels of *IFN-γ*. IFN-γ activates macrophages but, paradoxically, this hastens the spread of HIV into the macrophage population where it possesses mechanisms of cytolytic avoidance, as described above. Infected CD4+ T cells may not be so fortunate. NK activity directed against macrophages is also suppressed by HIV infection, as well as the HIV-infected macrophage *IL-12* production (which enhances NK activity). The pro-inflammatory cytokines *TNF-α, IL-1*, and *IL-6*, often released by *monocytes* and macrophages as an acute response to infection, tend to upregulate HIV replication in macrophages (IL-6) and T cells (TNF-α). In contrast, *TGF-β* and IFN-γ inhibit viral replication, but are steadily reduced during disease progression.

ACRYLATES

Acrylates are low-molecular-weight agents, which may cause *occupational asthma* or *contact dermatitis*. They are used in glues by surgeons and by dentists as fillers.

ACTIVATOR PROTEIN 1 (AP-1)

AP-1 is an inducible *transcription factor* that binds to *promoter* or enhancer regions of many *cytokine genes*, often in close association with the *nuclear factor of activated T cells* (NF-AT).

AP-1 is composed of c-fos and c-jun or c-jun/c-jun homodimers.

AP-1 binding has been demonstrated as obligatory for NF-AT-mediated *cytokine gene activation* in many cases. The *signal transduction* pathway responsible for AP-1 activation involves jun and p38 kinase (see *mitogen-activated protein kinase*). Cytokine genes known to have functional AP-1 binding motifs include *IL-2, IL-4, IL-5, TNF*, and *GM-CSF* promoter regions, as well as GM-CSF and *IL-3 enhancer* regions.

ACTIVATION-INDUCED APOPTOSIS

(See *T cell apoptosis*.)

ACUPUNCTURE

Acupuncture as a treatment for *allergic diseases* belongs to the *complementary procedures*.

ACUTE URTICARIA

Any form of *urticaria* lasting for less than 6 weeks. In contrast to chronic urticaria, acute urticaria is no indication for an in-depth general workup of a patient.

ADENINE

A purine base that is an essential component of *DNA*. When it is joined to ribose via a phosphate bond, it becomes adenyl-*nucleotide* or forms *adenosine*.

ADENOSINE

Adenosine is a nucleoside and consists of *adenine* in glycosidic linkage with ribose. Most adenosine is derived from cleavage of adenosine 5′-monophosphate (AMP) by membrane-associated 5′-nucleotidase. However, the majority of AMP is phosphorylated to ADP or ATP during the process of energy generation. All cells contain adenosine.

Some adenosine diffuses out of the cell and may then stimulate adenosine *receptors* on target cells.

Indeed, adenosine was shown to cause *airway obstruction* in patients with *asthma*. Moreover, increased adenosine concentrations were found in *bronchoalveolar lavage* (BAL) fluids of asthmatics. The adenosine-mediated bronchoconstriction in asthma is, at least partially, mediated via *mast cells*, where adenosine induces *signal transduction* pathways, which include activation of *phospholipase C* (PLC) and *calcium mobilization*. Of the known adenosine receptors A1, A2α, A2β, and A3, the latter three have been identified in *rat basophilic leukemia cells* (RBL-2H3) and *bone-marrow-derived mast cells* (BMMC). Activation of A2β and A3 receptors results in increased *mediator*-mediated *degranulation*. Besides transient activation of PLC, activation of adenosine receptor(s) leads to sustained *pertussis toxin*-sensitive activation of *phospholipase D* (PLD) and *protein kinase C* (PKC). The latter two events are believed to be important for the effects of adenosine agonists on degranulation of mast cells. Moreover, an extremely high expression of A3 receptors has been observed on the surface of *eosinophils*. *Antisense* molecules that abolished A1 receptor expression reduced *allergen*-induced bronchoconstriction in a rabbit *asthma* model.

ADENYLATE CYCLASE

Adenylate cyclase forms *cAMP* from ATP. It is a protein of the plasma membrane. Activation of *G protein-coupled receptors* activates not only *phospholipase C* (PLC), but often *adenylate cyclase*. For instance, binding of *catecholamines* such as fenoterol to *β-adrenergic receptors* increases cAMP levels.

> *Phosphodiesterase inhibitors* such as *theophylline* should act synergistically with *β2-agonists* that use cAMP as a second messenger.

ADHERENCE

The extent to which a patient follows an agreed plan of management, as distinct from *compliance*, which is following the doctor's instructions.

ADHESION MOLECULES

> Adhesion molecules allow the *migration* of inflammatory cells from the circulation to tissues and facilitate cell–cell interactions within tissues.

Adhesion molecules are inducible or constitutive proteins or glycoproteins expressed on the surface of many cell types, but are normally associated with lymphoid tissues. They play a major role in *leukocyte homing* to inflammatory lesions and initiate the process of transen-dothelial migration (diapodesis). As their name suggests, they mediate adhesion, including interactions between leukocytes and other cells of the *immune system*, and between leukocytes and *endothelial cells* as well as the *extracellular matrix*. Specific signals produced in response to wounding and infection control the expression and activation of certain adhesion molecules. The interactions and responses then initiated by the binding of adhesion molecules to their *receptors*/ligands play important roles in the mediation of the inflammatory and immune reactions that constitute one line of the body's defense against these insults. Most of the adhesion molecules characterized so far fall into three general families of proteins; the *immunoglobulin* (Ig) *superfamily*, the *integrin* family, or the *selectin* family.

The Ig superfamily of adhesion molecules — including *intercellular adhesion molecule-1* (ICAM-1), ICAM-2, ICAM-3, *vascular cell adhesion molecule-1* (VCAM-1), and the addressin MAdCAM-1 — bind to integrins on leukocytes and mediate their flattening onto the blood vessel wall with their subsequent extravasation into the surrounding tissue. *Chemo-kines* such as *MCP-1* and *IL-8* cause a conformational change in integrins so that they can bind to their ligands.

> Integrins serve as receptors for ICAMs and VCAMs.

The integrins are heterodimeric proteins consisting of an α- and a β-chain that mediate leukocyte adherence to the vascular endothelium or other cell–cell interactions. Different sets of integrins are expressed by different populations of leukocytes to provide specificity for binding to different types of adhesion molecules expressed along the vascular endothelium. For example, the $\alpha_4\beta_1$ integrin adhesion molecule, *very late antigen* (VLA)-4, expressed on *eosinophils, basophils*, and *T cells*, is the ligand for VCAM-1 on endothelial cells. Therefore, upregulation of specific adhesion molecules allows for modulation of the degree and type (neutrophilic or eosinophilic) of inflammatory response within a given tissue.

The selectin family members, *L-selectin, P-selectin*, and *E-selectin* are also involved in the adhesion of leukocytes to activated endothelium of postcapillary venules.

> Adhesion by selectins is characterized by weak interactions that produce the initial "rolling" motion of leukocytes on the endothelial surface before migration.

P-selectin and L-selectin, acting in concert, have been implicated in the mediation of weak initial interactions. Stronger interactions, probably involving E-selectin, follow the initial interactions, leading eventually to extravasation through the blood vessel walls into lymphoid tissues and sites of *inflammation*. These molecules mediate the adhesion and migration of different leukocytes through endothelial and epithelial barriers and are central in the development of *allergic inflammation* and *airway hyperresponsiveness*.

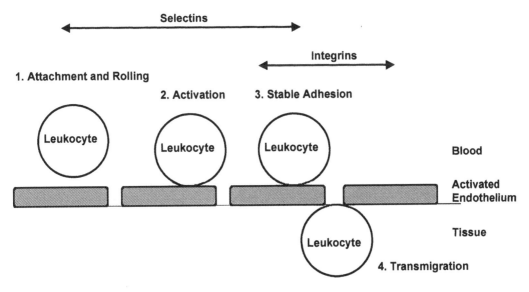

FIGURE 1 The four-step model of leukocyte recruitment into inflammatory tissues. Selectins and integrins expressed on leukocytes act in sequence with some overlap. Use of different molecules may generate some specificity in inflammatory cell recruitment. In addition, chemotactic factors are needed for both activation and transendothelial migration of leukocytes.

ADRENALINE

Adrenaline is a hormone produced by the adrenal medulla. It is a major component of the adrenergic inhibitory system of the lung (see also *nervous system*). Adrenaline is the drug of first choice for severe *anaphylactic reactions* and is also indicated for severe *airway obstruction*, laryngeal *edema*, severe *urticaria*, or *angioedema*. By stimulating α-adrenoceptors (see *adrenergic receptors*), it may reverse peripheral vasodilation observed in edema and urticaria. As a *β2-agonist*, adrenaline dilates the airways and suppresses *histamine* and *leukotriene* release.

High-risk allergy patients should be provided with easily injectable adrenaline or an *aerosol* inhaler for self-administration.

ADRENERGIC AGENTS

(See *β2-agonists.*)

ADRENERGIC RECEPTORS

Adrenergic *receptors* are divided into α, β1, and β2 subtypes. α-Receptors are found on vascular *smooth muscle* and induce vasoconstriction. β1-Receptors are present in the heart and induce tachycardia when stimulated. β2-Receptors are present on smooth muscle and cause relaxation when stimulated. *Adrenaline* and *noradrenaline* (see *nervous system*) stimulate all three receptors. *β2-Agonists* selectively activate β2-receptors. β2-Receptors are *G-protein-coupled receptors*, which stimulate *calcium mobilization*, *cAMP*, and *mitogen-activated protein kinase* (MAPK) pathways. The adapter protein *arrestin* has been identified to connect G protein-coupled receptors with *tyrosine kinase* pathways in β2-receptor *signal transduction*.

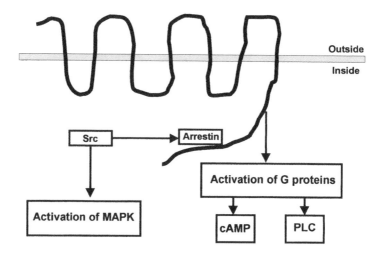

FIGURE 2   Signal transduction pathways initiated by β2-receptors.

ADULT-ONSET ASTHMA

A second age range in which *asthma* onset has been reported is in young adults. Unlike children with asthma, less than 50% of adult-onset asthmatics have an identifiable allergic trigger (see *intrinsic asthma*).

ADVERSE DRUG REACTIONS

Adverse drug reactions are unexpected, undesirable reactions and can be classified as (1) immunologic reactions due to humoral or cell-mediated reactions (see *drug allergy*), (2) *idiosyncrasy*, and (3) pharmacological reactions (see *intolerance*).

ADVERSE FOOD REACTIONS

Adverse reactions to food include toxic and nontoxic reactions after ingestion of food (see Table 1). Toxic food reaction may derive from the general toxicity to humans of substances that contaminate or are naturally present in the food. In contrast, nontoxic food reactions depend on an individual's susceptibility (see *food allergy* and *food intolerance*).

TABLE 1
Adverse Reaction to Food

1. Toxic
2. Nontoxic
   - Allergic
     – *IgE*-mediated
     – Non-IgE-mediated
   - Nonallergic
     – Enzymatic
     – Pharmacological
     – Undefined

AEROALLERGENS

Aeroallergens have special aerodynamic properties and are present in the air.

Indoor allergens

The aerodynamic properties of indoor allergens have been studied in experimental rooms and in homes using impactors (Cascade impactor or Anderson sampler), liquid impingers, or personal air samplers. *House-dust mite* feces contain high concentrations of the Group 1 allergens (~10 mg/ml) and become airborne following disturbance of the dust, e.g., by *vacuum cleaning*, bed-making, etc. These particles are about the same size as *pollen* grains (10 to 40 μm diameter). However, mite feces are only transiently present in the air.

Airborne mite allergen cannot be detected in the air under "undisturbed" conditions, and even after vigorous disturbance, the allergen falls rapidly and usually cannot be detected 30 to 40 min post-disturbance.

Cockroach allergen particles have aerodynamic properties similar to mite allergens in that they are >10 μm diameter and only detectable following disturbance. The precise nature of cockroach allergen particles is not known. Although some cockroach allergens are present in feces, the feces are too large to become airborne. Another possibility is that cockroach secretions contain allergen, which then becomes coated onto dust particles or forms dried flakes that can then become airborne.

Cat and *dog allergens* can usually be detected in houses under undisturbed conditions.

A significant proportion (20 to 50%) of both Fel d 1 and Can f 1 is found on smaller particles of ~5 μm diameter, which tend to remain airborne for longer periods (2 to 4 hours), depending on the air exchange rate in the house or apartment. This finding is thought to explain why cat- or dog-allergic patients often experience allergic symptoms within a short time of entering a house containing these pets, whereas this temporal relationship between exposure and symptoms is unusual in mite- or cockroach-allergic patients. Similarly, animal handlers who are allergic to mice or rats can have immediate symptoms on entering a vivarium containing these animals. Rat and mouse urinary allergens occur on particles ~7 μm diameter. Thus, it is possible that the buoyancy of cat and dog allergens is fundamentally different from those of mite and cockroach allergens, such that larger (10 μm) particles from cats and dogs are less dense and hence capable of easier deposition into the lung.

Outdoor allergens

Exposure to *grass*, *tree*, and *weed pollens*, as well as to *fungal allergens*, is assessed by counting pollen grains or spores in the air using Rotorod samplers, or Hirst or Burkard volumetric spore traps (see *pollen counting*). Most pollen grains are from 10 to 50 μm in diameter and reach concentrations of 200 to 300 grains/m^3 at the height of the grass pollen season, which can last from 2 or 3 weeks to several months. Some trees produce more copious amounts of pollen, exceeding 1000 grains/m^3 (e.g., olive). Pollen grains comprise an outer envelope or excine made up of a biogenic polymer called sporopollenin that is highly resistant to degradation. Fresh pollen contains a cellulose-rich middle layer or intine, as well as an inner protoplast containing starch granules, genetic material, and other organelles. The outer excine contains one or more pores (~2 to 10 μm diameter) for transfer of genetic material and 1 to 3 furrows. Pollen release by wind pollinated (anemophilous) plants is promoted by rapidly moving air of low humidity. Once airborne, pollen grains cause allergic symptoms by impacting onto the conjunctiva, nasal mucosa, and buccal cavity and rapidly releasing soluble allergens.

Fungal spores range from 2 to 100 μm in length and may be single celled or contain cross walls giving rise to multiple cells within a single spore. Spore shape can vary from almost spherical (e.g., conidial spores of *Aspergillus*, 2 μm) to elongated, club-like spores (e.g., Alternaria, ~50 μm). Common outdoor fungi include Cladosporium, Sporobolomyces, Aspergillus, Alternaria, Penicillium, Epicoccum, Fusarium, and Basidiospores. These species are most often involved in causing *IgE*-mediated *allergic disease*. Fungal spore counts can be extremely high, up to 30,000 spores/m^3, and these can increase considerably as a result of agricultural and farming practices, such as wheat or corn harvesting (over 10^8 spores/m^3). Similar high concentrations of fungal spores can occur as a result of occupational exposure, e.g., in the timber industry, processing of plant fibers, organic waste and sewage composting (recycling), mushroom farms, etc.

AEROALLERGEN NETWORKS

In the U.S. and Europe, *aeroallergen* networks have been established for monitoring *pollen* (see *pollen counting*) and fungal spore counts (see *fungal allergens*) in different geographic areas (European Aeroallergen Network [EAN] and National Pollen Network [NPN] in the U.S.). These networks issue daily pollen counts or "advisories" to the media so that *hay fever* patients may take steps to reduce their exposure or take *antihistamines* to reduce symptoms.

AEROSOL

A fine mist generated by nebulization (see *nebulizer*) or a *metered dose inhaler*. Droplets in the range of 2 to 10 μm will deposit in the larger airways. Larger particles will impact in the oropharynx or trachea. Smaller droplets may reach the alveoli but will mostly be breathed out without affecting the subject.

AFFINITY

The binding strength between two molecules at a single site, e.g., between an antigenic determinant (see *epitope*) and an *antibody* (see also *avidity*).

AFFINITY MATURATION

(See *antibody affinity maturation.*)

AGONISTS (β2-AGONISTS)

This group of drugs is particularly effective in the treatment of *asthma* (see *asthma treatment strategies*).

> β2-Agonists act principally by relaxing the *smooth muscles* in the airways and are very effective in the relief of asthma-associated *wheeze.*

The beneficial properties of *adrenaline* (epinephrine) in asthma were discovered in the 1940s. *Aerosol* preparations of adrenaline and isoprenaline were widely used during the 1960s and were blamed for the epidemic of *asthma deaths* that occurred during the 1960s. In retrospect, there is some uncertainty about the true role of isoprenaline in causing the epidemic of asthma deaths, and many clinicians and researchers now believe that they were incorrectly blamed. More selective agents, targeting the β2-receptor only (see *adrenergic receptors* and *nervous system*), were developed and entered clinical use from 1969 onward. Salbutamol (albuterol) may be regarded as the class standard, but terbutaline, fenoterol, pirbuterol, reproterol, and rimiterol are all effective β2-agonists and have replaced the less selective β-agonists, ephedrine, isophrenaline, and orciprenaline, in the treatment of asthma. Fenoterol was heavily used in patients with severe asthma, especially in New Zealand and Canada, and at one stage was thought to carry an additional risk of fatality. This has now been disproved, and it is clear that the association of fenoterol with asthma deaths was due to its selective use in patients with severe disease and not to any intrinsic property of the drug. Bambuterol is a pro-drug of terbutaline and can be used as a long-acting oral formulation. Eformoterol and salmeterol are long-acting β2-agonists with a duration of action between 12 and 15 hours, in contrast to the 3- to 4-hour duration of the short-acting β2-agonists. Despite their relative selectivity for the β2-receptor, β2-agonists may cause tremor, tachycardia, and hypocalemia, especially when given by mouth.

> The mechanism of action of β2-agonists is believed to be related to the opening of specific *potassium channels*, causing a reduction in intracellular calcium ion concentration (see *calcium mobilization*) and an increase in *cAMP.*

In addition to the symptomatic relief in human bronchial asthma, some β2-agonists inhibit the *mediator* release from *mast cells*, at least in vitro. However, these effects may not be relevant in vivo because of the short duration of action of the drugs. In contrast, long-acting β2-agonists may prevent both the *early* and *late-phase reaction*, indicating possible antiinflammatory effects. On the other hand, β2-agonists have been reported to reduce *IL-12* production, and therefore they may maintain *allergic inflammation*. Hence, it is still unclear whether and in which direction β2-agonists influence the inflammatory response in asthma.

AIANE

(See *European Network on Aspirin-Induced Asthma.*)

AIDS

(See *acquired immunodeficiency syndrome.*)

AIR CONDITIONING SYSTEM

Air conditioning systems can be important sources of *allergens*, especially *fungal allergens*. *Humidifier* fever has variously been attributed to *IgE*-mediated *allergy* and *alveolitis* (see *extrinsic allergic alveolitis*) caused by different airborne microorganisms derived from contaminated humidifiers.

AIR FILTERS

Although air filters significantly reduce particulate matter, clinical studies have shown no or only marginal effect on symptom scores in patients with perennial *allergic rhinitis* and *asthma*.

AIR POLLUTION

Pollutants have a variety of adverse effects on the health of exposed persons. The pollutants commonly monitored by governmental agencies include *sulfur dioxide* (SO_2), *nitrogen dioxide* (NO_2), *ozone* (O_3), particulate matter less than 10 microns in size (*PM10*), *lead*, and *carbon monoxide* (CO).

The term *smog* describes an extensive increase of *outdoor air pollutants*.

With the advent of unleaded gasoline, environmental lead exposure has decreased substantially. Likewise, in many areas, SO_2, NO_2, and O_3 have decreased as well. Besides outdoor air pollutants, people are also exposed to a wide variety of *indoor air pollutants*. Certain special subpopulations, including asthmatics, children, and the elderly, may experience increased risk of infectious diseases due to pollutant exposure (see *pollution and infectious diseases*). Air pollution is also frequently discussed as an adjuvant factor for allergic *sensitization*, and is perhaps responsible for increased prevalence rates of *allergic diseases* in industrialized countries. Table 2 summarizes published work that suggests an effect of pollutants on the initiation and maintenance of allergic diseases.

TABLE 2
Possible Role of Air Pollution in *Allergy*

1. Some organic substances may enhance *IgE* synthesis.
2. Some pollutants may enhance the production of inflammatory *mediators* (e.g., *histamine*, *leukotrienes*, etc.).
3. Some pollutants may decrease the *mucociliary clearance*, leading to decreased *allergen* clearance.
4. Some pollutants may increase the production of *cytokines*.
5. Some pollutants may enhance allergic sensitization due to *irritant* effects on skin and/or mucosa.

AIR TRAPPING

Air trapping is caused by widespread plugging of the airways. The plugging extends from the segmental and subsegmental airways to the smaller bronchi and bronchioles. It leads to hyperinflation of the lungs in severe *asthma exacerbation*.

AIRWAY ANATOMY

Airways

The upper portion of the respiratory tract includes the nose and its system of air *sinuses*, the pharynx, and two Eustachian tubes that maintain air in the middle ear. The lower portion extends from the larynx to the visceral pleura. The larynx functions as a valve protecting the lungs and as the organ of phonation. The larynx opens into the trachea, which divides into two main bronchi, successively branching in 8 to 23 generations. A single terminal bronchiolus with its succeeding branches of *bronchioles*, alveolar ducts, and their alveolar sacs form the acinus, the basic respiratory unit of the lung. The alveolar walls reach an area of 60 to 70 m².

Epithelium

Except the anterior nares, which are lined by stratified, keratinizing squamous *epithelial cells*, the epithelium of the upper respiratory tract is formed by ciliated (see *cilia*) columnar and *mucus*-secreting cells. The pharynx and parts of the larynx (anterior surface of the epiglottis, upper part of the aryepiglottic folds, and vocal cords) are covered by nonkeratinizing squamous epithelium. A ciliated and columnar epithelium is found in the trachea, bronchi, and bronchioli. The basement membrane acts as a barrier to the passage of macromolecules and cells. However, inflammatory cells are able to penetrate through the basement membrane into the epithelium by secreting *proteases*. Beneath the basement membrane is the lamina reticularis, which becomes thickened in *asthma* (see *subepithelial fibrosis*), bronchiectasis, tuberculosis, and chronic sinusitis. The *submucosal glands*, which can be found from the larynx to the small bronchi, produce both acidic and neutral mucus as well as lysozyme, lactoferrin, secretory IgA, and a low-molecular-weight antiprotease.

Vasculature

The nasal and tracheobronchial mucosa is highly vascular. The trachea is supplied by branches of the inferior thyroid arteries, which anastomose with bronchial arteries, derived from the descending aorta. Each airway is also accompanied by a branch of the pulmonary artery. The blood flow is controlled by innervation and the action of locally released *mediators* such as *histamine, bradykinin, platelet-activating factor* (PAF), and *prostaglandins* (PGs). The subepithelial capillaries of the nose are fenestrated and are presumably more permeable to water flux and exudation associated with *inflammation*. Those fenestrated capillaries can also be found in the bronchi of asthmatics.

Nerve control systems

The airways receive both autonomic (efferent) and sensory (afferent) nerve fibers. The efferent nerves supply and control the mucus-secreting cells, bronchial *smooth muscle*, and vasculature (see *nervous system*). There is a rich innervation of the surface epithelium from a subepithelial nerve plexus. The intraepithelial endings receive mechanical stimuli or those of *irritants* such as tobacco smoke (see *smoking*), ammoniac, *sulfur dioxide* (SO_2), ethyl ether, or *dust*.

Smooth muscle cells

Smooth muscle is found in the dorsal intercartilaginous gap of the trachea and the extrapulmonary bronchi, and it encircles the intrapulmonary bronchi in two opposing spirals. An increased muscle mass is a feature of the asthmatic bronchi due to an increase of muscle fiber number (see *smooth muscle hypertrophy*).

Defense mechanisms

There are a number of defense mechanisms to keep the airways free of *allergens, pollutants,* and infections: (1) nervous reflexes leading to *airway obstruction* and *cough*, (2) secretion of mucus containing bacteriostatic substances, (3) *mucociliary clearance*, and (4) humoral and cellular *immune response* (secretory IgA, *lymphocytes, mast cells, antigen-presenting cells*). The lymphoid tissue includes free immunocompetent cells — mainly *lymphocytes, plasma cells,* and *mast cells* — the lymphoreticular aggregates in the bronchi, interlobular septa and in the pleura, the *bronchus-associated lymphoid tissue*, and the *lymph nodes*, which are situated in the peribronchial tissue.

AIRWAY HYPERREACTIVITY

(See *airway hyperresponsiveness*.)

AIRWAY HYPERRESPONSIVENESS

Patients with *asthma* have irritable airways and will respond to a greater degree than normal subjects when they are exposed to solvents, aromatic compounds, perfumes, cigarette smoke (see *smoking*), etc. This phenomenon is responsible for some of the symptoms of asthma, in particular the coughing (see *cough*) and breathlessness that patients often exhibit when exercising.

Airway hyperresponsiveness might be due, at least partially, to alterations in the function of neuronal M_2 *muscarinic receptors* by *major basic protein* (MBP), an *eosinophil granule protein*.

Airway hyperresponsiveness can be measured by challenging the patient with *histamine* or *methacholine* (see *bronchial provocation tests*). These are agents that have a direct effect on *smooth muscle* cells and can be used to grade patients with mild, moderate, and severe disease. The degree of reactivity is measured by a provoking dose or provoking concentration of histamine/methacholine, which causes a 20% fall in *forced expiratory volume in first second* (FEV$_1$) (PD$_{20}$, PC$_{20}$).

Airway hyperresponsiveness is not specific for asthma (see *COPD*).

AIRWAY OBSTRUCTION

The conducting airways (trachea, *bronchi*, *bronchioles*) can become narrowed due to *smooth muscle* contracting, mucosal *edema*, or intraluminal *mucus*. In addition, the airways may narrow because of loss of elastic recoil due to destruction (see *airway remodeling*) or edema of the supporting tissue. All of these processes increase resistance to airflow and will cause the expiratory phase of breathing to be prolonged (see *lung function tests*). Airway obstruction may be measured by *spirometry*.

Airway obstruction is a characteristic feature of *asthma* and *COPD*.

AIRWAY REMODELING

As a result of the inflammatory process in *asthma*, which occurs within the airways' *epithelial cells* and submucosa, the physiology of the airway changes. This affects both the spontaneous variability of airway caliber and the responsiveness to medication. Components implicated in airway remodeling include *subepithelial fibrosis*, *edema*, cellular infiltration (see *allergic inflammation*), changes in the *extracellular matrix*, *smooth muscle hypertrophy*, and changes in the airways' autonomic innervation (see *nervous system*). *Eosinophils* and *mast cells* play an important role in this *inflammation*-mediated repair process.

AIRWAY RESISTANCE

Airway resistance is a parameter to evaluate *airway obstruction* in *lung function tests* (see *spirometry* and *body plethysmography*).

AIRWAY TONE

The caliber of the airway is maintained by the influence of the vagus nerve, which provides bronchoconstrictor (cholinergic, parasympathetic) stimulation (see *acetylcholine*) and *bronchodilator* influences from the sympathetic plexus (see *noradrenalin*).

ALBUTEROL

Albuterol is a *β2-agonist*.

ALDEHYDE

Aldehydes are a common cause of *occupational asthma*, especially in healthcare workers.

ALDER POLLEN

Alder belongs to the birch family of trees and is distributed across the northern hemisphere. Alder *pollen* may cause *allergic rhinitis* in early spring in sensitized patients (see *tree pollen*). The *major allergen*, Aln g 1, may cross-react with those of birch, hazel, and hornbeam (see *cross-reacting allergens*).

ALLELE

Alleles are alternative forms of a *gene* at a given locus.

ALLERGEN

An allergen can be defined as a protein, glycoprotein, or protein-haptenated ligand that is capable of causing primary *T cell sensitization* and subsequent allergic sensitivity on reexposure (see *sensitization*). The mechanism of allergenicity is defined as an *immediate hypersensitivity* reaction (see *Coombs and Gell classification,* type I), which by definition involves the interaction of allergen with *IgE antibody* bound to *high-affinity IgE receptors* on *mast cells* and *basophils. Cross-linking* of these *receptors* by a multivalent interaction between IgE and allergen results in *mediator* release from the effector cells that cause the signs and symptoms of IgE-mediated *allergic diseases.*

> *Common allergens* include *pollens, house-dust mites, animal dander,* body fluids, *mold* spores (see *fungal allergens*), insect components (see *hymenoptera allergy*), certain foods (see *food allergy*), latex (see *latex allergy*), and various chemicals and drugs (see *drug allergy*).

Allergens are of low molecular weight (5 to 50,000 daltons) and often have special aerodynamic properties (see *aeroallergens*). Many allergens have been *epitope* mapped to identify their major *T cell* reactive *peptides. Allergenic peptides* have formed the basis of several experimental *immunotherapy* trials, with some success (see *peptide immunotherapy*). There is little apparent *MHC restriction* between different allergens within individuals, but some allergens do exhibit a degree of MHC restriction across a number of subjects. Many allergens are pharmacologically active as enzymes in biological systems, while certain food allergens and small molecules (see *haptens*) such as *nickel* or platinum salts (see *metallic salts*) form complexes with inherent cytotoxicity (see *cytotoxicity of allergens*).

In general use, the term allergen can refer to these sources, to aqueous *allergen extracts* prepared from the source materials, or to highly purified or cloned allergen proteins. The systematic nomenclature for purified allergens (developed by the World Health Organization and International Union of Immunological Societies) uses the taxonomic name of the source material and an Arabic numeral to describe the allergen, in the chronologic order of identification (see *allergen nomenclature*). To be included in this nomenclature, newly described allergens have to have clearly defined molecular and allergenic properties. In most cases, multiple allergenic proteins have been purified from a given source. Thus more than 10 different allergens have now been isolated or cloned from house-dust mites or grass pollens.

> Many important allergens from pollens, dust mites, animal danders, insects, and foods (e.g., *peanut,* shrimp) have been cloned (see *cloning of allergens*) and expressed as *recombinant allergens.*

Amino acid sequence data derived from these studies has been used to establish the structure and biologic function of allergens, to identify the epitopes that are involved in IgE responses, and to investigate cellular mechanisms of inflammatory responses in *asthma* and *atopic dermatitis*. Recombinant allergens are being introduced for the diagnosis of allergic diseases and for developing therapeutic products. Allergens are one of the most well-defined groups of biomedically important proteins.

ALLERGEN AVOIDANCE

Allergen avoidance is an approach to the prevention and/or management of *IgE*-mediated *allergic diseases* by reducing or eliminating exposure to allergens. Primary allergen avoidance is designed to prevent the development of allergic *sensitization* in subjects who are thought to be at high risk of becoming sensitized (see *genetic predisposition*). Secondary allergen avoidance is intended to reduce the risk of a sensitized person developing allergic diseases such as *asthma, allergic rhinoconjunctivitis*, etc. Tertiary allergen avoidance is intended to reduce the symptoms and extent of disease in patients who have allergic illnesses.

> There is now overwhelming evidence that *sensitization* to allergens is the single most important *risk factor* for the development of asthma.

Greater emphasis on the role of indoor *aeroallergens* in causing the disease has focused attention on the need to reduce allergen exposure in houses. Measuring allergen exposure in houses using *monoclonal antibody*-based *ELISA* tests has established levels at which patients become sensitized (typically exposures of 1 to 2 μg allergen per gram dust) and at which they are likely to develop *asthma exacerbations* (~10 μg/g). Allergen avoidance studies carried out at high altitude (see *climate therapy*) or in hospital rooms have shown that reducing allergen exposure to <1 μg/g can reduce *airway hyperresponsiveness* and alleviate asthma symptoms. Studies are now being designed to assess whether allergen avoidance protocols can be developed for routine use and whether early allergen avoidance procedures (in the first 3 years of life) will reduce the prevalence of asthma.

Reducing the exposure to allergens might be achieved by the following means:

- To reduce *animal dander* exposure, either remove the animal from the home or keep it out of the patient's bedroom and seal or cover with a dense filter any air ducts leading to the bedroom. Remove products made from feathers from the home and consider limiting the pet's contact with upholstered furniture and carpets. Washing the animal weekly may reduce the amount of dander and dried saliva it sheds into the environment.
- To reduce *house-dust mite* exposure, it is essential to encase the patient's mattress in a cover impermeable to allergens, encase the pillow as well or wash it weekly; wash the patient's bedding in hot (>130°F/55°C) water. It is desirable to reduce indoor humidity to less than 50%, remove carpets from the patient's bedroom, remove carpets laid directly on concrete, minimize the number of stuffed toys in children's beds and wash the toys weekly in hot (>130°F/55°C) water, and avoid sleeping or lying on upholstered furniture. Mite allergen exposure can be reduced in high-altitude areas.
- To reduce *cockroach allergen* exposure, control them with poison bait or traps, keep surfaces free of crumbs and moisture, and store food and rubbish in sealed containers. No human or animal food should be left exposed overnight.
- To reduce exposure to outdoor *pollens* and *molds*, stay indoors with windows closed, especially during the afternoon. Conduct outdoor activities just after dawn to minimize pollen exposures.
- To reduce exposure to indoor molds, fix leaks and eliminate water sources associated with mold growth; clean mold off surfaces. Consider reducing indoor humidity to less than 50%.

The effectiveness of allergen avoidance is disputed. Most evidence relates to tertiary allergen avoidance, and it seems that the degree of improvement is proportionate to the degree of sensitization. Patients who are monosensitized are more likely to improve than those who show *polysensitization.*

ALLERGEN CHALLENGE

The symptoms of *allergic rhinoconjunctivitis* or *asthma* can be induced by exposing the nose or lungs, respectively, to relevant *allergens*. Allergen challenge methods are now well standardized and safe, but they are cumbersome and only one allergen can be tested on a given day.

> In clinical practice, allergen challenges are usually performed only in cases of suspected *occupational asthma.*

Allergen challenge is a useful tool in clinical research and has provided a great deal of information on the pathophysiology and pathogenesis of asthma (see *bronchial provocation tests*). In bronchial allergen challenge, a dose of allergen is inhaled and the patient's *spirometry* is followed over 15 minutes. If the *forced expiratory volume in first second* (FEV_1) drops by 20%, then the dose of allergen that causes this drop is termed the PD_{20} (provoking dose for 20% fall in FEV_1). If the drop in FEV_1 is less than 20%, then a larger dose of allergen is given until the patient reacts. The PD_{20} is calculated by cumulating the dose given and, if necessary, interpolating to obtain an estimate of the dose which, when given as a single dose, would achieve a 20% fall in FEV_1. This *early asthmatic reaction* may be followed by a *late-phase asthmatic reaction* 3 to 12 hours after the early response. Allergen challenge can also be performed in a single segment of the airways (see *local allergen challenge*). The tendency to show late asthmatic reactions is correlated with disease severity, and the pathophysiology of the late asthmatic reaction is thought to be closer to that of the real disease as opposed to the early asthmatic reaction. Nevertheless, this is an artificial model of the disease and does not entirely mimic the real disease.

> Allergen challenge is also frequently used to diagnose patients with *hymenoptera allergy* and *food allergy* (see *food challenge*).

ALLERGEN CLONING

(See *cloning of allergens.*)

ALLERGEN EXTRACTS

Preparations of an *allergen* obtained by extraction of the active constituents from animal or vegetable substances used for diagnostic or therapeutic purposes. Highly purified allergen extracts have been prepared by numerous techniques. Purified allergens have been used for skin testing (see *skin tests*), and allergen-specific hyposensitization by *immunotherapy.* In immunotherapy, the term "allergen vaccine" is used to indicate that vaccines modify the immune response (see *allergen-induced immune responses* and *allergic inflammation*). Aqueous vaccines are used for both venom (see *hymenoptera allergy*) and inhalant allergen (see *hay fever*) immunotherapy. In an attempt to reduce side effects and to make immunotherapy more effective, allergenic extracts have been modified by physical or chemical procedures. Allergenic vaccines should be standardized for total allergenic potency, biologic activity, and *major allergen* contents. Problems of standardization are still encountered. Production of *recombinant allergens* and the development of *peptide immunotherapy* are now common, but rational and effective protocols for their clinical use remain to be determined.

ALLERGENIC PEPTIDES

These are *antigenic peptides* derived from *allergens* after processing by *antigen-presenting cells* (APCs). They represent *T cell epitopes*. *Allergen challenge* of patients with *asthma* results in a *delayed hypersensitivity* reaction without an immediate allergic reaction (see *Coombs and Gell classification*). This indicates that *IgE*-mediated *immediate hypersensitivity* reactions are not a prerequisite for the development of asthma.

ALLERGEN-INDUCED IMMUNE RESPONSES

> Individuals with IgE-mediated *allergic diseases* make *IgG*, IgA, and *IgE antibodies* against *allergens* in both serum and nasal secretions.

IgE antibodies to *pollen* allergens can account for >20% of the total IgE. IgE antibody responses to food allergens (see *food allergy*) develop within the first few months of life, whereas antibody responses to inhaled allergens develop over the first 2 to 3 years of infancy. IgG antibody levels rise (up to 50-fold) in patients being treated by *immunotherapy* using aqueous *allergen extracts*. A rise in IgG antibodies correlates with clinical efficacy in patients with *hymenoptera allergy*, but is not necessarily associated with clinical improvement following immunotherapy in pollen or *house-dust-mite*-allergic patients (see *immunotherapy: effects on IgE and IgG isotypes*). Asymptomatic individuals may also have positive *skin tests* and allergen-specific serum IgE antibodies (see *RAST, Phadiatop,* and *CAP-System*), but do not have clinical IgE-mediated symptoms. The levels of allergen-specific IgG antibodies in nonallergic individuals are usually lower than in allergic patients, and there is also evidence to suggest that the *affinity* of these IgG antibodies is lower.

> *T cells* are major regulators of the *allergic inflammation*.

Proliferative T cell responses can be demonstrated in vitro using peripheral blood T cells from allergic patients or *T cell clones* specific for house-dust mite, pollen, and *cat allergens* (see *lymphocyte transformation test*). Assessing T cell responses to allergens is difficult because many patients, even with high antibody levels, make weak or inconsistent T cell responses. For these reasons, studies have often focused on small numbers of highly selected patients, and there are few large population studies.

> T cell clones derived from allergic individuals have a predominantly *Th2* phenotype and secrete *IL-2, IL-4,* and *IL-5*.

T cell clones have also been obtained from nonallergic individuals, and these are *Th1* cells secreting *IFN-γ*. *Epitope* mapping studies with Der p 1, Der p 2, Fel d 1, Bet v 1, and other allergens, suggest that most allergens have multiple *T cell epitopes*, which are not HLA restricted (see *MHC restriction*). Allergen-specific T cells have inflammatory effects in vivo. *Patch tests* with purified mite allergens result in the recruitment of *basophils, eosinophils,* and mononuclear cells into the skin of *atopic dermatitis* subjects and the production of eczematous lesions (see *eczema*) at 48 hours. The frequency of allergen-reactive T cells in the skin of these lesions is higher than in the peripheral blood.

> *Allergen challenge* in the lung results in recruitment of inflammatory cells and is thought to be T-cell-mediated.

Now that the *amino acid* sequences of many allergens are known (see *cloning of allergens*), strategies are being developed for new forms of allergen-specific immunotherapy involving

T cell epitopes and specifically designed molecules which no longer bind IgE. The key advantage of these approaches is that the peptides can be synthesized, and any alterations in allergen structure can be clearly defined (see *peptide immunotherapy*). One approach is to design allergen vaccines containing a cocktail of *recombinant allergens* or variants, which have been modified by mutagenesis so that they have marked reduced binding to IgE. The rationale here is to deliver a broad spectrum of T cell epitopes and to reduce the possibility for IgE-mediated side effects (see *anaphylaxis*).

> The most recent strategies involve using plasmid DNA vaccines (see *DNA immunotherapy*) to act as Th1 adjuvants and elicit Th1 responses to allergens, leading to IgG, but not IgE, antibody production.

Plasmid DNA vaccines have been studied in experimental animals, but there have been no trials as yet in humans.

ALLERGEN NOMENCLATURE

An *allergen* nomenclature subcommittee was established under the auspices of the World Health Organization and the International Union of Immunologic Societies (WHO/IUIS). The objective of the subcommittee was to develop a systematic nomenclature to replace the arbitrary descriptions of allergens that occurred previously. The committee adopted a system whereby allergens were described using the first three letters of the genus, followed by the first letter of the species name and an Arabic numeral to indicate the chronologic order of allergen purification. Thus, the ragweed allergen known as "Antigen E" became Ambrosia artemisifolia allergen 1, or Amb a 1. *Grass pollen* allergen "Rye 1" became Lolium perenne allergen 1, or Lol p 1, etc. A key part of the systematic WHO/IUIS nomenclature is that the allergen should satisfy biochemical criteria, which define the molecular structure of the protein (see *cloning of allergens*), and immunologic criteria, which define its importance as an allergen (see Table 3).

TABLE 3
Criteria for Inclusion of Allergens in the WHO/IUIS Nomenclature

1. The molecular and structural properties should be clearly and unambiguously defined, including:
   - Purification of the allergen protein to homogeneity.
   - Determination of molecular weight, pI, and carbohydrate composition.
   - Determination of *nucleotide* and/or *amino acid* sequence.
   - Production of *monoclonal antibodies* against the allergen.
2. The importance of the allergen in causing *IgE* responses should be defined by:
   - Comparing the prevalence of serum IgE antibodies in large population(s) of allergic patients. Ideally, at least 50 or more patients should be tested.
   - Demonstrating biologic activity; e.g., by skin testing (see *skin tests*) or *histamine* release assay.
   - Investigating whether depletion of the allergen from an *allergen extract* (e.g., by immunoabsorption) reduces IgE binding activity.
   - Demonstrating, where possible, that *recombinant allergens* have comparable IgE antibody binding activity to the natural allergen

---

Many allergens have biochemical names, which describe their biologic function and may have preceded the allergen nomenclature. Examples include egg allergens (ovomucoid and ovalbumin), insect allergens (see *bee venom phospholipase A_2*), and shrimp tropomyosin. In the *allergy* literature, it is preferable to use the systematic allergen nomenclature. However, in other contexts, such as comparisons of biochemical activities or protein structure, it may be appropriate or more useful to use the biochemical names.

ALLERGEN VACCINATION

(See *immunotherapy.*)

ALLERGIC ALVEOLITIS

Farmer's lung is the most commonly seen form of *extrinsic allergic alveolitis*, sometimes referred to as hypersensitivity pneumonitis. The disease is caused by frequent exposure to *mold* spores in inhaled air. An *immediate hypersensitivity* reaction is not the cause of its pathology. In fact, there is no involvement of *IgE*. Pathology results from *Th1*-type reactivity to carbohydrate *antigens* and lectins and the production of high titers of *IgG*. The IgG *antibodies* react with the inhaled *antigen* in the alveolar wall of the lung (see *Coombs and Gell classification*, type III), causing alveolar wall *inflammation* and compromising *gas exchange*. A granulomatous reaction also occurs around spores, the presence of which may impair lung function or even result in permanent lung damage.

ALLERGIC ASTHMA

Asthma in which the patient is sensitized to *allergens* and in which these allergens are thought to be relevant to the causation of the disease. Almost all children with asthma are sensitized, but fewer adults with asthma are sensitized (see *sensitization*). Confirmation of the allergic basis of asthma may be sought by *skin tests*, but while every patient with allergic asthma is sensitized and shows positive skin tests, not everyone with positive skin tests who has asthma necessarily has an allergic basis for their disease. The attribution of their disease depends ultimately on the clinical history, both of the onset and progression of the disease.

ALLERGIC BRONCHOPULMONARY ASPERGILLOSIS (ABPA)

A condition with features of *allergic asthma* and *allergic alveolitis* in which the patient is sensitized to the *mold Aspergillus* fumigatus (see also *fungal allergens*). All patients with ABPA show positive *skin tests* to aspergillus extract (see *allergen extracts*). Most will show precipitating *IgG antibodies* against aspergillus (aspergillus precipitins, see *immune complex*), but these are not a mandatory requirement for diagnosis (see Table 4). In contrast to other forms of allergic asthma, patients with ABPA show intermittent pulmonary shadowing on their chest X-ray and do not usually respond satisfactorily to *β2-agonists*.

ABPA patients require systemic *corticosteroid* treatment. No treatment results in pulmonary *fibrosis*.

TABLE 4
Diagnostic Criteria of ABPA

1. Asthma
2. Positive skin test to Aspergillus
3. Elevated total serum *IgE level* (>1000 ng/ml)
4. Elevated Aspergillus-specific serum IgE
5. Current or previous pulmonary infiltrates
6. Peripheral blood *eosinophilia* (>1000/mm^3)
7. Serum precipitins to Aspergillus
8. Central bronchiectasis

Note: The first four criteria are the minimal criteria for ABPA diagnosis.

The differential diagnosis to allergic asthma is often difficult. Therefore, several diagnostic criteria for the disease have been developed. The currently accepted diagnostic criteria are shown in Table 4.

Significant progress regarding the ABPA diagnosis has recently been made. Cloning and production of aspergillus allergens (see *cloning of allergens*) revealed more than 10 different *recombinant allergens* that bind IgE from sera of patients. The measurements of specific Asp f 4 and Asp f 6 IgE levels allow a clear-cut discrimination between Aspergillus-allergic asthma and ABPA.

ALLERGIC CONJUNCTIVITIS

(See *conjunctivitis*.)

ALLERGIC CONTACT DERMATITIS

(See *contact dermatitis*.)

ALLERGIC DISEASES

The terms *allergy* and *hypersensitivity* describe the situation of an adverse clinical reaction to an exogenous *antigen* or *allergen*. Such clinical responses may have different pathogenic mechanisms, but are all called allergic diseases.

> It is not correct to restrict allergic diseases to *IgE*-mediated diseases.

If an endogenous antigen causes an adverse clinical reaction, we call it an autoimmune disease (see *autoimmunity*). In 1963, Coombs and Gell classified the mechanisms of hypersensitivity (see *Coombs and Gell classification*). This classification relates mechanisms to disease entities. For instance, *type I reactions* are important in *hay fever*, whereas in allergic *contact dermatitis*, *type IV reactions* are prominent. *Type III reactions* are of pathogenic relevance in *extrinsic allergic alveolitis* and in *allergic vasculitis*. However, it is possible that many different kinds of allergic processes are involved. For example, *asthma* and *atopic dermatitis* are often characterized by type I and type IV reactions. However, both diseases can also occur as selective type IV reactions (see *intrinsic asthma* and *intrinsic atopic dermatitis*), indicating that *IgE*-mediated mechanisms may not be essential for the development of these diseases. Allergic diseases, such as hay fever, asthma, and atopic dermatitis, affect 10 to 20% of the population (see Table 5). Asthma is the most common chronic disease of children in Western countries, and the prevalence is still increasing (see *asthma epidemiology*).

TABLE 5
Prevalence of Hay Fever in Switzerland
(SAPALDIA study, 1995)

Year	Prevalence (%)	
1926	0.8	(whole population)
1958	4.8	(whole population)
1986	9.6	(whole population)
1993	11.6	(whole population)
	17.3	(< 15 years)

ALLERGIC GRANULOMATOSIS

A synonym of *Churg–Strauss syndrome*.

ALLERGIC INFLAMMATION

Introduction

The mechanisms of *IgE*-mediated allergic *inflammation* have been studied extensively in *asthma*. Although in 1892 Osler had already referred to asthma as a special form of inflammation of the smaller *bronchioles*, only in the 1960s were the cellular components in asthmatic death (see *death from asthma*) studied. The airway wall was found to be infiltrated by a mixture of mononuclear cells and *granulocytes*, especially *eosinophils*. With the application of bronchoscopy, it became clear that even in mild asthma there is an inflammatory response. Both circulating (*monocytes, lymphocytes, basophils, eosinophils, neutrophils*) and resident inflammatory cells (*macrophages, dendritic cells, mast cells*) are involved.

Allergic inflammation is a manifestation of either *immediate hypersensitivity* as defined by *Coombs and Gell* (1963) or, as in the case of asthma or *atopic dermatitis*, a more complex combination of immediate (*type I reaction*) and *delayed hypersensitivity* (*type IV reaction*). However, allergic inflammations can also be the consequence of non-*IgE*-mediated mechanisms, as seen in allergic *contact dermatitis* (type IV reaction) or *allergic alveolitis* and *allergic vasculitis* (both *type III reactions*).

The immediate reaction is characterized by activation of *high-affinity IgE receptors* or other surface molecules on mast cells or basophils, leading to *mediator* release such as *histamine* and *leukotrienes*. For allergen-induced immediate hypersensitivity, the individual has to be sensitized (see *sensitization*) by initial exposure to that *allergen* or a *cross-reacting allergen*.

Primary T cell sensitization

This process generally occurs at mucosal surfaces or, in experimental or occupational situations, through the skin (contact dermatitis). Allergens are taken up by *antigen-presenting cells* (APCs), which later present *allergenic peptides to T cells*. The processes of *antigen* uptake and antigen presentation are performed by lung *macrophages* in *mucosa-associated lymphoid tissues* (MALT) of the respiratory tract, by *Langerhans cells* in the skin, or by *M cells* located in the Peyer's patches of *gut-associated lymphoid tissues* (GALT).

Under normal circumstances, primary allergen reactions with *CD4*+ T cells result in the induction of *anergy*, and immune homeostasis is maintained.

This is thought to occur as T cells require co-stimulatory signals to achieve a state of activation.

In allergic inflammation, APCs are activated and upregulate the necessary molecules for *co-stimulation*.

In this scenario, CD4+ T cells are activated via the *T cell antigen receptor* and co-stimulatory receptors (e.g., *CD28*), resulting in a proliferative response of allergen-specific T cells (see *T cell proliferation*) and *cytokine* production.

T cell cytokines

In order to understand how allergic hypersensitivity follows from initial *T cell sensitization*, it is first necessary to consider how *T helper (Th) cell differentiation* affects the nature of an ongoing immune reaction. Two major subsets of CD4+ T cells (and probably also *CD8*+ T cells) can be induced to secrete distinct sets of cytokines with broadly opposing or antagonistic effects on target cells, depending on how they are activated and on the local cytokine environment in which they develop.

The cytokine-secreting profiles of T cells can be separated into two well-defined and mutually exclusive categories, *Th1* and *Th2 cells*. Th1 cells secrete *IFN-γ, TNF-β,* and *IL-2,* whereas Th2 cells secrete *IL-4, IL-5, IL-6,* and *IL-13.*

There are some cytokines such as *IL-3, TNF-α,* and *GM-CSF* that are common to both Th1 and Th2 subsets. Between the Th1 and Th2 extremes is another recognized category, *Th0,* which can secrete a mixture of Th1 and Th2 cytokines and which may represent a differentiation stage, or be a committed antigen-specific phenotype in its own right. All IgE-mediated *allergic diseases* are associated with the development of pathologic Th2 cells.

Development of Th2 cells

This step plays a central role in allergic sensitization and subsequent development of allergic sensitivity. However, how Th2 cells develop is not entirely clear (Table 6).

One factor that might favor Th2 cytokine expression could be low antigen concentrations.

It has been shown that a 10 to 50 times lower *threshold* amount of antigen is required for induction of IL-4 than of IFN-γ. Increasing antigen concentrations favors IFN-γ production, whereas IL-4 generation decreases at higher antigen doses (see *antigen dose responses*). Another important factor appears to be the local cytokine environment in which T cells mature.

T cells exposed to an antigen in the presence of Th2 cytokines develop into Th2 cells. Conversely, Th1 cytokines induce Th1 cytokine production from reactive T cells.

The nature of the local cytokine environment may also determine whether anergic cells develop into Th1 or Th2 cells (see *immunotherapy*). IL-4 is inhibitory to IFN-γ and *IL-12,* which may explain the lack of IFN-γ that is often observed in allergic diseases (see Figure 3). A third important factor that may favor Th2 cytokine expression is the form of co-stimulation the T cell may receive.

It appears that *CD86,* but not *CD80* (both ligands for CD28) co-stimulatory signals from APCs, stimulates Th2 differentiation.

Moreover, the *genetic predisposition* of an individual is an important factor. In addition, environmental factors such as the presence of subclinical bacterial or viral infections, particularly early in life, probably also enhance predisposition to allergic sensitization.

TABLE 6
Factors that Favor Th2 Cell Development

1. Low antigen concentration
2. Th2 cytokine environment
3. High CD86 and low IL-12 expression of APCs
4. Genetic predisposition
5. Environmental factors

IgE production and immediate hypersensitivity

This characteristic feature of IgE-mediated allergic diseases is the first important consequence of increased Th2 cytokine *gene* expression. IL-4 and IL-13 together with *CD40* stimulation have the ability to induce *immunoglobulin class switching* in *B cells*. This results in antigen-specific IgE *isotype* selection that is of major functional significance in the development of allergic inflammation.

> IgE binds directly to high-affinity receptors on mast cells and basophils, and *cross-linking* of these receptors by multivalent interactions between IgE and antigen (allergen) initiates *degranulation* and the release of inflammatory mediators of allergy.

These pathogenic steps are responsible for allergic symptoms such as rapid skin irritation (the classic wheal and flare), rhinitis, sneezing, and itchy eyes. Besides mediators, which are responsible for this immediate hypersensitivity reaction, mast cells can contain considerable amounts of IL-4. Therefore, mast cells create a Th2-dominated cytokine microenvironment, which maintains and, perhaps, amplifies the development of Th2 cells, leading to chronic allergic inflammation (see Figure 3).

Eosinophilia

Besides elevated IgE levels, increased numbers of eosinophils is another important feature of many allergic diseases. Eosinophils and Th2 cells are the main players of the delayed hypersensitivity reaction in asthma and atopic dermatitis. Two mechanisms are important for the accumulation of these cell types in allergic tissues: (1) recruitment and (2) prolonged survival. Both mechanisms are at least partially mediated by Th2 cytokines. For instance, IL-4 and IL-13 upregulate certain *adhesion molecules* that help to recruit T cells and eosinophils into the inflamed tissue.

> IL-5 prevents *eosinophil apoptosis*, which probably represents the most important mechanism responsible for tissue eosinophilia.

Besides Th2 cytokines, *chemotactic factors* such as *chemokines* (e.g., *eotaxin*), *complement factors* (e.g., *C5a*), leukotrienes, and other lipid mediators (e.g., *platelet-activating factor*) are involved in the recruitment of eosinophils. The role of the eosinophil in asthma remains enigmatic, but it does have a primary effector function during inflammation, with the secretion of cytotoxic proteins (see *eosinophil granule proteins*), lipid mediators, and *oxygen metabolites*. Moreover, eosinophils express, like mast cells, large amounts of Th2 cytokines such as IL-4, IL-5, and IL-13, which maintains and amplifies the development of Th2 cells (see Figure 3).

Role of CD8⁺ T cells

There is good evidence that *CD8⁺* T cells may be another source of IL-5 in asthma. Furthermore, there is circumstantial evidence that CD8⁺ T cells have functionally responsive phenotypes, which can polarize into Th1- and Th2-like cytokine-secreting cells. These have been tentatively named *Tc1* and *Tc2* cells.

Limitation of the inflammatory response

As described above, T-cell-derived cytokines have a major influence on the priming, activation, and function of inflammatory cells.

> T cells produce powerful immunosuppressive cytokines, such as *IL-10* and *TGF-β*.

Moreover, IL-12 induces IFN-γ production, and IFN-γ generally downregulates Th2 cytokine gene expression. In the chronic phase of several allergic diseases, increased expression of Th1 cytokines has been reported. IL-10 is induced in anergic T cells, especially during high allergen concentrations. Activated T cells also express death factors such as *Fas ligand* that

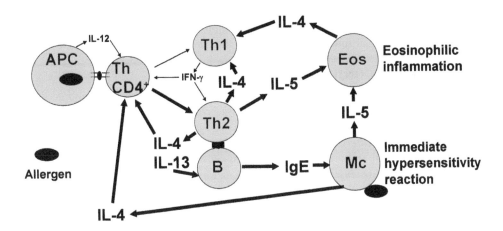

FIGURE 3 Simplified model of IgE-mediated allergic inflammation. Th2 cytokines, such as IL-4, IL-5, and IL-13, are overexpressed. In contrast, IL-12 and IFN-γ activities are usually low. Mast cell (Mc) and eosinophil (Eos) activation leads to mediator release, resulting in immediate hypersensitivity reaction and chronic eosinophilic inflammation. These two cell types maintain allergic inflammation by the generation of immunoregulatory cytokines themselves.

induce *apoptosis* in these cells in an autocrine or paracrine manner. Moreover, inflammatory cells such as mast cells and eosinophils that express functional *Fas receptors* may undergo apoptosis as a consequence of cellular interactions with Fas ligand-expressing T cells (see also *immunosuppressive mechanisms*).

ALLERGIC KERATOCONJUNCTIVITIS

Two forms of allergic keratoconjunctivitis can be distinguished, the vernal and the atopic. Vernal keratoconjunctivitis is a serious ocular *allergy* which occurs during the spring and the summer, and affects children, predominantly boys, before the age of 14 years. Most of these patients have a personal or family history of *atopy*. In contrast, atopic keratoconjunctivitis is seen in adult patients with *atopic dermatitis* and persists throughout the year. In both diseases, a dense cellular infiltrate of the conjunctiva is characteristic, consisting of *mast cells, lymphocytes, macrophages, plasma cells, neutrophils,* and *eosinophils*. Their role in the pathogenesis is not clear. *Immediate* and *delayed hypersensitivity* reactions, *IgE-* and *complement factor*-mediated mechanisms have been postulated.

ALLERGIC RHINITIS

Rhinitis is defined as *inflammation* of the lining of the nose and is characterized by nasal discharge, blockage, sneezing, itching, impaired sense of smell, and is often associated with *conjunctivitis* (see *allergic rhinoconjunctivitis*). Seasonal rhinitis can be caused at different times of the year by a number of *allergens* including *tree pollens, grass pollens, weed pollens,* and *molds. Perennial rhinitis* is a chronic *IgE*-mediated *allergic inflammation* which occurs primarily as a result of *allergy* to *house-dust mite*, but can also be caused by cats (see *cat allergen*), dogs (see *dog allergen*), horses, other animals (see *animal dander*), or chemical allergens to which there is a relatively continuous exposure. The immunological mechanism is believed to be mediated by *Langerhans cells* (but not *macrophages*) in the nasal mucosa presenting allergen to *T cells. T cell proliferation, Th2 cytokine* secretion, IgE production, and activation of *mast cells* on exposure to a specific allergen form the positive feedback for continued reactivity. Treatment of allergic rhinitis is by avoidance of the precipitating allergen where possible (see *allergen avoidance*), drug therapy with *antihistamines* and topical *corticosteroids*, and, in selected cases, specific *immunotherapy* can be very effective. Chronic inflammation of the nasal mucosa can extend to the *sinuses* and may cause *nasal polyps*.

ALLERGIC RHINOCONJUNCTIVITIS

This rhinoconjunctival *hypersensitivity* reaction is the most common of the atopic diseases (see *atopy*). In addition to the symptoms of *allergic rhinitis*, there is redness, swelling, and itching of the conjunctiva and tearing of the eyes. The *pollen* from trees, grass, and ragweed are the most important *allergens* in spring and summer. Upon contact with the nasal mucosa, the pollen grains swell and release their allergens onto the nasal mucosa. In addition to the seasonal allergens, *house-dust mite* allergens may cause a perennial form of allergic rhinoconjunctivitis. Allergen-specific *IgE*, bound to mucosal *mast cells* via the *high-affinity IgE-receptor*, is cross-linked (see *cross-linking*) by the allergens, which leads to release of vasoactive substances (i.e., *histamine*). A careful patients' history of seasonal or perennial rhinoconjunctivitis, *skin tests* (e.g., *prick tests*), and nasal provocation tests (see *allergen challenge* and *nasal lavage*) with *allergen extracts* are helpful in identifying the relevant allergen. If there are no contraindications, *immunotherapy* with allergen extracts is a useful therapeutic approach. In addition, symptomatic therapy with topical or systemic *antihistamines*, mast cell stabilizers (see *cromones*), or *corticosteroids* may be beneficial.

ALLERGIC SENSITIZATION

(See *sensitization*.)

ALLERGIC SUSCEPTIBILITY

(See *genetic predisposition*.)

ALLERGIC URTICARIA

Urticaria can be caused by allergic and nonallergic mechanisms. Possible allergic mechanisms include *IgE*-, anti-IgE-, and *immune complex*-mediated pathologies.

ALLERGIC VASCULITIS

Allergic *vasculitis*, also known as *immune complex* vasculitis, vasculitis allergica, or leukocytoclastic vasculitis, is defined as a symmetrical hemorrhagic exanthem caused by an immune complex vasculitis (see *Coombs and Gell classification*, type III) of the small vessels, usually veins.

The deposition of circulating immune complexes in the vessel wall, which may be demonstrated in subendothelial location by direct immunofluorescence microscopy, is the central pathogenetic event.

The formation of immune complexes and subsequent activation of the *complement system* leads to the accumulation of *granulocytes*, release of lysosomal enzymes, and subsequent destruction of the vessel wall. *Purpura*, as proven by diascopy, is the diagnostic hallmark of this disease. The lower legs are consistently involved in a symmetrical distribution pattern by petechiae. Polyarthralgia and renal hemorrhage are frequently associated with the cutaneous findings. Depending on the morphology of the additional skin lesions, five subtypes are differentiated (see Table 7).

There are many antigenic components that are considered as causes of allergic vasculitis. If there is no obvious causative event (e.g., streptococcal infection) present, a thorough examination for causative *antigens* has to be performed. This includes a screening for neoplasms

TABLE 7
Subtypes of Allergic Vasculitis

Subtype	Features
1. Hemorrhagic type (Schönlein–Henoch purpura or purpura rheumatica)	• Frequently observed • Renal involvement with hematuria • Hyperpigmentation from hemosiderin deposits may persist in the predilection sites
2. Hemorrhagic-necrotic type	• Purpuric macules • Flat red–black necroses
3. Papulonecrotic type	• Red, inflammatory, and hemorrhagic papules, which may later become necrotic • Healing with varioliform scars • Hyperpigmented atrophic scars in the predilection sites.
4. Polymorphous-nodular type	• Macular, urticarial, papular, or nodular lesions • Some lesions may even resemble those of *erythema multiforme*
5. *Urticaria vasculitis*	• Urticarial exanthem with wheals persisting for longer than a day • Hemorrhage detectable on diascopy

as well as for hepatitis, chronic focal, or *parasitic diseases*. Most important, a careful drug history should be taken and allergy testing for *drug* and *food allergies* should be performed.

> *NSAIDs* and *antibiotics* are considered to be the most common causes of allergic vasculitis.

Following discontinuation of all drugs as far as possible and in combination with an elimination of all other suspected causes (treatment of foci of infection or current infections), and systemic administration of *corticosteroids* is the most promising therapeutic regimen.

ALLERGOID

(See *modified allergen vaccines*.)

ALLERGY

In medical parlance, allergy means a condition in which there is an altered immune response (see *allergen-induced immune responses*) to a foreign *antigen* (see *allergen*), causing *sensitization* and clinical disease (see *allergic diseases*). Most commonly this involves *IgE antibodies* and *immediate hypersensitivity* (see *Coombs and Gell classification*, type I). Allergic reactions do not resemble the pharmacological (toxic) effects of a substance, and there is always an immunological background of the reaction. The term "allergy" is also applied to certain forms of *delayed hypersensitivity* (*type IV reaction*) in which patients demonstrate a *contact dermatitis*. Other patients develop vasculitic rashes (see *allergic vasculitis*) and certain forms of *immune complex* (*type III reaction*) *hypersensitivity*. These include allergic reactions to certain drugs (see *drug allergy*) and allergic reactions to inhaled proteins such as *extrinsic allergic alveolitis*, bird fancier's lung, farmer's lung, etc.

> The term "allergy" should not be used as a synonym for immediate hypersensitivity.

It is a general term to describe adverse clinical reactions to an antigen. However, certain other conditions involving altered reactions to foreign substances are not regarded as allergic disease, a good example being coeliac disease (see *gluten-sensitive enteropathy*) in which a form of cell-mediated immunity develops to wheat proteins. Logically this should be regarded as an allergic disease, but in practice it is not. The term "allergy" has also passed into general use as meaning that the individual has an aversion to or dislike of something, e.g., "I'm allergic to Monday mornings."

ALLERGY DIET

Many *allergic diseases* may be triggered by the uptake of a specific kind of food (see *food allergy*). Avoidance of this food may positively influence the course of the allergic disease (see *allergen avoidance*). Commonly used standard schemes include a diet free of additives and preservatives, a hypoallergenic diet, and the ultima ratio of a diet from cooked potatoes and cooked rice. Other specifically designed diet forms are those with a low *nickel* content and those avoiding a specific kind of food, e.g., seafood, milk and milk products, hens' eggs, or soy bean. However, there is no point in instituting dietary regulations without a proven *hypersensitivity* reaction (see *food challenge*).

An unnecessarily severe dietary regimen may lead to social isolation of the patient or even cause severe malnutrition.

ALLOGENIC

Any mixture of cells, tissues, or *antibodies* derived from two different subjects of the same species. Co-culture of allogenic *lymphocytes* (mixed lymphocyte reaction) has shown that about 1 to 10% of all lymphocytes from an individual are reactive to allogenic stimulation (see *lymphocyte transformation test*).

ALTERED PEPTIDE LIGANDS (APL)

A novel and potentially therapeutic strategy of *peptide immunotherapy* is emerging whereby APLs are administered in appropriate delivery systems, taken up and presented by *antigen-presenting cells* (APCs). These APLs, which may differ from the original *peptide* by only one or two *amino acids*, are able to down-regulate the *T cell* response toward the original *antigen*. The exact mechanisms of this action are unclear but may be caused by a more rapid dissociation of the *T cell antigen receptor* (TCR)/peptide/*major histocompatibility complex* (MHC) than usual. This would result in a qualitatively different signal from the TCR (kinetic theory), or may result from an inappropriate structural modification of the *receptor* complex, which again is unable to provide a fully activating signal (conformational model).

ALTERNARIA

(See *fungal allergens*.)

ALTERNATIVE MEDICINE

(See *complementary procedures*.)

ALTERNATIVE SPLICING

Alternative splicing is a means of forming several proteins from one *gene*. This can be done by different arrangements of *exons*. Some *receptors* can occur as soluble receptors. There are two ways to generate such soluble receptors: (1) the receptor is cleaved by *proteases*, and (2) the exon encoding the membrane-anchoring domain of the receptor is not transcribed (see *transcription*).

ALVEOLITIS

Alveolitis is an *inflammation* of the alveolar wall. The amount of inflammatory cells in the *bronchoalveolar lavage* (BAL) correlates well with findings obtained by histology. Therefore, the differential cell count in the BAL fluid may provide evidence for the underlying disease. Further diagnostic help can be obtained by immunophenotyping of the BAL *lymphocytes* (see *flow cytometry*). Depending on the inflammatory cells infiltrating the lungs, three forms of alveolitis are differentiated (see Table 8). However, please note that in clinical practice, mixed types are frequently observed.

TABLE 8
Subtypes of Alveolitis

Subtype	Associated Inflammatory Diseases
1. Lymphocytic type	• *Extrinsic allergic alveolitis*
	• *Sarcoidosis*
	• Tuberculosis
	• Asbestosis
	• Lymphangiosis carcinoma
	• M. Crohn
	• *AIDS*
	• Berylliosis
	• Drug-induced alveolitis
	• Viral pneumonia
	• BOOP
2. Granulocytic type	• *Cryptogenic fibrosing alveolitis*
	• *Collagen* diseases
	• Acute respiratory distress syndrome
	• Asbestosis
	• Infectious diseases
	• M. Wegener
3. Eosinophilic type	• *Eosinophilic pneumonia*
	• *Asthma*
	• *Churg–Strauss syndrome*
	• *ABPA*
	• Cryptogenic fibrosing alveolitis
	• Drug-induced alveolitis
	• *Hypereosinophilic syndrome*
	• Pneumocystis carinii

AMINO ACID

Amino acids are the basic structural units of proteins. Interestingly, all proteins in all species are constructed from the same set of 20 amino acids. Amino acids are often designated by either a three-letter abbreviation or a one-letter symbol (see *codon*) to enable concise communication (see Table 9).

4-AMINOPYRIDINE

This is *a potassium channel* blocker.

AMPLIFICATION

This term is used when molecules or signals increase in their numbers and/or function. For instance, *cDNA* molecules can by amplified by *polymerase chain reaction* (PCR). Moreover, activation signals are amplified during *signal transduction* events. The term is also used for the production of multiple copies of a *DNA* sequence.

TABLE 9
Abbreviations for Amino Acids

Amino acid	Three-Letter Abbreviation	One-Letter Symbol
Alanine	Ala	A
Arginine	Arg	R
Asparagine	Asn	N
Aspartic acid	Asp	D
Asparagine or aspartic acid	Asx	B
Cysteine	Cys	C
Glutamine	Gln	Q
Glutamic acid	Glu	E
Glutamine or glutamic acid	Glx	Z
Glycine	Gly	G
Histidine	His	H
Isoleucine	Ile	I
Leucine	Leu	L
Lysine	Lys	K
Methionine	Met	M
Phenyalanine	Phe	F
Proline	Pro	P
Serine	Ser	S
Threonine	Thr	T
Tryptophan	Trp	W
Tyrosine	Tyr	Y
Valine	Val	V

α-AMYLASE

α-Amylase from *Aspergillus* oryzae is used in the baking industry to standardize the enzymatic activity of flour. It can cause *bakers' asthma* (see also *occupational asthma*).

α-AMYLASE INHIBITOR PROTEIN

α-Amylase inhibitor protein has been identified as a *major allergen* of wheat flour. It may cause *bakers' asthma* (see also *occupational asthma*).

ANALGESIC-INDUCED ASTHMA

(See *aspirin-sensitive asthma*.)

ANAPHYLACTIC REACTION

This is an *IgE*-mediated *immediate hypersensitivity* reaction (see *Coombs and Gell classification*, type I). Symptoms range from cutaneous wheal and flare reactions (see *urticaria*) and subcutaneous *angioedema* to cardiovascular reactions with complete anaphylactic shock (see *anaphylaxis*). Relevant *allergens* may range from venoms of the hymenoptera (see *hymenoptera allergy*), drugs (see *drug allergy*), and various food allergens (see *food allergy*) up to the natural latex allergens (see *latex allergy*). The demonstration of an IgE-mediated reaction by *skin tests* or in vitro IgE tests (see *RAST, Phadiatop, CAP-System*) is required to establish the diagnosis.

ANAPHYLACTOID REACTION

This is a *hypersensitivity* reaction clinically resembling an *anaphylactic reaction*, but without an *IgE*-mediated pathogenesis (see *idiosyncrasy*). For instance, the complement protein fragments *C3a* and *C5a* can bind to specific *receptors* on the surface of *mast cells* and *basophils*, and can trigger *mediator* release, leading to the same clinical manifestations as seen in *anaphylaxis*. Moreover, certain hyperosmolar solutions (*dextran*, mannitol, opiates) may stimulate mast cells in a receptor-independent way. In addition, increased production of *leukotrienes* in *aspirin*-sensitive patients (see *aspirin-sensitive asthma*) can lead to anaphylactoid reactions.

ANAPHYLATOXINS

The *complement factors C3a*, *C4a*, and *C5a* cause *mast cell* and *basophil degranulation*, and elicit *anaphylactoid reactions* through their specific *receptors*.

ANAPHYLAXIS

Systemic *IgE*-mediated allergic responses (see *immediate hypersensitivity*) can occur throughout the body, causing hypotension, *urticaria*, *angioedema*, *asthma*, gastrointestinal upset, and, at least sometimes, death.

Anaphylaxis represents the most dramatic clinical manifestation of an immediate hypersensitivity reaction (see *Coombs & Gell classification*, type I). It may also occur as a side-effect of *immunotherapy.*

Anaphylaxis was first seen in dogs, which were immunized with *antigen*. Instead of the expected protection, the animals developed a paradoxical fatal reaction. This observation is described in the name for this phenomenon (Greek: ana = backward, phylaxis = protection). The onset of symptoms is seen within seconds after exposure to the responsible *allergen*. *Penicillin* hypersensitivity is the most frequent cause of anaphylaxis (see *drug allergy*), followed by hymenoptera venom (see *hymenoptera allergy*), latex, and food allergens (peanuts, nuts, fish, and eggs; see *food allergy*). In extremely sensitized individuals, even the smell of fish causes anaphylaxis.

Prompt treatment with *adrenaline, antihistamines, corticosteroids*, oxygen, and plasma expanders will usually abort the attack. It is important to note that up to 20% of the patients treated for the initial episode may have a further life-threatening event after 6 to 8 hours (biphasic reaction, see *late-phase response*). All patients with anaphylaxis should be investigated to determine the cause.

Mast cells and *basophils* can be activated by *nonimmunological mechanisms* (other than via the *high-affinity IgE receptor*), leading to the same clinical manifestations as seen in anaphylaxis. These are called *anaphylactoid reactions.*

ANERGY

T cell anergy can be defined as an induced state of unresponsiveness to an *antigen* following primary *T cell* sensitization. It has long been known that antigen-specific T cells can be anergized by exposure to high doses of the specific antigen but in the absence of either cognate or noncognate simultaneous *co-stimulation* (see *cognate/noncognate interactions*). An example of a cognate mechanism involves the interaction of *CD28* expressed on the surface of T cells with its ligands *CD80* and *CD86* on professional *antigen-presenting cells* (APCs) or *B cells*. There are several possible mechanisms that may disturb these molecular interactions (see Table 10).

TABLE 10
Mechanisms that Prevent Optimal
CD28 Stimulation in T Cells

1. Decreased CD28 ligand(s) expression
2. Decreased CD28 expression
3. Increased *CTLA-4* expression
4. Interruption of CD28 *signal transduction*

Successful immunotherapy is associated with the induction of anergy in allergen-specific T cells that appears to be mediated by *IL-10*.

IL-10 may cause anergy by disruption of CD28-induced signal transduction pathways.

Moreover, blocking other important co-stimulatory interactions such as *CD40* (B cell) with *CD40 ligand* (T cell), or *CD30* with its unknown ligand can also anergize T cells. An example of a noncognate interaction is that between *IL-2* and its *receptor* (or any other *cytokine* with its specific *cytokine receptor*). In particular, failure of antigen-responsive T cells to secrete IL-2 results in almost total anergy, which, however, can be overcome by the addition of exogenous IL-2.

Anergy shares some features with *apoptosis*.

There are two major characteristics that link these phenomena. Anergy and apoptosis are both induced by specific immunological recognition (see *T cell antigen receptor*), and they both occur as a result of a lack of, or inappropriate, co-stimulatory signals. The functional result of both mechanisms is specific immunological unresponsiveness.

ANESTHETIC ALLERGY

Hypotension and *anaphylactic reactions* are relatively common during general anesthesia. In some cases, the hypotension is due to blood loss or primary cardiac abnormalities, but several anesthetic agents are known to cause *allergies*, especially neuromuscular relaxing agents and certain induction agents (see *drug allergy*). Antibiotics (e.g., *penicillin*) and opiate analgesics (e.g., *morphine*) given at the time of anesthesia can also induce *anaphylaxis* and *anaphylactoid reactions*, respectively. In recent years, *latex allergy* has accounted for an increasing number of patients who experience adverse reactions during anesthesia. Patients with anesthetic anaphylaxis should be referred to and investigated by a specialist.

ANGIOEDEMA

Angioedema, first described by Quincke in 1882, is an urticarial reaction (see *urticaria*) inside the subcutaneous tissue, preferentially of the face and neck area. Sometimes, a grotesque swelling of the face may be associated with mucosal involvement down to the laryngeal area, causing a life-threatening obstruction. If trunk and extremities are involved, the term *urticaria profunda* is preferred. *IgE*-mediated *immediate hypersensitivity* reactions (see *Coombs and Gell classification*, type I) are the most common cause of angioedema, but a nonallergic pathogenesis (see *pseudoallergy*) as well as a hereditary form (*C1 inhibitor* defect) have been described. Blockers of the *angiotensin-converting enzyme* (ACE) may also induce angioedema. A complete workup of patients includes all diagnostic procedures for urticaria as well as a screening for quantitative and qualitative C1 inhibitor alterations.

ANGIONEUROTIC EDEMA

A synonym of *angioedema*.

ANGIOTENSIN

Angiotensin I is cleaved to angiotensin II by the *angiotensin-converting enzyme* (ACE), but also by other *proteases*, such as *chymase* from *mast cells*. Angiotensin II plays a role in the control of blood pressure. Just as angiotensin I is cleaved not only by ACE, ACE is also not specific with respect to its targets.

ANGIOTENSIN-CONVERTING ENZYME (ACE)

ACE is a *protease* with multiple targets. Besides *angiotensin* I, ACE cleaves molecules such as *IL-1* precursor or *bradykinin*.

> ACE blockers, which are frequently used to normalize blood pressure in patients with hypertension, may increase bradykinin concentrations.

For instance, ACE blockers may cause *airway obstruction* and/or *cough* in patients with *asthma*. Moreover, ACE blockers may also induce *angioedema* due to decreased bradykinin degradation.

ANIMAL DANDER

In addition to *house-dust mites*, animal dander is an important indoor *allergen*. Cats are the most common pets in the Western world, but allergens may also come from dogs, guinea pigs, rabbits, and horses. In addition to dander, pelt, serum, urine, and saliva have also been shown to exhibit allergenic activity. Animal-derived particles are usually found in house dust. The *cat allergen* is commonly airborne (see *aeroallergens*). Because cat hairs are passively transferred to the clothing of people, the allergen can also be found in places where cats are not found.

> Animal allergens are small particles which can be inhaled and therefore preferentially provoke respiratory *IgE*-mediated *allergies*.

After direct skin contact with an animal, some sensitized persons will develop *contact urticaria*. Animal dander as the trigger for skin lesions in *atopic dermatitis* has also been reported. Allergies to rodents, rabbits, cows, and horses may also play a role in *occupational asthma*.

ANNEALING

Pairing of single-stranded complementary *DNA*, resulting in a double strand. The term is also used for *primers*, which bind to *cDNA* during the *polymerase chain reaction* (PCR).

ANTI-ALLERGIC/ANTI-ASTHMATIC DRUGS

There are several groups of drugs with anti-allergic/anti-asthmatic potency, but with different modes of action. Table 11 lists currently used and possible future drug types. Since *T cells* are important regulatory cells in *allergic diseases*, their direct effects on T cells are indicated.

ANTI-ANTIBODIES

Anti-*immunoglobulin antibodies* are antibodies to immunoglobulin constant domains that are useful for detecting bound antibody molecules in *immunoassays*, *immunohistochemistry*, *flow cytometry*, and other applications. Antibodies directed against *idiotypes* of other antibodies are called anti-idiotypic antibodies.

TABLE 11
Groups of Anti-Allergic/Anti-Asthmatic Compounds

Drug Type	Action	Effect on T cells
Antiadenosines	*Bronchodilators*	?
Anticholinergic agents	Bronchodilators	–
Anticytokine therapy	Immunomodulation	–/+(+)
Antihistamines	H1 receptor antagonists	–
Anti-IgE therapy	IgE reduction	–
Antileukotrienes	*Leukotriene* synthesis blocker, *leukotriene receptor antagonists*	–
β2-Agonists	Bronchodilators	–
Corticosteroids	Antiinflammatory, immunosuppressive	++
Cromones	*Mast cell* stabilizers	?
Cyclosporin A	Immunosuppressive	++
Cytokine therapy	Immunomodulation	++
Immunotherapy	*Anergy*	++
Phosphodiesterase inhibitors	Bronchodilators	+
Potassium channel openers	Bronchodilators	?
Xanthines	Bronchodilators	–

ANTIBIOTICS

Antibiotics are a group of drugs given to control bacterial infections. In cases of *asthma exacerbations*, antibiotics should not be given routinely, but rather prescribed when there is specific evidence of a bacterial infection.

Most antibiotics may potentially act as *allergens*.

Antibiotics are low-molecular-weight substances (*haptens*) requiring carrier proteins such as serum globulins before they are capable of inducing an *immune response*. *Penicillin* and related antibiotics (β-lactam drugs) are the most important allergenic compounds. *Type 1-4 reactions*, which were described by Coombs and Gell (see *Coombs and Gell classification*), can occur in penicillin *allergy*.

ANTIBODY

An antibody is a molecule that is produced and secreted by *B cells/plasma cells* and specifically binds to *antigens*. Antibody molecules bind to and neutralize pathogens or prepare them for uptake and destruction by *phagocytes*. Each antibody molecule has a unique structure that allows it to bind to its specific antigen, but all antibodies have the same overall structure and are known collectively as *immunoglobulins* (Ig). Some patients have a genetically determined or an acquired defect and cannot synthesize sufficient amounts of antibodies, resulting in humoral immunodeficiency. Such patients are often treated with *intravenous immunoglobulin (IVIG) preparations*.

Moreover, surface Ig serves as the specific antigen *receptor* of B cells (see *B cell antigen receptor*). *IgE* is bound via *high-affinity IgE receptors* on *mast cells* and *basophils*, and plays an important role in a subgroup of *allergic diseases*. Many molecules are made up in part by blocks of proteins known as immunoglobulin domains, because they were first described in the structure of antibody molecules (see *immunoglobulin superfamily*). Antibodies are often used to detect specific antigens (see *flow cytometry*, *immunohistochemistry*, and *immunoassay*).

ANTIBODY AFFINITY MATURATION

B cells stimulated during *secondary immune responses* undergo a second proliferative phase (see *B cell proliferation*), during which the *genes* encoding *immunoglobulin* variable domains undergo somatic *mutations* before the B cell differentiates into *plasma cells*. The extensive somatic mutation leads to the selection of high-*affinity* precursor cells, which undergo clonal expansion. The resulting high-affinity antibodies are much more efficient than the antibodies produced during *primary immune responses*.

ANTIBODY THERAPY

Antibodies or *immunoglobulin* (Ig) preparations are given to patients for therapeutic purposes. These therapies have either nonspecific or specific influences on the *immune system* (see Table 12).

TABLE 12
Antibody Therapies

Type of Therapy	Application
Nonspecific antibody therapy	
• *Intravenous immunoglobulin (IVIG) preparations*	Humoral immunodeficiencies, several bacterial infections, thrombocytopenic purpura, Kawasaki syndrome
• *Anti-IgE-therapy**	*IgE*-mediated *allergic diseases*
Specific antibody therapy (see *anticytokine therapy*)	
• Anti-*IL-4*-therapy*	IgE-mediated allergic diseases
• Anti-*IL-5*-therapy*	Eosinophilic *inflammations*
• Anti-*IL-6*-therapy	Myeloma
• Anti-*TNF*-therapy	Rheumatoid arthritis
• Anti-*CD2*-therapy	Transplant rejection
• Anti-*CD3*-therapy	Transplant rejection
• Anti-*CD4*-therapy	Rheumatoid arthritis
• Anti-*CD25*-therapy	Leukemia
• Anti-LPS-therapy	Sepsis
• Anti-VEGF-therapy	Diabetic neuropathy
• Anti-HER2/Neu	Breast cancer

* Currently in clinical trials.

ANTICHOLINERGIC AGENTS

In normal health, the airways are under the influence of cholinergic, vagal tone (see *airways tone* and *nervous system*). Anticholinergic agents will open up the airways and can be particularly useful in the management of older patients with *asthma* (see *asthma treatment strategies*) or patients with *chronic obstructive pulmonary disease* (COPD).

> The mechanism of action of anticholinergics is the neutralization of the muscarinic actions of *acetylcholine* by blocking *muscarinic receptors*.

Anticholinergics are also recommended to control asthma symptoms in patients with *pollutant*-mediated bronchoconstriction or when side effects of an adrenergic *bronchodilator* cannot be tolerated. After administration of anticholinergic drugs, the onset of *bronchodilation* develops more slowly compared to a short-acting *β2-agonist*.

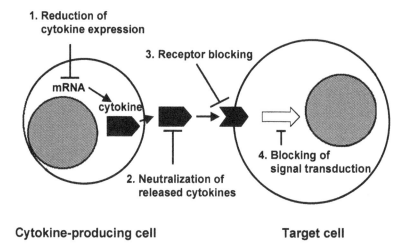

Cytokine-producing cell   **Target cell**

FIGURE 4 Anticytokine therapy may be performed at the following levels: (1) reduction of cytokine gene expression, (2) neutralization of released cytokines, (3) blocking of cytokine receptors, and (4) inhibition of cytokine receptor signaling.

ANTICYTOKINE THERAPY

Cytokines and *cytokine receptors* have been targeted as potential areas for therapeutic intervention in a number of diseases where abnormal cytokine production occurs. Cytokine action can be inhibited at several possible levels (see Figure 4).

Reduction of cytokine gene expression

Several pharmacological agents have been used as immunosuppressive drugs with a high degree of success, particularly in transplant rejection. These agents include *cyclosporin A* and *FK506* as well as *corticosteroids* that have potent downregulatory effects on cytokine *gene* activation and cytokine secretion. The strategy of *antisense* oligonucleotides might be useful to specifically inhibit cytokine generation.

Neutralization of released cytokines

Monoclonal antibodies (mAbs) against *TNF-α* have proven to be clinically efficacious in inflammatory disorders such as *rheumatoid arthritis*. Neutralizing anti-*IL-4* and anti-*IL-5* mAbs have been developed for clinical studies in *IgE*-mediated *allergic diseases* including *asthma* (see *antibody therapy*). In addition, soluble cytokine receptors have been used to reduce the levels of specific circulating cytokines including *IL-1*, *IL-2*, IL-4, and *IL-6*.

Blocking of cytokine receptors

The inhibition of receptor ligation through the use of mAbs is one possibility. For instance, immunosuppression has been achieved through mAb against the *IL-2* receptor. Moreover, several cytokine receptor antagonists have been used successfully to block the effects of cytokines. One such molecule is the *IL-1 receptor antagonist* (IL-1Rα) that blocks the action of IL-1. IL-1 plays an important role in the initiation and maintenance of inflammatory responses. Administration of IL-1Rα inhibits the influx of inflammatory *leukocytes* (e.g., *neutrophils* and *eosinophils*) by downregulation of endothelial *adhesion molecules*. IL-1Rα has been used successfully in the treatment of diabetes, arthritis, and septic shock.

Inhibition of cytokine receptor signaling

Cytokine signaling pathways (see *signal transduction*) including *transcription* and *translation* can be blocked by pharmacological agents.

> Cytokine and anticytokine therapies for allergic diseases have been tried, but with equivocal results. Much of the problem with this approach probably lies in the built-in *redundancy* of the cytokine system and the pluripotent nature and cross-reactive functionality of many cytokines (see *pleiotropism*).

However, recombinant human *IL-10* and *IL-12* therapy (see *cytokine therapy*) and anti-IL-4 treatment is now being tried, with some success, after the rather discouraging results of treating IgE-mediated allergic diseases (e.g., *house-dust mite allergy*) with the *Th1* cytokine *IFN-γ*. Other possible targets for anticytokine therapy in asthma might be IL-5 and *IL-13*.

ANTIGEN

An antigen is able to induce an *immune response*. It reacts with *antibodies* or specific *B cell* or *T cell antigen receptors*. The name has arisen from its ability to generate antibodies. The antigenic determinant is called an *epitope*, which is the portion of the antigen bound by a given antibody or antigen *receptor*. If the antigen induces an *allergic disease*, it is called an *allergen*.

ANTIGEN DOSE RESPONSES

The concentration of an *antigen* presented to a *T cell* can determine the differential production of *Th1* and *Th2 cytokines*. In a number of experimental models, it has been demonstrated that exposure of T cells derived from atopic donors (or donors specifically sensitive to a particular stimulating *allergen*) to incremental doses of a specific allergen can qualitatively and quantitatively alter the production and secretion of *T cell cytokines*. In Figure 5, the effect of increasing concentrations of bee venom on *cytokine* production by *peripheral blood mononuclear cells* (PBMC) of a bee-venom-allergic subject (see *hymenoptera allergy*) is shown.

> At doses just above those where no response can be detected, the first demonstrable cytokine production is that of *IL-2*.

This would appear to be a purely "empirical" phenomenon, resulting from low-level antigen presentation by *antigen-presenting cells* (APCs) to a sensitized T cell population that undergoes the first stages of activation and induction of proliferation (see *T cell antigen receptor*). If this low-dose exposure is maintained, no *T cell proliferation* occurs and the response is downregulated (see *anergy*) such that a significantly higher allergen dose is required to elicit the same IL-2 response. A higher allergen dose will elicit a small but significant proliferative response, but again no other *T cell cytokine* is produced. When the allergen concentration is raised a little further, evidence of the production of the pro-inflammatory cytokines *IFN-γ* and *TNF-α* becomes apparent. The peak production of IL-2, IFN-γ, and TNF-α occur at the same allergen dose that causes maximum cellular proliferation. This represents a classic Th1 profile and is evident even from donors sensitive to the eliciting allergen.

> As the concentration of allergen rises, IFN-γ and TNF-α production rapidly declines to undetectable levels and is replaced by *IL-4* and *IL-10*, while IL-2 and a proliferative response are still evident, albeit at lower levels.

This *Th2* profile would dominate the response of T cells activated in vivo and be responsible for the induction of *IgE*.

> Under conditions of high allergen concentrations, T cell proliferation ceases and Th2 cytokines disappear, to be replaced by transiently high levels of pro-inflammatory "stress" cytokines and *chemokines*, such as IFN-γ, TNF-α, and *RANTES*, before cytotoxic mechanisms kill the cells.

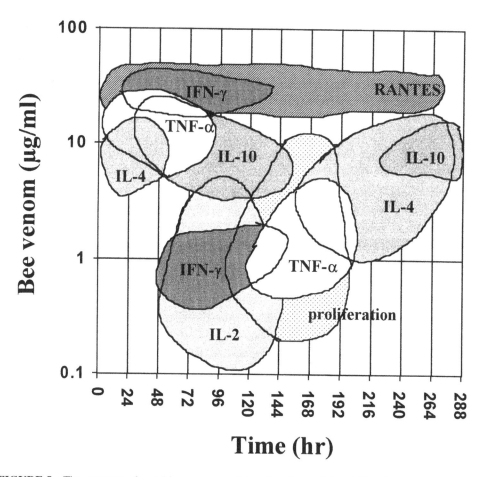

FIGURE 5 The amount of cytokines generated in vitro by peripheral blood mononuclear cells (PBMC) depends on the antigen dose.

The mechanisms that underlie this ability of T cells to apparently switch their cytokine-secreting profiles in response to changes in antigen dose are not clearly understood. There is limited evidence that the T cell antigen receptor can transduce differential signals depending on the occupancy by allergen of the complementary *MHC class II molecules* on APC. In addition, induced expression of co-stimulatory molecules by T cells such as *CD28* has also not been observed after interaction with allergen. However, there is more compelling evidence that these responses may be linked to the ability or inability of the APC to secrete *IL-12* after being activated during the process of antigen recognition, uptake, processing, and presentation.

ANTIGENIC PEPTIDES

Following *antigen* uptake by *antigen-presenting cells* (APCs) by *phagocytosis, pinocytosis,* or internalization of *receptor*-bound molecules, *antigenic peptide* fragments are generated by the action of enzymes in endosomal compartments (see *antigen processing*). The *peptides* are selected by their respective affinities for *major histocompatibility complex* (MHC) molecules, either occupying empty sites or displacing molecules with a lower affinity. The peptide MHC complexes are transported to the cell surface, where they are recognized by the *T cell antigen receptor* (TCR) of *CD4+ T cells*, and co-receptor ligation between the MHC and CD4 molecules occurs (see *T cell–APC interactions*). In order to be presented by *MHC class I* or *II molecules* and be recognized by the TCR, there are quite stringent structural requirements on peptide antigens.

> Peptides cannot greatly exceed the length of the antigen-binding groove, and yet cannot be too short, because both circumstances result in steric hindrance and inability of the co-receptor CD4 or *CD8* molecules to bind to the MHC.

This limitation has facilitated the investigation of *antigen recognition*, where sequence-overlapping synthetic peptides have been used for *epitope mapping*. Large peptides or antigen (*allergen*) fragments, which are unable to bind, require further processing by relevant APCs, but are often the most efficient at eliciting *T cell proliferation*.

ANTIGEN-PRESENTING CELLS (APCs)

Antigen presentation is the process by which antigens become associated with cell surface proteins of the *major histocompatibility complex* (MHC), for recognition by *T cells*. *CD4+ T helper cells* recognize *peptides* of exogenous antigens that have been internalized and processed by APC (see *T cell–APC interactions*) including *monocytes, macrophages, dendritic cells, B cells, Langerhans cells* and, under certain conditions, *T cells* (see *T cell antigen presentation*). Through specific proteolytic machinery, antigens are degraded into peptide fragments of 10 to 12 amino acids (see *antigenic peptides*), which are "loaded" into the cleft of *MHC class II molecules*, and the complex is shuttled to the cell surface and presented to CD4+ T cells. In contrast, *CD8+* cytotoxic T cells recognize peptides from endogenous antigens (e.g., from virus-infected cells) in the cleft of *MHC class I molecules*, found on the surface of all nucleated cells. Moreover, the APC has considerable importance in determining the *cytokine* profile of responding T cells (see *T helper cell differentiation*). Factors that favor *Th2 cell* development include low *IL-12*, but high *CD86* expression by APCs. In addition, low antigen doses presented by the APC preferentially induce Th2 cytokines (see *antigen dose responses*).

ANTIGEN PROCESSING

Following *antigen* uptake via *phagocytosis, pinocytosis,* or *receptor*-mediated *endocytosis* into *antigen-presenting cells* (APCs) (for detailed information, see also *Langerhans cells*), the extracellular fluid containing intracellular vesicles are called early *endosomes*. Here, at an acidic pH, cellular *proteases* cleave the intact protein *antigens* into smaller oligopeptide strands. Subsequently, the endosomes fuse with the *major histocompatibility complex* (MHC) class II-rich vesicles, where Ii (see *invariant chain*) is released from the *MHC class II molecules* and the *antigenic peptides* are loaded to the MHC molecules. Finally, the late endosomes undergo fusion with the plasma membrane, and the loaded MHC molecules are expressed on the cell surface (see *antigen recognition* and *T cell antigen receptor*).

ANTIGEN RECEPTORS

(See *T cell antigen receptor, B cell antigen receptor,* and *high-affinity IgE receptor*.)

ANTIGEN RECOGNITION

> In order to achieve *antigen*-specific activation of *T cells* via the *T cell antigen receptor* (TCR), the current dogma is that *antigenic peptides* are presented in the groove of *MHC class I* or *MHC class II molecules* of *antigen-presenting cells* (APC) to the T cell. This process also involves *CD4* or *CD8* molecules associated with the TCR (see *T cell–APC interactions*).

The TCR comprises two highly variable α and β chains that are associated with the stable *CD3* γ, δ, ε chain complex and with an accessory *signaling* molecule, the ζ chain. During the binding of antigen to the α/β complex, the CD4 or CD8 molecules act as co-receptors, binding to the invariant portion of the interacting MHC molecule.

Studies demonstrating the allelic polymorphism of MHC molecules suggest that T cell (TCR) restriction is brought about by positive selection in the *thymus*, with immature T cells being deleted by apoptosis, having failed to acquire antigenic specificity and the necessary co-receptor molecules necessary for MHC recognition. Having acquired an antigenic specificity and an *MHC restriction*, the TCR becomes a functional *receptor* able to transduce signals (see *signal transduction*), following the extracellular recognition of antigen, into the interior cytoplasmic regions of its transmembranous chains.

It is apparent that an additional co-stimulatory signal (see *co-stimulation*) or signals are required for *T cell activation*, following recognition of the antigen and signaling via the TCR.

Co-stimulatory signals may be provided by one or a combination of several receptor–ligand interactions. The co-stimulatory molecule most closely associated with the TCR is *CD45* and its ligand CD22 expressed on *B cells*. However, other molecules with known facultative co-stimulatory activity include *CD28*, *CD30*, and *CD40* with their respective ligands. There is also evidence that engagement of *CD2*, CD5, and certain *cytokine receptors* can provide co-stimulation. This requirement for co-stimulation is important in allowing an adaptive *immune response* to discriminate self from potentially pathogenic non-self antigens and, as TCR recognition and co-stimulation are required at the same time, in preventing separate and unrelated signals from inappropriately activating a T cell. If a T cell receives a signal via the TCR, but no simultaneous co-stimulation, that cell will become unresponsive to further antigenic stimulation (see *anergy*) or will undergo apoptosis. In contrast to normal antigens, the activation of the TCR by *superantigens* is not MHC-restricted.

The TCR/antigen/MHC/co-receptor/co-stimulatory mechanism (Figure 6) has a remarkable feature — its ability to provide differential or modulated signals in response to varying concentrations of an antigen.

This may well be associated with the type of APC that presents antigen to the T cell. For example, *dendritic cells* exposed to low doses of antigen induce a predominantly *Th2* type of *cytokine* production from activated T cells in a mixed population, whereas when exposed to high doses of antigen the T cell response becomes predominantly *Th1* in nature (see *antigen dose responses*). This may be an effect of the relative activity of the dendritic cell and its ability to secrete *IL-12*. IL-12 is a powerful enhancer of Th1 responses and, conversely, an inhibitor of Th2 cytokine production. These observations may have clinical relevance in the induction of *allergic diseases* as well as in the mechanisms of *immunotherapy*.

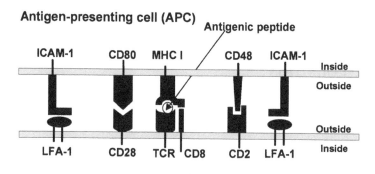

FIGURE 6   The TCR/antigen/co-receptor/co-stimulatory mechanism in T cell activation.

ANTIHISTAMINES

Antihistamines are a group of anti-allergic drugs (see *anti-allergic/anti-asthmatic drugs*) that competitively block the biological effects of *histamine* at the different *histamine receptors*. H_1-antagonists are the relevant subclass of molecules for anti-allergic effects at the different mucocutaneous sites. The sedative side effects of the classical molecules (e.g., dimentiden) are beneficial for some indications such as *atopic dermatitis*, but must be considered as unwanted. The newer nonsedating antihistamines (e.g., *loratadine, cetericine*) are widely used in chronic *urticaria, allergic rhinoconjunctivitis*, and atopic dermatitis, but are not generally useful for treating *asthma*. H_2-antagonists block acid production in the stomach.

ANTI-IgE THERAPY

Various strategies have been considered that aim at the selective inhibition of *IgE antibody* functions and production. An alternative approach has been the use of anti-IgE antibodies to inhibit the IgE response.

Initial studies found that treatment of neonatal mice with polyclonal anti-IgE antibodies specifically reduced serum *IgE levels*.

Secondary IgE responses could be inhibited if anti-IgE was administered during immunization. This effect was not only due to clearance of IgE, since the numbers of IgE-producing *B cells* were also reduced. The approach using anti-IgE antibodies also targets the inhibition of IgE interaction with *high-affinity IgE receptors* (FcεRI). The target structure has been located within the Cε3 domain of IgE.

Using this information, a murine antibody has been developed, and to avoid *antigenicity* of a murine mAb in humans, a humanized version has been made. This antibody was shown to block passive sensitization of human *basophils* and lung *mast cells*. In addition, it inhibited IgE production by human B cells in vitro.

Various human and monkey studies have confirmed that anti-IgE does not *cross-link* IgE receptors on basophils and mast cells.

Administration of anti-IgE results in complex formation with IgE. The maximal size of complexes was two to three IgE molecules and anti-IgE each. An important safety feature of this antibody is that these small *immune complexes* do not activate the *complement system*.

Based on the animal studies data, a series of human clinical trials have been undertaken. In these studies, the anti-IgE antibodies were well tolerated and resulted in a dose-dependent decrease in serum IgE levels. It has been shown that treatment with a single injection of this anti-IgE antibody reduced serum IgE to undetectable levels for more than 2 months. Anti-IgE antibodies did not induce any detectable antibody response in the human, and a marked decrease in FcεRI levels on basophils was also observed. These data demonstrate that FcεRI expression is regulated by plasma IgE levels. The anti-IgE treatment reduced seasonal ragweed *allergy* by reducing symptom scores. In *asthma*, anti-IgE administration produced a significant attenuation of the *early-phase response* as well as the *late-phase response*, indicating a role for IgE not only in immediate, but also in *delayed hypersensitivity* reactions.

Anti-IgE treatment may represent a promising new strategy for the treatment of IgE-mediated *allergic diseases*.

ANTIINFLAMMATORY MECHANISMS

(See *immunosuppressive mechanisms*.)

ANTILEUKOTRIENES

(See *leukotriene receptor antagonists*.)

ANTIMUSCARINIC AGENTS

(See *anticholinergic drugs*.)

ANTINUCLEAR ANTIBODIES (ANA)

Several systemic autoimmune diseases (see *autoimmunity*) are associated with increased levels of ANAs in serum. The profile of ANA can be correlated to defined disease entities.

ANTIOXIDANT

During *inflammation*, *phagocytes* (e.g., *macrophages*, *neutrophils*, or *eosinophils*) generate reactive *oxygen metabolites*, which cause tissue damage. *Glutathione* is an important natural antioxidant. Reduced levels of antioxidants not only increase tissue damage, but also allow *fibroblast* activation by oxidants, leading to an excess formation of *extracellular matrix* proteins and *fibrosis*. Therefore, antioxidant treatment strategies include the normalization of glutathione levels. *N-Acetylcysteine*, a precursor of glutathione biosynthesis, might be able to restore decreased glutathione concentrations in epithelial lining fluid.

ANTISENSE

Antisense oligonucleotides are molecules designed to hybridize to specific sequences of target *mRNAs*. The resulting heteroduplex is cleaved by RNase H. This mechanism appears to play an important role in synthetic antisense oligonucleotide inhibition of *gene* expression both in vivo and in vitro. However, other mechanisms (e.g., inhibition of *translation*) might also play a role. Antisense oligonucleotide drug development therapeutic potential has been illustrated by impressive successes in animal models and in selective clinical trials. For instance, *adenosine* A1 receptors were reduced in the lungs of allergic rabbits, which served as an experimental model of *asthma*, following specific antisense therapy. In the future, this strategy might be helpful to specifically reduce *cytokine* expression in *allergic diseases* (see *anticytokine therapy*).

AP-1

(See *activator protein 1*.)

APOPTOSIS

Apoptosis is the most common form of physiologic or *programmed cell death* (PCD). It is essential for organ development during embryogenesis. After development completion, a multicellular organism must renew many lineages. For instance, red and white blood cells (see *leukocytes*) are constantly generated from hematopoietic progenitor cells in the *bone marrow*. Therefore, a physiologic cell death is a necessary process to maintain correct cell numbers. Apoptotic cells are removed by neighboring *phagocytes* without the induction of an inflammatory response. In contrast to apoptosis, *necrosis* is always a pathologic form of cell death resulting from acute cellular injury that is always associated with *inflammation*.

Apoptosis is defined by characteristic morphologic changes in the dying cell.

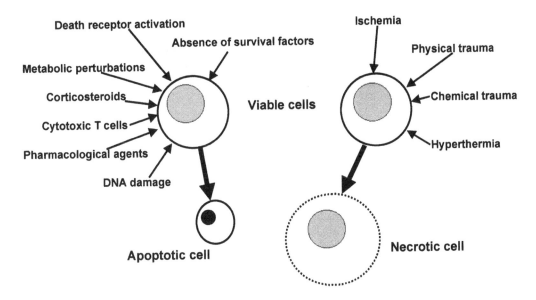

FIGURE 7   Stimuli and morphological features of apoptosis and necrosis.

The most readily observed morphologic features involve the nucleus, where the chromatin becomes extremely condensed before a complete collapse of the nucleus can be observed. Secondly, a loss of cell volume is clearly detectable (see Figure 7).

In addition to morphological changes, apoptosis is characterized by controlled autodigestion of the cell.

Intracellular *proteases* are essential players in the apoptotic death machinery.

These proteases are called *caspases* and belong to one protein family. The caspases-mediated proteolysis results in cytoskeletal disruption, cell-shrinkage, and membrane blebbing. Caspases also activate endonucleases, which degrade nuclear *DNA*. These endonucleases are responsible for nucleus condensation and the internucleosomal *DNA fragmentation* that is often observed in apoptotic cells. This specific type of DNA fragmentation is actually used to demonstrate an apoptotic death in many cellular systems.

All the above-mentioned morphologic changes can be explained by the proteolytic activity in apoptotic cells.

Besides caspases, apoptosis is also controlled by members of the *Bcl-2* family within cells. Since the process of apoptosis participates in the control of cell numbers, its (dys)regulation (see Figure 8) plays an important role in inflammatory processes (see *T cell apoptosis*, *B cell apoptosis*, *eosinophil apoptosis*, *neutrophil apoptosis*, and *mast cell apoptosis*).

APPLE ALLERGEN

Fresh apples may cause *oral allergy syndrome* (OAS). There is a sequence *homology* between the apple *allergen* and the *major allergen* of *birch pollen*, Bet v 1.

ARACHIDONIC ACID (AA)

AA (5,8,11,14-eicosatetraenoic acid) is a fatty acid and is stored in cell membranes as a glycerolipid. Activated cytosolic *phospholipase A_2* (PLA_2) specifically hydrolyzes nuclear

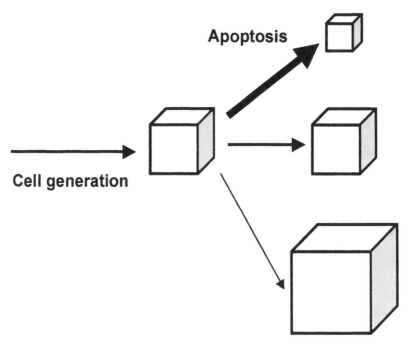

FIGURE 8 Cell numbers are regulated by both cell generation and apoptosis. Under normal conditions apoptosis is an important mechanism to maintain cellular homeostasis. The figure illustrates the effect of decreased (thin arrow) or accelerated (thick arrow) apoptosis on cell numbers.

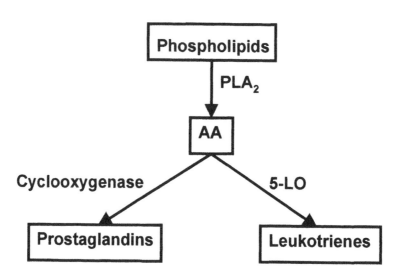

FIGURE 9 Metabolism of arachidonic acid (AA).

membrane phospholipids to generate AA. As shown in Figure 9, there are two major pathways by which AA is metabolized, the *cyclooxygenase* (COX) pathway (which eventually leads to production of *prostaglandins*), and the *5-lipoxygenase* (5-LO) pathway (which leads to production of *leukotrienes*).

ARRESTIN

Arrestin is a molecule that is believed to act as a deactivator of *signal transduction* initiated via activation of *G-protein-coupled receptors*. Arrestin binds to G-protein-coupled receptors, and is thought to sterically prevent *G protein* interaction, thereby quenching the catalytic activity of the *receptor*. However, recent data suggest that arrestin, at least in *β2-adrenergic receptor* signaling, may act as an adapter molecule between G proteins and the *mitogen-activated protein kinase* (MAPK) pathway.

ARTHUS REACTION

This is a descriptive term of an *immune complex* reaction (see *Coombs and Gell classification,* type III).

ARYLSULFATASE

This enzyme belongs to the group of *acid hydrolases* and exists in two isomeric forms, A and B; both are present in *mast cells, eosinophils,* and *fibroblasts*. The arylsulfatase type B is also present in *basophils, neutrophils,* and *monocytes*. Upon *IgE*-mediated activation, only the A isomer is released (together with *histamine*) from mast cells, suggesting that type B is stored in secondary *granules*, which are not accessible to secretion. Arylsulfatase cleaves sulfate esters of aromatic compounds.

ASCERTAINMENT

This is the identification of individuals or families with an inherited condition.

ASCORBATE

Ascorbate (vitamin C), vitamins A and E, as well as selenium are nutritional *antioxidants* involved in various host-defense mechanisms. Some patients with *asthma* report *wheeze* after ingestion of ascorbate.

ASPERGILLUS

Aspergillus is a fungus that is ubiquitously distributed. There are several known species. Among these, Aspergillus fumigatus appears to be the most important strain involved in pathogenic processes. It can cause several diseases depending on the susceptibility of the host. For instance, aspergillus is an important *fungal allergen* and can cause *IgE*-mediated *allergic diseases*, such as *allergic rhinitis* and *allergic asthma*, but can also cause *allergic bronchopulmonary aspergillosis* (ABPA). A complete spectrum of aspergillus-induced diseases is given in Table 13.

ASPIRIN

Aspirin is an important *nonsteroidal antiinflammatory drug* (NSAID) that blocks the activity of *cyclooxygenase* by acetylating the terminal amino group of this *prostaglandin* (PG)-producing enzyme. PGs enhance inflammatory effects; therefore, aspirin is a potent antiinflammatory agent. Because aspirin has side effects on the gastrointestinal tract, there are now new compounds available (see *cyclooxygenase-2 inhibitors*). Recent data suggest that aspirin is also a blocker of *nuclear factor-κB* (NF-κB) and a trigger of *lipoxins*.

Aspirin does not reduce *allergic inflammation*, but may induce *asthma* in sensitive patients (see *aspirin-sensitive asthma*).

TABLE 13
Aspergillus-Induced Diseases

Allergic diseases
- Allergic rhinitis
- Allergic *sinusitis*
- Allergic asthma
- *Extrinsic allergic alveolitis*
- ABPA

Saprophytic diseases
- Pulmonary aspergillus intracavitary colonization
- Aspergilloma

Invasive diseases
- Tracheobronchitis
- Chronic necrotizing pulmonary aspergillosis
- Invasive pulmonary aspergillosis
- Disseminated aspergillosis
- Aspergillus pleural empyema
- Orbital aspergillosis

ASPIRIN-INDUCED ASTHMA

This is a synonym of *aspirin-sensitive asthma.*

ASPIRIN-SENSITIVE ASTHMA

A substantial minority of adult asthmatic patients report worsening of their symptoms after taking *aspirin* or other *nonsteroidal antiinflammatory drugs* (NSAIDs). The mechanism of aspirin-sensitive *asthma* involves increased sensitivity to *leukotrienes*, and excessive production of leukotrienes after ingestion of drugs that block the *cyclooxygenase* (COX) pathway of *arachidonic acid* (AA) metabolism. Clinical features of aspirin-sensitive asthma include *nasal polyps, eosinophilia,* and *adult-onset asthma.* In the past, aspirin-sensitive asthma was thought to be more common in nonallergic asthmatics (see *intrinsic asthma*), but recent data suggest that it is, in fact, equally common in both allergic (see *allergic asthma*) and nonallergic patients. Management is by avoidance of aspirin and NSAIDs, and patients normally respond well to *leukotriene receptor antagonists* (see also *European Network on Aspirin-Induced Asthma*).

ASSOCIATION

This term is used to describe direct interactions between molecules, e.g., during *signal transduction* cascades. The term is also frequently used when certain measurable parameters correlate with a functional response (e.g., symptoms of a patient). In a population, the occurrence together of two or more different phenotypes or the occurrence of a phenotype together with *alleles* more often than expected by chance is also called association.

ASTEATOSIS

(See *dry skin.*)

ASTHMA

Asthma is becoming increasingly common throughout the Western developed world, and there is a huge amount of literature devoted to the epidemiology (see *asthma epidemiology*), genetics (see *genetic predisposition*), pathophysiology (see *allergic inflammation, cytokines, eosinophils, IgE, mast cells, mediators, T cells*, etc.) and therapy (see *asthma treatment strategies*) of the disease. Much of this is of limited relevance to the practicing clinician, who wants a simple guide to the strategies that work for diagnosis, treatment, and long-term management of the condition. From 1988 onward a series of *management guidelines of asthma* have been issued: at first these encapsulated existing best practices, but subsequently guideline developers have started to address the evidence underpinning existing practices. This process has revealed a number of interesting areas of disagreement between evidence and practice, and the guidelines have been modified accordingly.

Definition
Asthma is a heterogeneous lung disease (see *allergic asthma, aspirin-sensitive asthma, exercise-induced asthma, intrinsic asthma*, etc.) with the following characteristics: (1) *airway obstruction* that is reversible (but not completely so in some patients) either spontaneously or with treatment, (2) *inflammation* of the airway mucosa, (3) *airway hyperresponsiveness* to a variety of stimuli.

Diagnosis
In clinical terms, asthma may be defined as a disorder in which there is variable narrowing of the airways, with changes of airway caliber occurring over short periods of time. The baseline lung function may be normal, but serial recording of *peak expiratory flow rate* (PEFR) will usually show variation throughout the day. Variability may be expressed as the difference between the maximum and minimum PEFR values in a given day, divided by the maximum PEFR value. If this proportion exceeds 15%, then the patient is automatically regarded as asthmatic. In patients who do not fulfil this criterion, asthma may still be diagnosed if the patient shows a good response to inhaled *β2-agonist* (again 15% or greater), or responds to a course of oral or inhaled *corticosteroids* with a similar degree of improvement. Finally, some patients only show bronchoconstriction after exercise or when suffering from respiratory infections (see *asthma exacerbation*). In adults with *occupational asthma*, the pattern of PEFR variability may differ from the usual "morning dips." If the patient is sensitized to *allergens* encountered in the workplace, then the PEFR may be lowest toward the end of the day (or after the shift), and there may be different patterns at the beginning and end of a working week (see *questionnaire*).

The principal differential diagnoses of asthma are *chronic obstructive pulmonary disease* (COPD) and heart disease.

In COPD, there is usually a degree of fixed air flow obstruction and often some *emphysema*, which may be detected by formal *lung function tests*, including a carbon monoxide *transfer factor*. Particular diagnostic difficulties arise in patients with a history of *child-onset asthma*, those who have smoked, and those who have worked in industries that are associated with occupational asthma.

Therapy
The present *asthma treatment strategies* are built on three guiding principles: (1) treat the inflammation, and the other symptoms will come into line, (2) start with high doses, and step down as you achieve control, and (3) help patients to manage their asthma themselves through self-management plans rather than relying on medical support.

ASTHMA DEATH
(See *death from asthma*.)

ASTHMA EPIDEMIOLOGY

For all age groups, the incidence of *asthma* has been estimated to range from 2.65/1000/year to 4.00/1000/year. Prevalence estimates for asthma in the U.S. range from 3.0 to 10.5%. Occurrence of asthma is generally thought to be lower in less developed areas. These estimates are difficult to make because asthma is often under-diagnosed. Of interest is the increased prevalence of asthma in Australia and New Zealand. Children born to parents with asthma have a threefold increased risk of developing asthma than children born of non-atopic parents (see *genetic predisposition*). Many have suggested that a more accurate assessment of asthma may be made from examination of specific symptoms (*wheeze, cough*) rather than the diagnosis of asthma. There are two primary ages during which asthma may have its onset: before age 5 and in adulthood (see *risk factors*).

ASTHMA EXACERBATION

This is an episode of destabilization of *asthma*, often associated with increased *cough* and *sputum*, prolonged *airway obstruction*, and dyspnea.

> Exacerbations may be triggered by viral infection, especially in children.

The viruses most frequently associated with asthma exacerbation are *rhinovirus* and *respiratory syncytial virus*. Consequently, subjects with asthma may be more likely to have exacerbations during the fall, when viral respiratory tract infections are more likely to occur. *Allergen* exposure, chemicals, or tobacco smoke (see *smoking*) may also exacerbate asthma. Outdoor environmental *pollutants*, especially *ozone* and particulate matter, also are associated with increased asthma symptoms, hospital and emergency room visits, and medication use.

Most patients are advised to double their dose of *inhaled corticosteroids* (ICS) at the first sign of deterioration, although there is little evidence that this makes much difference. In any significant exacerbation, the most useful measure is to start oral *corticosteroids* (e.g., *prednisolone* 30 to 40 mg daily). Conventional inhalers may become ineffective, due to complete *airway obstruction* by *mucus* plugs, and nebulized *bronchodilators* (see *nebulizer*) are useful to ensure that the drugs are delivered to all ventilated airways. The role of intravenous aminophylline (see *theophylline*) remains controversial, with most studies showing little or no benefit above that conferred by nebulized *salbutamol*. *Antibiotics* are not routinely needed, but should be given if there is evidence of bacterial infection. In severe exacerbations, the arterial *blood gases* will show *hypoxemia*, with a reduced p_aCO_2, but if the exacerbation is prolonged, and the patient becomes exhausted, the p_aCO_2 may start to rise. This is an indication for assisted ventilation, because if left untreated, the patient will rapidly succumb.

ASTHMA PREVENTION

Outside of *occupational asthma*, primary prevention of *asthma* onset through avoidance of asthma-inducing *allergens* or *pollutants* is unproven. Recent research suggests that avoidance of *house-dust mite* allergen and *smoking* can reduce asthma incidence in infants. Secondary prevention of asthma in patients with *allergic rhinoconjunctivitis* might be achieved by *allergen avoidance*, early *immunotherapy* (before *polysensitization*), and optimal antiinflammatory therapy.

ASTHMA TREATMENT STRATEGIES

Treating inflammation to control asthma

Patients with infrequent symptoms (*wheeze* or using *β2-agonists* fewer than three times per week) are probably best managed on a β2-agonist *bronchodilator*, used on an as-required basis. These patients do have airways *inflammation* on biopsy, but their symptoms are so infrequent that it would be impossible to achieve *compliance* with regular medication, even if there was any evidence of long-term benefit from regular therapy.

> Most adult patients with mild persistent *asthma* should be started on *inhaled corticosteroids* (ICS).

This is typically done by using beclomethasone 400 to 800 mg/day, and then adjusting to achieve a maintenance dose that keeps the *peak expiratory flow rate* (PEFR) stable and minimizes or abolishes symptoms.

> Breakthrough symptom relief is achieved by providing a β2-agonist as required.

Evidence from Finland would suggest that there may be some long-term advantage in starting ICS early, in that patients who started ICS at presentation ended up with better lung function than patients who were managed for the 2 years with a β2-agonist as required before receiving ICS. There have been criticisms of this study, in that there were many drop-outs in the β2-agonist only group, but until better data are provided, the indications are that we should aim to start ICS earlier rather than later.

> Patients who do not settle on standard doses of ICS (typically they will show persistent variability of PEFR, persistent nocturnal waking, or excessive use of a β2-agonist) should be given a long-acting bronchodilator as well as their ICS.

At present, there seem to be few criteria to use in choosing between salmeterol and eformoterol. Eformoterol has some theoretical advantages in speed of onset of action, but physicians have greater familiarity with salmeterol. Some patients may prefer an oral bronchodilator such as *theophylline* or bambuterol. The usefulness of oral bronchodilators may be limited by tremor and other systemic toxicity: blood monitoring and tailoring of doses is advisable when using theophylline preparations. *Anticholinergic agents* are recommended to control asthma symptoms in patients who cannot tolerate the side effects of an adrenergic bronchodilator. *Intravenous immunoglobulin* (*IVIG*) *preparations* may have a steroid-sparing effect.

Start high and step down

The initial sets of asthma management guidelines implied that one should start low and step up the level of therapy gradually until one achieves "good control." However, at the moment, it is clear that many clinicians use a different approach, starting patients on high-dose ICS or even oral *corticosteroids*, and then stepping down to the maintenance dose. To start with, this debate was largely based on opinion, but there is now some evidence that the "start high, step down" approach is superior to the "start low and step up" approach. One advantage of the "start high, step down" approach is that the illness will come under control more quickly, so the patient may be more inclined to trust the doctor and follow future therapeutic advice!

Self-management plans

Alongside the development of guidelines (see *management guidelines of asthma*), many clinicians recognized that in the practical day-to-day management of asthma it would be better to involve the patient, in the form of a self-management plan.

> The key elements of self-management are (1) empowering patients to monitor their disease; (2) providing them with the tools to make planned adjustments to the therapy; (3) providing a safety net in the form of ready access to advice if they reach the limits of their competence or confidence to manage problems.

The first part of this process can be achieved by providing patients with their own *peak flow meters*. Following an initial period when they make regular recordings and bring these to the asthma clinic for verification and discussion, patients are then given a written plan of what to do if their PEFR drops to a specified level. Typically the patient and doctor, or the patient and the asthma specialist nurse, will agree on a "usual best" level, a level at which the dose of ICS should be increased, a level at which oral corticosteroids should be commenced, and a level at which urgent medical attention should be sought. The patient is then educated in the rationale of asthma therapy, both for maintenance and for *asthma exacerbations*, and is given a supply of *prednisolone* for emergency use. The patient is encouraged to be responsible for ordering further supplies of medication and negotiates an agreed level of supervision with the primary care team who are in overall charge. Arrangements are made for contact with the clinic or practice in the event of an emergency.

> *Education* and cooperation are the most successful means of achieving compliance.

For the doctor and asthma specialist nurse, the price of self-management includes the need to be available and nonjudgmental when patients reach the limits of their knowledge and competence. It is not enough to say "phone me if you have any queries"; you have to respond positively when you are phoned about what may seem to you to be trivial matters. They are not trivial to the patient, otherwise they would not have phoned you.

New developments/strategies
Due to intensive research, our understanding of asthma pathogenic mechanisms is constantly improving. Consequently, new drugs and treatment strategies are frequently developed (see *leukotriene receptor antagonists, phosphodiesterase inhibitors, anti-IgE therapy, cytokine therapy, anticytokine therapy, antisense, gene therapy, DNA immunotherapy, peptide immunotherapy, IL-10, CD86,* and *interferon-α*).

ATOPIC DERMATITIS

Atopic dermatitis is one of the most common skin diseases in developed countries, and its incidence is still increasing. The predisposition to develop atopic dermatitis, the atopic diathesis (see *atopy*), is also a predisposition for *allergic asthma* and *allergic rhinoconjunctivitis* (see *genetic predisposition*).

Definition
Atopic dermatitis may be defined as a chronic or chronic recurrent inflammatory skin disease with marked pruritus, variability in lesion morphology and overall course, and characteristic immunological phenomena. Diagnostic criteria for atopic dermatitis have been established by *Hanifin-Rajka*. These criteria are frequently used in clinical trials.

Clinical features
The clinical morphology of atopic dermatitis is highly variable, and the characteristic findings depend on the patient's age.

> In neonates, crusted lesions resembling scalded milk, the milk scurf (*Crusta lactea*), are the first manifestations of atopic dermatitis.

Scalp, cheeks, and arms are commonly affected, but widespread involvement of the entire skin is common as well. There is a high tendency toward exudative lesions and superinfection. Later on in childhood, the involvement changes to the characteristic flexural eczema. *Lichenification*, which is uncommon in neonatal life, becomes the characteristic hallmark of the disease.

> In adolescents and young adults, symmetrical involvement of the flexures, back of the hands, head, neck, and upper thorax is characteristic of atopic dermatitis.

In addition, many *stigmata* of the atopic constitution, such as *Hertoghe's sign* and *Dennie–Morgan infraorbital fold* become apparent. Agonizing *pruritus*, frequently occurring in paroxysmal attacks, causes insomnia, exhaustion, and impaired performance at school and work. The rubbing and scratching leads to the characteristic, reactive lichenification of the skin. Intolerance to wool and itch sensations during sweating are typical. Exposure to relevant *allergens* such as *animal dander* or *house-dust mite* may trigger acute phases of atopic dermatitis. Most of all, patients react to environmental stress with worsening of the atopic dermatitis. Atopic dermatitis tends to decrease in intensity after the age of 30 years.

> Pruritic nodules in otherwise unaffected skin may predominate the symptoms of atopic dermatitis in later life.

This *prurigo*-form of atopic dermatitis is extremely difficult to treat and may persist for decades. In addition, special forms of atopic dermatitis may be present at different locations: scalp lesions with some hemorrhagic crusts in areas of pityriasiform scaling are seen from time to time, especially in patients with pityrosporon colonization at the scalp and positive *prick test* reactions toward pityrosporon ovale. Moreover, earlobe involvement with minor inflammatory reactions at the lower attachment of the earlobe with a single, deep fissure is often observed. Pronounced creasing of the lips, especially during winter time, leads to an exfoliative cheilitis sicca. Pulpite sèche is the occurrence of reddened skin at the fingertips with fine, firmly attached scaling sometimes accompanied by fissures and reminiscent of tinea manuum. Nummular atopic dermatitis is a clinically defined subgroup with coin-shaped lesions otherwise resembling classical atopic dermatitis, the reasons for which remain unclear.

Pathogenesis
The exact pathogenesis of atopic dermatitis is still unclear. However, some features of the underlying immune dysregulation have been identified. Atopic dermatitis patients are mounting *IgE*-responses against environmental *aeroallergens*, *food allergens*, and autoantigens of the skin, leading to increased serum *IgE-levels*. CD1a-positive epidermal cells (i.e., *Langerhans cells* and *IDEC*) show an upregulation of *high-affinity IgE-receptors*. There is evidence for an IgE-mediated and facilitated *antigen* presentation of *aeroallergens* in atopic dermatitis patients. The skin lesions demonstrate dense lymphocytic infiltrates (see below). Besides this, atopic dermatitis patients have a tendency toward cutaneous infections and frequently exhibit disturbances of cellular and humoral immunity. The genetic background of atopic dermatitis has been thoroughly investigated, and there is evidence with a linkage to some *candidate genes*.

Histopathology and immunohistochemistry
The histopathology of atopic dermatitis is uncharacteristic; the predominant features reflect the clinical characteristics of the biopsied lesions. *Acanthosis*, a few spongiotic vesicles, and a perivascular lymphohistiocytic infiltrate predominate the acute form in children.

> Chronic lesions of atopic dermatitis show the characteristic thickening of the *epidermis* with hyper- and parakeratosis.

Histopathology cannot differentiate atopic dermatitis from allergic *contact dermatitis*. Immunohistochemical investigations (see *immunohistochemistry*) have revealed that both *CD4+* and *CD8+ T cells* infiltrate into the skin. The majority of these cells are CLA+ (see *cutaneous lymphocyte antigen*). Besides T cells, significant numbers of *B cells* are part of the lymphocytic infiltrate. The lymphocytes express large amounts of *IL-5* and *IL-13*, but only marginal levels of *IFN-γ*. However, some authors reported that the IFN-γ *gene* is induced in chronic lesions.

Diagnostic procedures

The diagnosis of atopic dermatitis is easy when typical skin lesions such as flexural eczema and stigmata of the atopic constitution are present. However, atypical cases with minimal or uncharacteristic symptoms may be a diagnostic problem even for experienced dermatologists. The differential diagnosis from chronic allergic contact dermatitis, psoriasis vulgaris, pityriasis rubra pilaris, or cutaneous *T cell lymphoma* may sometimes require a biopsy. Histological or immunohistological examination and eventually Langerhans cell phenotyping might be useful to support the clinical diagnosis.

> Upon diagnosis of atopic dermatitis, a number of additional diagnostic procedures must be undertaken, not to formally establish the diagnosis, but to identify the relevant provocation factors for the individual patient.

The basis of all diagnostic procedures is a carefully taken history, which should include the family and personal history of *allergic diseases*, and all aspects of provocation factors from the private and occupational environment. Quite often, patients report worsening of the atopic dermatitis from *food allergens*, contact with animals, or psychological stress.

Laboratory investigations should include a differential blood count, total serum *IgE levels*, allergen-specific IgE (see *RAST, Phadiatop, CAP-System*), anti-streptolysin, and anti-staphylolysin serum titers. If possible, a prick test should be done as a screening test for aeroallergen or food allergen *sensitization*, whereas *delayed hypersensitivity* reactions against ointment bases or other contact allergens should be assessed by a *patch test*. Sometimes, oral *provocation tests* are needed to clarify the clinical relevance of a positive prick test reaction for the atopic dermatitis.

Therapy

The therapy of atopic dermatitis is an art. Scientifically based information and motivation to follow the guidelines of treatment are the only bases for long-term success in the management of atopic dermatitis. Every patient's lesions change over time, and every patient shows a unique, individual response to various treatment options.

> There is no standard treatment for atopic dermatitis, not even in a single patient over time. The basis for each atopic dermatitis therapy is proper skin care, including the frequent application of an emollient. In addition to the emollient therapy of unaffected skin, inflammatory skin lesions should be treated with an antiinflammatory drug.

For a given patient at a given timepoint, the experienced dermatologist will decide on the optimal therapy. Every patient should have a semi-fatty cream and a fatty ointment available at home for daily selection of "what feels best." Bath oils can be used to prevent additional drying of the skin, while frequent bathing, especially in hot water, should be avoided. Emollients containing urea (5 to 10%) are good moisturizers, but have a stinging effect if applied to inflamed skin, especially in children. Glycerol is a good moisturizer too, but has limitations for inflamed skin.

Topical *corticosteroids* are the most commonly prescribed therapy, since they have few side effects and are easy and convenient to use. The experienced dermatologist will choose an ointment with the desired antiinflammatory strength and ointment base characteristics from the various products available in his country. Coal tar products are no longer frequently used, because they are less effective than newer treatments and have cosmetic disadvantages. Liquor carbonis detergens formulations provide an optimal ratio between antiinflammatory effects and cosmetic acceptance. Various *UV light* modalities (e.g., UV-A, UV-A/UV-B, UV-B, 311 nm UV-B, PUVA, and recently photo-sole therapy) have been used with success in atopic dermatitis. Disadvantages include photo-aging of the skin, especially for UV-A therapy, and a possible increased risk of skin cancer, especially for UV-B and PUVA-treated patients. Topical immunosuppressive *macrolides* (e.g., *tacrolimus* and ascomycin ointments) are highly promising.

Many different drugs are used as supportive therapies in atopic dermatitis. For instance, *antihistamines* may help to control the itch, especially at night. Antiseptics and antibiotics are needed in case of clinically apparent superinfection, and help to reduce the amount of antiinflammatory drugs needed to control the atopic dermatitis. Bufexamac is a topical *nonsteroidal antiinflammatory drug* (NSAID) which may help for a time, but is limited in use because of the frequently occurring *contact sensitization*.

> Systemic treatment of atopic dermatitis should be considered only if topical treatment fails.

Cyclosporin A, *azathioprine*, and *methotrexate* have been used with success in severe, recalcitrant cases. Extracorporal photopheresis is another effective, but cost-intensive therapy. The benefit of this regimen should be weighed against the known (and yet unknown) side effects.

> The elimination of identified provocation factors is crucial for the long-term course of atopic dermatitis.

House-dust mites should be effectively removed by a combination of *acaricides*, frequent use of *vacuum cleaners*, dust-mite-tight covers for mattresses, blankets, and pillows, as well as removal of carpets, curtains, and sofas (see *allergen avoidance*). Unspecific atopic dermatitis diets (see *allergy diet*) without proper diagnosis are not recommended, as their effects are more than questionable; they may even lead to malnutrition. Only those food items should be avoided that have been proven to cause flare-up reactions in oral provocation tests. If the disease is worsened by the presence of domestic animals (cats, dogs, birds), they should be removed from the house. Removal of certain plants (e.g., Ficus benjamina) from the house, and especially from sleeping rooms, may be beneficial as well. *Climate therapy*, especially in high-altitude areas (in the European Alps over 1500 m, there are no house-dust mites) or a sea climate, is helpful. Due to its location below sea level, a therapy at the Dead Sea gives a combination of sole therapy and UV-A-enriched heliotherapy. The relief from stress at work or in private life may also help.

ATOPIC DIATHESIS

(See *atopy*.)

ATOPIC ECZEMA

A synonym of *atopic dermatitis* that is more frequently used in Europe.

ATOPIC KERATOCONJUNCTIVITIS

This is a form of *allergic keratoconjunctivitis*.

ATOPY

The word "atopy" (atopia = strangeness) was coined to describe the phenomenon of *allergy* and reactivity to foreign material (*allergens*) causing the cluster of *asthma*, *allergic rhinitis*, and *atopic dermatitis*.

> No overall accepted definition exists for *atopy*. Atopy could be defined as the *genetic predisposition* toward the development of *immediate hypersensitivity* reactions against common environmental *antigens*.

Traditionally, atopy was know to be associated with large amounts of tissue-sensitizing *IgE antibodies*. Over the years, the term has been modified and, in some cases, has lost its link to IgE *sensitization*. For instance, atopic dermatitis is a clinical definition and not based on IgE measurements. In general, allergy is the process underlying *allergic diseases*, whereas atopy is the state that the patient is in. Atopy predisposes the patient to become allergic.

Atopy occurs in about 30% of the general population in industrialized countries (see *risk factors*). Several studies show that men have an increased risk of developing asthma and of being sensitized to common *aeroallergens* such as *house-dust mite* and *cat allergen* as assessed by skin *prick test* and specific IgE measurements (see *RAST*, *Phadiatop*, and *CAP-System*) compared to women. These gender differences are more prominent in children than in teenagers or young adults. Moreover, total *IgE levels* are higher in men compared to women independently from *smoking*.

ATOPY PATCH TEST

(See *patch test*.)

ATOPY STIGMATA

Constitutional stigmata associated with *atopic dermatitis*. These include *dry skin* (*xerosis*, *sebostasis*), *hyperlinear palms* and soles, a doubled infraorbital fold (*Dennie–Morgan fold*), thinning or complete absence of the eyebrows in their lateral aspects (*Hertoghe's sign*), *keratosis pilaris*, white *dermographism*, facial pallor, orbital darkening, and a low hairline.

ATROPINE

Atropine is a naturally occurring alkaloid found in high concentrations in the leaves, seeds, stems, and roots of Datura genus plants. It is well absorbed from mucosal surfaces. It is highly selective for *muscarinic receptors*, and may counteract all physiologic functions of the parasympathetic system (see *acetylcholine*). It causes relaxation of *smooth muscle* in the airways (see *bronchodilation*), in the gastrointestinal and biliary tracts, the iris, peripheral vasculature, as well as in the bladder and ureters. Moreover, atropine causes mild bradycardia in small doses and tachycardia in higher doses. It also inhibits *mucociliary clearance* in the airways.

> Because atropine acts as a *bronchodilator*, several anticholinergic agents have been developed to treat *asthma* and *COPD*.

Ipratropium and *oxitropium* are quaternary ammonium compounds derived from atropine. They are poorly absorbed, while retaining their local anticholinergic actions after inhalation (see *asthma treatment strategies*).

ATS

American Thoracic Society.

AUTOALLERGY

Identical *IgE*-mediated immune reactions (see *allergen-induced immune responses*) caused by different *antigens* can be observed as a consequence of *cross-reacting allergens*. Such a phenomenon could also occur when *epitopes* of human proteins are identical or very similar to those found in *allergens*. Indeed, some allergens may have the capacity to induce autoimmune reactions (see *autoimmunity*). For instance, there is a high degree of similarity between the Mn-superoxide dismutases (this is an allergen of Aspergillus fumigatus, see *fungal allergens*) across species. Therefore, a possible autoallergy has been proposed in *allergic bronchopulmonary aspergillosis* (ABPA). There are many more examples where allergens and human proteins are highly homologous. Future work will determine the importance of autoallergy in the pathogenesis of IgE-mediated *allergic diseases*.

AUTOIMMUNITY

Autoimmune diseases are diseases where the *immune response* is directed against self-*antigens*. Pathologic immune reactions may arise as a consequence of autoantibody production (see *Coombs and Gell classification*, type II). Other autoimmune diseases are associated with *delayed hypersensitivity* (type IV) with aberrant *Th1* and/or *Tc1 cell* activity. For instance, a polarized Th1 response is implicated in *multiple sclerosis*, insulin-dependent diabetes mellitus (IDDM), and *rheumatoid arthritis* (RA). In these diseases, a failure of *T cell–APC interactions* results in the presentation and recognition of self-antigens.

AUTOSOME

An autosome is any *chromosome* other than the sex chromosomes. They exist in pairs in an individual, regardless of the sex. There are 22 pairs in the human *genome*.

AVIDITY

Avidity is the total strength of binding of two molecules (e.g., between an *antigen* and an *antibody*) or cells to one another at multiple sites. It is distinct from *affinity*, which is the strength of binding of one site on a molecule to its ligand.

AVOIDANCE OF ALLERGENS

(See *allergen avoidance*.)

AVOIDANCE OF INDOOR AIR POLLUTANTS

Several methods are useful to decrease indoor *allergens* (*aeroallergens*) and *pollutants* exposure (see *allergen avoidance, air conditioning, air-duct cleaning, dehumidifiers, humidifiers, indoor air cleaning devices, vacuuming*).

AZATHIOPRINE

This is an *immunosuppressive drug*.

AZELASTINE

This is a long-acting *antihistamine* of the second generation. It inhibits both *immediate* and *delayed hypersensitivity* reactions in *allergic rhinitis* patients. There is evidence that azelastine also inhibits *histamine* release in *mast cells* and *basophils*. It may also block *leukotriene* synthesis in mast cells and *neutrophils*.

B

B7.1

(See *CD80*.)

B7.2

(See *CD86*.)

BACTERIAL EXPRESSION SYSTEM

Protein expression from a cloned *gene* using a bacterial host. Expression of a cloned gene is under the control of *plasmid DNA* sequences flanking the gene of interest. These sequences include a *promoter* region, where the DNA-dependent *RNA polymerase* initiates *transcription* of *mRNA* from the gene. mRNA is subsequently translated to protein (see *translation*) by bacterial protein synthesis machinery (ribosomes, tRNA). Promoters may be constitutive (always available to polymerase) or inducible (availability to polymerase is controlled, usually by a competitive inhibitor molecule). Bacterial expression systems for allergens have been developed in E. coli. The advantages of using bacterial systems include simple culture conditions, rapid generation times, and large yields at low production costs.

BAKERS' ASTHMA

People working with flour can often develop *occupational asthma*. The most common agent implicated is the enzyme *α-amylase*, which is added to the flour to improve it. Moreover, the water-soluble albumin and globulin fractions as well as wheat *α-amylase inhibitor protein* were identified as *major allergens* of wheat flour. Individuals with *asthma* are excluded from joining the baking trade. Therefore, most cases of bakers' asthma are obviously induced by occupational exposure. In Western countries, for example, during a working period of 20 years, 20% of bakers become sensitized.

BAMBUTEROL

Bambuterol is a *β2-agonist*.

BANANA

IgE-mediated allergic reactions have been reported in patients with *latex allergy* (see *cross-reacting allergens*).

BARE LYMPHOCYTE SYNDROME

A disease caused by defective MHC class II transactivator, where a lack of *MHC class II molecule* expression is observed on all cells.

BASE PAIR (bp)

Measure of the length of a double-stranded *DNA* molecule by the pairs *adenine* (A) and *thymine* (T) or *cytosine* (C) and *guanine* (G).

BASOPHIL

Basophils, like *eosinophils* and *neutrophils*, belong to the *granulocyte* subpopulation of *leukocytes*. Like *mast cells*, these cells express *high-affinity IgE receptors* on the surface. Therefore, they play a major role in *immediate hypersensitivity* reactions of *IgE*-mediated *allergic diseases*. Although basophils also generate and release *histamine*, they appear to be more functionally related to eosinophils than to mast cells. Basophils and eosinophils share most of their surface *receptors* (see *eosinophil surface molecules*) and respond to *cytokines, chemokines*, and other agents in a similar fashion. Since they express large amounts of *IL-4* and *IL-13*, basophils may play a major role in the development of *Th2 cells* in these diseases. However, their exact role and contribution in the development of allergic diseases is still unclear.

B CELL

B cells belong to the *lymphocyte* subpopulation of *leukocytes*, which they share with *T cells*. B cells are generally located in the circulation and in lymphoid tissues. They are derived from *bone marrow* stem cells. In their immature state, they are smooth, spherical cells of about 15 to 20 μm in diameter. They are characterized by the expression of surface-bound IgM that is part of the *B cell antigen receptor* (positive for CD19). B cells can recognize and present *antigen* to T cells (see *B cell antigen presentation*) and, when activated, develop into large polymorphous *antibody*-producing *plasma cells* (negative for CD19). *Antibody affinity maturation* and *gene rearrangement* result in *isotype* selection and expression of antigen-specific antibodies of five main classes: IgM, IgA, IgD, *IgE*, and *IgG*. Activation (see *B cell activation*), maturation, differentiation (see *B cell differentiation*), and survival (see *B cell apoptosis*) are strongly enhanced by *cytokines* such as *IL-2, IL-4, IL-6*, and IL-11.

B CELL ACTIVATION

> *B cells* can specifically be activated by *antigens* via the *B cell antigen receptor*, resulting in *B cell proliferation* and IgM production without *T cell* help.

In contrast to specific activation, nonspecific activation of B cells is defined as polyclonal B cell activation. This could be achieved by *antibodies* to or natural ligands of CD19, CD21, or *CD40*. In addition, anti-*immunoglobulin* treatment induces a polyclonal B cell activation in vitro. Many other agents can also act as polyclonal activators, the so-called mitogens. For instance, lipopolysaccharide (from cell walls of Gram negative bacteria), pokeweed mitogen, and dextran sulfate are polyclonal B cell activators.

> B cells can also be activated by *T cell cytokines*. Such T cell help is needed for *IgG* production during *secondary immune response*.

Strong *IL-4* and/or *IL-13* stimulation may result in *immunoglobulin class switching* and increased *IgE* production.

B CELL ANTIGEN PRESENTATION

Following *cross-linking* of *B cell antigen receptors*, further surface *immunoglobulins* move on the cell surface to the side where the *antigen* meets the cell. This process is called "capping." The antigen is then internalized by receptor-mediated *endocytosis*. During the next 5 to 7 hours, antigen is proteolytically digested into short *peptide* sequences (see *antigen processing*). The processed *antigenic peptides* are bound to *MHC class II molecules* and transported to the cell surface. The antigenic peptide (see *T cell epitope*) is then presented to the *T cell*.

> Presentation of antigen to resting T cells by *B cells* is not an effective mechanism of *T cell activation*. In fact, this method of presentation is likely to lead to T cell *anergy*. However, presentation of antigen by B cells to activated T cells does augment humoral immune responses.

The T cell is stimulated by the antigenic peptide via the *T cell antigen receptor* (TCR) and co-stimulatory ligands (see *co-stimulation*). Although B cells are not the only cell type that present antigen to T cells (see *antigen-presenting cells*), B cell antigen presentation appears to be very important in *antibody* responses.

> Specific B cells with surface immunoglobulins that recognize the antigen and present it to T cells during a *secondary immune response* are more relevant than nonspecific antigen-presenting cells.

In contrast, nonspecific antigen uptake and processing by B cells is not as efficient compared to macrophages. This is because B cells have fewer lysosomes and cannot degrade antigens as efficiently as *macrophages*.

B CELL ANTIGEN RECEPTOR

The surface *B cell* antigen *receptor* complex is composed of an *immunoglobulin* associated with heterodimers of the transmembrane proteins Ig-α and Ig-β. The Ig-α and Ig-β subunits have cytoplasmic sequences that contain *signaling* motifs also found in the *T cell antigen receptor* ζ, γ, and δ subunits (see *tyrosine-based activation motifs*).

> Activation of the B cell antigen receptor occurs by *cross-linking* two adjacent surface immunoglobulins.

An *antigen* or an *antibody* specific for surface immunoglobulins can trigger *B cell activation*. Immediately after cross-linking, a number of biochemical changes are induced in the B cell. *Tyrosine kinases* such as *Lyn*, Syk, and Blk and, as a consequence, *phospholipase Cγ* (PLCγ) are activated. PLCγ cleaves *phosphatidylinositol-4,5-biphosphate* (PIP$_2$) to the second messengers *inositol-1,4,5-triphosphate* (IP$_3$) and *diacylglycerol* (DAG). IP$_3$ leads to the *calcium mobilization* from intracellular stores. DAG activates *protein kinase C* (PKC). PKC phosphorylates intracellular proteins on serine and threonine residues. Interestingly, these *signal transduction* pathways initiated via B and T cell antigen receptors are very similar (see *T cell antigen receptor*, Figure 47; compare with Figure 10). Within an hour following B cell receptor activation, *transcription* of the cellular protooncogenes c-myc and c-fos is stimulated. Further stimulation of B cells via *cytokine receptors* and other *surface molecules* induces *B cell proliferation*. Whereas B cell antigen receptor activation leads to increased production of IgM and *IgG*, *IgE* synthesis is downregulated. This phenomenon may explain, at least partially, the efficacy of *immunotherapy*. B cell antigen receptor activation is negatively regulated by the *tyrosine phosphatase* SHP-1. SHP-1-deficient B cells produce large amounts of antibodies, including *autoantibodies*.

B CELL APOPTOSIS

Programmed cell death or *apoptosis* of *B cells* is a highly regulated process. Some of the *receptors* initiating apoptosis are characteristic for developmental stages.

> *Cross-linking* of surface *immunoglobulins* induces apoptosis in immature B cells. However, the same stimulus induces proliferation (see *B cell proliferation*) in mature B cells. Interestingly, very strong activation of the *B cell antigen receptor* also induces apoptosis in mature B cells.

Death following B cell antigen receptor activation occurs relatively slowly compared to other cellular systems (16 to 18 hours), and requires protein synthesis. *IL-4* receptor and *CD40*

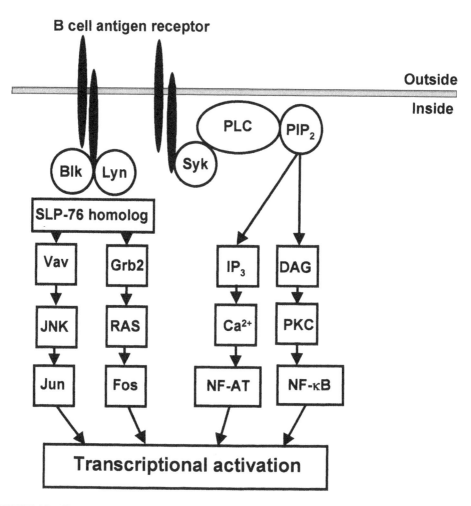

FIGURE 10 Signal transduction pathways initiated via the B cell antigen receptor.

triggering counteract B cell antigen receptor-induced apoptosis and may play a role in B cell tolerance. Therefore, autoreactive B cells (see *autoimmunity*) might be prevented from deletion in the presence of activated T cells that supply *IL-4* and *CD40 ligand*. In addition, concurrent activation of CD21 can prevent apoptosis induced via the B cell antigen receptor in immature and mature B cells.

B cell apoptosis is also regulated through the *Fas receptor* (*CD95*).

Mature B cells express little Fas receptor protein, and its expression is increased upon B cell antigen receptor activation. Moreover, B cell stimulation as a result of CD40 engagement is accompanied by the induction of the Fas receptor *gene* as well as increased susceptibility to Fas-receptor-mediated apoptosis. In contrast, IL-4 induces resistance to Fas-receptor-mediated apoptosis. In addition, suboptimal doses of anti-IgM and IL-4 act in synergy to produce enhanced resistance. These data suggest differential regulation of B cell death and survival by *Th1* and *Th2* cells. Th1 cells express *Fas ligand* and may kill B cells in the absence of IL-4.

However, Th2 cells, which produce IL-4 and express very little or no Fas ligand protect B cells from Fas-receptor- and B cell antigen-receptor-mediated apoptosis.

Fas-receptor-deficient (lpr) mice are characterized by increased *autoantibody* production. In this model, autoreactive B cells are found within T cell areas. This suggests that in the absence of T-cell-mediated apoptosis, autoreactive B cells survive and produce autoantibodies. Therefore, Fas-receptor-mediated apoptosis represents a principal mechanism for eliminating autoreactive B cells. Moreover, a set of intracellular gene products has been associated with resistance to B cell apoptosis. The anti-apoptotic protein *Bcl-2* was first identified in a B cell lymphoma.

B CELL CO-RECEPTOR

The *B cell* co-receptor is a complex of three proteins: CD21 (complement receptor 2), CD19, and TAPA-1. Co-receptors (see *co-stimulation*) enhance *signaling* of *antigen receptors* by activating more *Src*-family *tyrosine kinases*. Thus, when the co-receptor is triggered at the same time as the *B cell antigen receptor*, a lower amount of *antigen* is needed to activate the cells (see *threshold*). Engagement of CD21 and other molecules also modulate *B cell apoptosis* depending on the activation (see *B cell activation*) and differentiation (see *B cell differentiation*) stage.

B CELL DIFFERENTIATION

The differentiation of hematopoietic stem cells to immature *B cells* occurs in the *bone marrow*. Before *immunoglobulin gene rearrangement* takes place, "early pro-B cells" appear. The immunoglobulin *genes* rearrange in subsequent stages, and *surface molecules* change depending on growth factors. The following steps are "late pro-B cell" stage with diversity and junction genes joining, and "pre-B cell" stage with heavy chain production. The light chains undergo rearrangement, and complete IgM molecules are expressed on the surface of immature B cells. Upon reaching maturity, they leave the bone marrow to migrate through the B-cell-rich areas of peripheral lymphoid tissues, such as the follicles of *lymph nodes* and spleen. Such mature B cells survive by *survival signals* provided mostly by *T cells*.

B CELL EPITOPES

Antigenic determinants, or *epitopes* of *B cells* are those sites of an *antigen* which are recognized by *antibodies*. The immunogenic regions of an antigen are determined by inherent features, e.g., its surface accessibility. On the other hand, the resulting *immune response* is also dependent on the genetic characteristics of the responder (see *genetic predisposition*). Protein antigens have multiple determinants, and it has been proposed that the antigen surface presents a continuum of epitopes to the immune system. *X-ray crystallography* of antigen–antibody complexes has provided a structural view of the interface. These studies have shown that an epitope is composed of an array of *amino acids* on the surface of the protein that form an area of 700 Å^2 to 900 Å^2. The amino acids within this area are held in place by the tertiary folding of the protein (see *tertiary structure*).

B cell epitopes are mostly discontinuous in the primary amino acid sequence of the antigen (see *conformational epitopes*).

Residues comprising the epitope contribute to the stability of the antigen–antibody complex by participating in salt-bridges, H-bonding, and by van der Waals interactions with the complementary residues of the antibody combining site. Although most *allergens* are proteins, carbohydrate antigens can also mediate *hypersensitivity*. Food (see *food allergy*) and *pollen* allergens are often glycoproteins, and a portion of the *IgE* response is directed to the polysaccharide moiety. The antigenic determinants consist of short oligosaccharides at the ends of the polysaccharide chains.

B CELL PROLIFERATION

Naive *B cells*, like naive *T cells* (see *naive lymphocytes*), must undergo clonal expansion before they can differentiate into effector cells. In *primary immune responses*, B cells do not need the help of T cells when stimulated by polymeric *antigens* via the *B cell antigen receptor*. However, for an efficient proliferative response in *secondary immune responses*, B cells need to be additionally stimulated by *CD40* ligand (see *CD154*) and *IL-4*, which are both provided by T cells.

B CELL SURFACE MARKERS

Surface molecules expressed by *B cells* (see Table 14). Some of these molecules are used to specifically detect B cells in mixed cell populations (see *CD antigens*).

TABLE 14
B Cell Surface Markers

CD No.	Molecular Weight (kDa)	Expression and Function
CD5	67	B cell subset, B chronic lymphoid lymphoma, activated B cells
CD10	100	Common acute lymphoblastic leukemia antigen, pre-B-cell subset
CD19	95	B cell development, activation, differentiation, pro-B and B cells
CD20	33-35-37	Three isoforms, all B cells
CD21	145	Epstein–Barr virus and complement receptor 2, mature B cells
CD22	130-140	Two isoforms, cytoplasm of B cell precursors, surface of mature B cells
CD23	45	Low-affinity *IgE* receptor (FcεRII), activated B cells
CD24	35-45	Pro B cells, mature B cells
CD40	44-48	B cell growth, differentiation, mature B cells
CD53	32-40	B cell activation, membrane transport
CD72	42	CD5 ligand, early B cell differentiation
CD74	33-35-41	Several isoforms, invariant chain associated with *MHC class II molecules*
CD75		Neurominidase sensitive carbohydrate antigen
CD79ab	33-40-45	Part of *B cell antigen receptor* complex associated with membrane *immunoglobulins*
CD80	60	Ligand for *CD28* and CD152, provides co-stimulatory signals to *T cells*, increased after *B cell activation*
CD86	80	Ligand for CD28 and CD152, provides co-stimulatory signals to T cells, increased after B cell activation

B CELL TOLERANCE

B cell tolerance is a state of unresponsiveness following *B cell antigen receptor* activation and the consequent inability to produce *antibodies*. Although mechanisms in B and *T cell* tolerance are different, B cell tolerance is mainly related to T cell tolerance. A T cell tolerance always effects B cell antibody production, and without T cell help, B cells are not able to produce *IgG* antibodies to T-cell-dependent antigens. Low amounts of antibody production are always present; however, since self-reactive T cells are deleted in the *thymus*, they can no longer assist B cells to increase self-reactive antibody titers. Similarly, *anergy* is also a state of unresponsiveness. However, this term is usually used to describe a regulated suppression of T cells.

B CELL ULTRASTRUCTURE

Electron microscopy studies have shown that resting *B cells* have no granules. However, scattered ribosomes and rough endoplasmic reticulum are seen in the cytoplasm. Upon *B cell antigen receptor* activation, B cells develop a machinery for *immunoglobulin* synthesis. High amounts of Golgi apparatus, rough endoplasmic reticulum, and free ribosomes are seen in the cytoplasm.

Bcl-2

Bcl-2 was first identified as an oncogene implicated in *B cell* lymphoma. Subsequently, a number of related proteins were identified (see *Bcl-2 family*). It is now clear that Bcl-2 is an intracellular protein that regulates *apoptosis*. High expression of Bcl-2 may prevent cells from apoptosis even when they receive death stimuli.

The regulation of Bcl-2 expression is critical for many functions of the *immune system*.

Upregulation of Bcl-2 appears to be the normal mechanism for positive selection of developing *T cells* in the *thymus*. In contrast, Bcl-2 is not significantly expressed in mature *neutrophils* and *eosinophils*, which may explain, at least partially, their short life span. However, Bcl-2 is expressed in eosinophils from a subgroup of patients with the *hypereosinophilic syndrome*. *Eosinophil apoptosis* is markedly delayed in eosinophils expressing Bcl-2.

Bcl-2 FAMILY

Several *genes* encoding proteins are homologous to *Bcl-2* and belong, therefore, to the Bcl-2 family. All these gene products are involved in the regulation of *apoptosis*. Bcl-2 family proteins function as cell death antagonists (e.g., Bcl-2, Bcl-x$_L$, Mcl-1) or agonists (e.g., Bcl-x$_S$, Bax, Bak, Bid, Bad). Bcl-2 family members interact with each other to form various heteromeric and monomeric complexes. Apoptosis appears to be regulated by the expression of anti-apoptotic and pro-apoptotic members of the Bcl-2 family (see Figure 11). For example, high expression of Bcl-2 or Bcl-x$_L$ protects cells from death induced by a wide range of agents. In contrast, high levels of Bax accelerate apoptosis. In eosinophilic *inflammation*, delayed *eosinophil apoptosis* occurs mainly by overexpression of *IL-5*, which upregulates the expression of Bcl-x$_L$ in *eosinophils*. In *neutrophils*, delayed apoptosis is mediated by *cytokine*-dependent downregulation of Bax during bacterial infections.

BECLOMETHASONE DIPROPRIONATE

This is an *inhaled corticosteroid*.

BEE VENOM ALLERGY

Bee venom *allergy* is a subtype of *hymenoptera allergy*.

BEE VENOM PHOSPHOLIPASE A$_2$ (PLA$_2$)

PLA$_2$ is the *major allergen* of bee venom (see *hymenoptera allergy*) and is highly toxic to cells in higher concentrations. At lower concentrations, it is a powerful *antigen*. More than 90% of subjects with bee venom *anaphylaxis* produce *IgE antibody* to it. It is a relatively small, complete allergen whose crystal structure (see *X-ray crystallography*) has been resolved. In common with mammalian *phospholipase A$_2$* (PLA$_2$), bee venom PLA$_2$ has a calcium binding site and, as its name suggests, it hydrolyzes the 2-ester bond of L-glycerophospholipids. PLA$_2$ causes direct release of preformed *IL-4* from *mast cells* by local cellular disruption as a result of concentration-dependent cytotoxicity by hydrolyzing certain membrane phospholipids (see *cytotoxicity of allergens*). This may create a microenvironment that favors the development of *Th2 cells*. *T cell epitope mapping* has revealed three important *linear epitopes* that stimulate T cells. Such *antigenic peptides* have been used to treat bee venom *allergy* in clinical trials (see *peptide immunotherapy*).

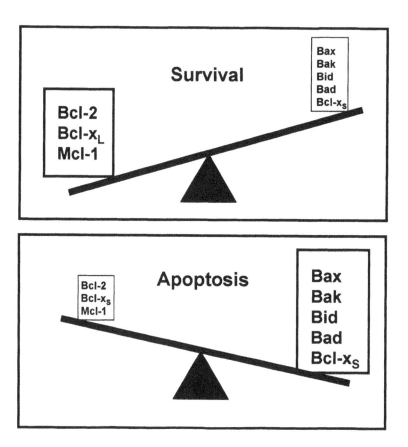

FIGURE 11 Apoptosis is regulated by the expression of anti-apoptotic and pro-apoptotic members of Bcl-2 family proteins.

BENZALKONIUM CHLORIDE

Benzalkonium chloride is a bactericidal compound that is added to some *nebulizer* solutions. In some patients, benzalkonium chloride may cause *airway obstruction*. This airway obstruction is thought to be due to the release of *mediators* due to a nonspecific effect on the cell membrane of *mast cells*.

β2-AGONISTS

(See *Agonists*.)

β-BLOCKER ASTHMA

β-Blocker drugs oppose the action of *adrenaline* on *smooth muscle* and can induce *bronchospasm*. Some patients with *asthma* are very sensitive to β-blockers, and a small dose can precipitate catastrophic *asthma exacerbation*, which may prove fatal (see *death from asthma*). This extreme sensitivity seems to be due to a deficit of *β-receptors* (see *adrenergic receptors*) on the post-muscarinic *acetylcholine* receptor.

β-blockers should not be used in any patient known to have asthma.

BIORESONANCE

Bioresonance is a treatment method of *allergic diseases* that belongs to the *complementary procedures*.

BIRBECK GRANULES (BG)

BG are the most specific identification signs of a *Langerhans cell* (LC). Invisible by light microscopy, they are identified by electron microscopy as cytoplasmic, tennis-racket-shaped organelles with a characteristic, trilamellar handle. BG were first described in 1961 by Michael S. Birbeck, a British scientist who studied the ultrastructure of LCs in vitiligo. The function of BG is still unclear at present; however, some data suggest a role in *antigen processing* by the LC. The *LAG protein* is a BG-specific protein, detected by an anti-LAG *monoclonal antibody*. The absolute specificity of BG for LCs was questioned by two recent observations: (1) BG-like structures are present in EDTA-treated *platelets*, and (2) a healthy individual was identified who demonstrated complete BG absence inside all LCs. In spite of these findings, BG are still regarded as the most specific LC identifying feature.

BIRCH POLLEN

Birch *pollen* is a common cause of *allergic rhinoconjunctivitis* throughout the Northern Hemisphere, especially in northern and central Europe. Birch trees shed large amounts of windborne pollen (see *aeroallergens*). The *major allergen* Bet v 1 shows strong *amino acid* sequence *homologies* to Aln g 1 (*alder pollen*) and Cor a 1 (hazel pollen) (see *cross-reacting allergens*). There is also cross-reactivity to numerous foods, including apples (see *apple allergen*), pears, cherries, plums, *celery*, and kiwi. *Profilin* is another *allergen* (Bet v 2) that has high homology to profilins found in other trees, grasses, fruits, and vegetables (see *oral allergy syndrome*).

BLATTELLA

Genus of cockroach (order Cursoria, class Hexapoda). The primary species associated with respiratory *allergy* is *Blattella germanica*, the German cockroach. Studies of *sensitization* to *cockroach allergens* from *Blattella germanica* and *Periplaneta americana* have demonstrated that increased concentrations of *IgE antibodies* specific to these *allergens* represent an important *risk factor* for *asthma*, especially in urban areas.

BLATTELLA GERMANICA

German cockroach (see *cockroach allergens*). A small cockroach, approximately 3/4" in length, that sometimes infests houses in the U.S. A single pair can produce up to 30,000 offspring in a few months. Kitchens and bathrooms are favored sites for infestation.

BLEPHAROCONJUNCTIVITIS

In a few patients, *atopic dermatitis* is associated with blepharoconjunctivitis, which is a chronic and serious form of *conjunctivitis*. The eyelids and the periorbital skin show dryness, scaling, induration, and *erythema*, as well as exudative and crusted lesions. In addition, thickening of the palpebral conjunctiva and giant papillary hypertrophy occur. A thick mucous exudate is seen. The lesions may lead to ectropion. Moreover, colonization of the lid margin with *Staphylococcus aureus* is a frequent finding. In contrast to *atopic keratoconjunctivitis*, the cornea is not affected. Treatment involves *cromoglycates*, short courses of topical *corticosteroids*, topical *antibiotics*, tear substitutes, and mucolytics. Topical *cyclosporin A* (CsA) has been shown to be very effective in controlling symptoms.

BLOMIA

Genus of *house-dust mite* (order Acarina, class Arachnida, family Glycyphagidae). Mites of the genus Blomia are found in tropical and subtropical areas of the world, including Central and South America, the southeastern United States, Malaysia, Hong Kong, Taiwan, India, and Egypt. Allergenically important species include B. tropicalis and B. kulagini.

BLOOD GASES

Measurement of the oxygen (O_2) and carbon dioxide (CO_2) gas tensions in arterial blood. Conventionally, the blood bicarbonate and pH are also included. In acute *asthma*, the arterial oxygen pressure (p_aO_2) falls due to *ventilation–perfusion mismatch* (see *hypoxia*). In worsening asthma, the p_aO_2 will fall further, and the p_aCO_2 will rise if the patient tires. This is a very dire prognostic sign and is regarded as an indication for *ventilation*.

BODY PLETHYSMOGRAPHY

The body plethysmograph can be used to measure thoracic gas volume by exploitation of Boyle's law. The patient sits in the body box and breathes freely while the lung volumes are measured. At an appropriate point in the respiratory cycle a shutter mechanism is activated to close the airway. At this point, inspiration against the obstruction will result in a change in intrathoracic pressure and decompression of the gas within the thorax. Simultaneously, the pressure in the body box will rise due to the expansion of the thoracic gas. The change in volume can be calculated from the two pressure changes, and that allows the beginning thoracic gas volume to be calculated. Body box measurements are particularly useful in patients with severe *airway obstruction* and those with pulmonary bullae, since in these cases air can become trapped and will not mix freely with inspired gas. This means that the helium dilution techniques underestimate the residual volume, whereas the body box measurements give a direct measurement of the total gas volume that is unaffected by mixing. In addition, *airway resistance* can also be measured using a body box, but for routine clinical use simple *spirometry* suffices (see also *lung function tests*).

BONE MARROW

The cells of the *immune system* originate in the bone marrow, where many of them also mature. *Leukocytes*, *platelets*, and erythrocytes derive from the same pluripotent hematopoietic stem cell. From these cells, precursors of erythrocytes, platelets, and myeloid and common lymphoid progenitors develop in the bone marrow (see Figure 12). The differentiation from immature into mature cells is controlled by *cytokines*. Some of these cytokines are also generated at inflammatory sites and may reach the bone marrow via the circulation. In such a scenario, it is likely that the generation of inflammatory cells is increased.

> Indeed, increased *IL-5* expression in *allergic inflammation* is associated with increased production of *eosinophils* in the bone marrow, leading to blood *eosinophilia*.

Under these circumstances of excessive cell generation, it is possible that progenitors are also released into the blood. These cells may develop into mature cells at inflammatory sites. For instance, it has been demonstrated that *eosinophil progenitors* develop into mature eosinophils within *nasal polyps*.

BONE-MARROW-DERIVED MAST CELLS (BMMC)

Mast cells are derived from *bone marrow* stem cells. They undergo part of their differentiation in the bone marrow and complete it in peripheral mucosal or connective tissue microenvironments, which are rich in *fibroblasts* or stromal cells. Therefore, BMMC represent immature

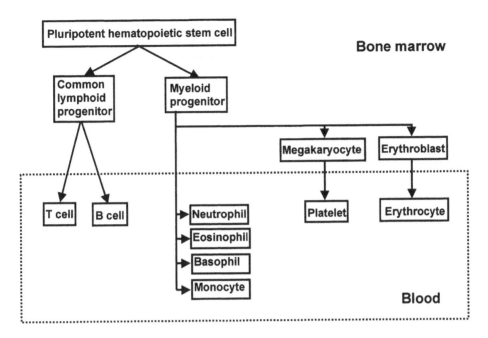

FIGURE 12 The development of leukocytes and other blood cells from hematopoietic stem cells in the bone marrow.

cells, which are driven by appropriate signals to differentiate to either *mucosal mast cells* (MMC) or *connective tissue mast cells* (CTMC).

BMMC are an important tool for in vitro studies.

Mouse BMMC undergo maturation toward CTMC-type mast-cell-like phenotype after co-culture with 3T3 fibroblasts and exposure to *stem cell factor* (SCF). Rat BMMC co-cultured with 3T3 fibroblasts also require SCF for their survival and differentiation. *IL-3, IL-4*, and *IL-10* also promote proliferation and differentiation of rodent BMMC. Human BMMC differentiate under the influence of SCF to mature mast cells. In contrast, IL-3, IL-4, *IL-9*, and M-CSF are not able to induce maturation of human BMMC (see *basophils*).

BOVINE ALLERGENS

(See *cow allergens*.)

bp

(See *base pair*.)

BRADYKININ

Inhaled bradykinin causes *bronchoconstriction* in asthmatic patients. Therefore, it is considered a *mediator* involved in *asthma*. Blockers of the *angiotensin-converting enzyme* (ACE) may increase bradykinin concentrations in the airways and can cause *cough* in asthmatic patients. Bradykinin belongs to the *kinins*, a family of vasoactive *peptides*. The contribution of bradykinin to asthma is unclear but will be determined by potent and specific bradykinin antagonists in clinical studies. However, it is unlikely that they will be as effective as *β2-agonists* or *corticosteroids*.

BREAST FEEDING

Breast feeding may decrease allergic *sensitization* by reducing both exposure to and intestinal absorption of food *allergens* (see *food allergy*). Breast milk includes a number of components with anti-infectious, antiinflammatory, and immunomodulating effects. The protective role of breast milk includes *immunoglobulins*, especially secretory IgA.

> In infants with a high risk (see *risk factors*) for *atopy*, breast feeding in combination with avoidance of cow's milk and solid food for over 4 months has resulted in a significant reduction of the cumulative *prevalence* of *cow's milk allergy* during the first 1 to 2 years of life.

Some studies also indicate a preventive effect of breast feeding against the development of *atopic dermatitis* that can be enhanced by avoiding major food allergens (see *allergen avoidance*) such as peanuts (see *peanut allergy*), tree nuts, fish, milk, eggs, and soybeans (see *soybean allergy*) in the maternal diet during lactation. However, breast feeding has not been associated with a decreased incidence of *asthma* (see *childhood asthma*). Moreover, no study could demonstrate any protective effect of maternal *diet* during pregnancy.

BRITTLE ASTHMA

A minority of patients show unstable lung function and may present with catastrophic drops in lung function following a period of being asymptomatic. The pathophysiological mechanisms involved in brittle *asthma* have not been well defined. Management is along standard lines, but patients often require continuous parenteral *β2-agonists* and are usually provided with the opportunity to self-admit to the hospital in the event of an *asthma exacerbation*.

BROMELIN

Bromelin is a protease derived from pineapple. It may be a cause of *occupational asthma*.

BRONCHIAL HYPERRESPONSIVENESS–HYPERREACTIVITY

(See *airway hyperresponsiveness*.)

BRONCHIAL PROVOCATION TESTS

These include specific challenges with *allergen* (see *allergen challenge*) and nonspecific challenges with *histamine, methacholine, acetylcholine,* or *carbachol* to measure *airway hyperresponsiveness*. In both types of test, baseline lung function is assessed by *forced expiratory maneuvers*, and a control challenge with isotonic saline is performed. The post-saline *forced expiratory volume in first second* (FEV$_1$) is taken as the baseline for the *provocation test*. The subject then inhales increasing amounts of the challenge substance. This may be achieved by a dosimeter or by inhaling a known concentration for a fixed period of time. The test is terminated when the FEV$_1$ falls by 20% or more from the post-saline baseline. The sensitivity can be expressed in terms of the dose of allergen, methacholine, or histamine, which causes a 20% drop in FEV$_1$ (PD_{20} for dose, PC_{20} for concentration). If alternative measures of lung function are chosen, e.g., specific *airway resistance*, the percentage change will be different. For example, a 20% fall in FEV$_1$ equates roughly to a 50% fall in specific *airway resistance*. For comparability purposes it is necessary to specify the agent used, the delivery system, and the *spirometer* used to assess responsiveness.

BRONCHIOLE

This is one of the thousands of small airways into which the bronchi (see *bronchus*) split, forming a tree-like network inside the lung (see *airway anatomy*). In *asthma, allergic inflammation* of the bronchioles is associated with *airway hyperresponsiveness*.

BRONCHITIS

This is an *inflammation* of the bronchi (see *bronchus*) resulting in persistent *cough* (see *chronic bronchitis* and *COPD*).

BRONCHOALVEOLAR LAVAGE (BAL)

BAL is a technique for washing out part of the lung via a bronchoscope. The tip of the bronchoscope is wedged in the small segmental airway, and warm isotonic saline is washed into the segment, then aspirated back into a receiver pot. The volume of fluid used varies and can influence the composition of the return fluid. Typically, 60 to 120 ml will be washed out of a single segment. This technique permits us to sample cells that are not firmly anchored to the lining of the lower respiratory tract.

> BAL cells can be used for differential diagnosis of inflammatory lung diseases (e.g., *sarcoidosis* or *extrinsic allergic alveolitis*) by analysis of differential cell counts, total lavage cell counts, cell morphology, and lymphocyte surface markers (see *CD antigens* and *flow cytometry*).

Moreover, BAL is a research method that allows scientists to obtain biochemical constituents of the fluid lining the conducting airways and alveoli. For instance, the technique has been of great value for studying toxicological effects of *pollutants* (see *pollutants and bronchoalveolar lavage*) instilled or inhaled into the lung, as a number of histopathological changes have been correlated with changes in the constituents of BAL fluid. BAL fluid can be analyzed using techniques such as *enzyme-linked immunoassay* (ELISA) for the presence of *cytokines* or substances in small concentration on the *epithelial cell* surface. Constituents of BAL fluid may also be cultured for in vitro experimentation.

BRONCHOCENTRIC GRANULOMATOSIS

A destructive granulomatous condition in which the granulomas are centered on the bronchi rather than the small blood vessels. The prognosis of bronchocentric granulomatosis is much better than that of vasculitis granulomatosis. Patients with bronchocentric granulomatosis fall into two distinct groups: those with *asthma* and those without. Those with asthma are generally younger; they have marked *eosinophilia* and have fungal growth within the *mucus* plugs in the airways. Bronchocentric granulomatosis has been considered a variant of *allergic bronchopulmonary aspergillosis* (ABPA), but aspergillus cannot always be detected. Patients may respond to *prednisolone* or *azathioprin* but may also resolve without specific therapy. Relatively little is known about the natural history of the condition, but in general it appears to follow a relatively benign course.

BRONCHOCONSTRICTION

(See *airway obstruction*.)

BRONCHODILATION

Opening up the airways by relaxation of *smooth muscle* (see *bronchodilators*).

BRONCHODILATORS

Bronchodilators may relax contracted *smooth muscle* and prevent contraction of smooth muscle by various stimuli in patients with *asthma*. Various anti-asthmatic drugs (see *asthma treatment strategies*) act as bronchodilators (see *β2-agonists*, *theophylline*, and *anticholinergic agents*). Some *neuropeptides* such as *vasoactive intestinal polypeptide* (VIP) and *calcitonin-gene-related peptide* (CGRP), as well as *nitric oxide* (NO), also have relaxant effects on airway smooth muscles.

BRONCHOPROTECTION

The ability of a drug to protect against *airway obstruction* due to challenge with *allergen, histamine,* etc.

BRONCHOSPASM

Narrowing of the airways (see *airway obstruction*) caused by contraction of airway *smooth muscles* or by a combination of airway smooth muscle contractions plus intraluminal *inflammation* and *mucus*.

BRONCHUS

A bronchus is any of the larger air passages that connect the trachea to the lungs.

BRONCHUS-ASSOCIATED LYMPHOID TISSUE (BALT)

BALT is formed of follicular lymphoid tissue and is closely related to bronchial *epithelial cells*. It is distributed along distal *bronchi* and *bronchioles*, especially at sites where inhaled *antigens* or *pollutants* may impinge in greatest concentrations (e.g., at bifurcation points). The precise role of BALT is not completely understood. BALT is uncommon in normal fetuses and infants, but can occur in human fetal or infant lung as a consequence of intrauterine or neonatal antigenic stimulation. The lymphoid follicles of BALT comprise mainly *B cells* that can generate *antibodies*, especially IgA.

BUCKLEY'S SYNDROME

(See *hyper-IgE-syndrome*.)

BUDESONIDE

Budesonide is an *inhaled corticosteroid*.

BULLOUS DRUG REACTION

This is a rare subtype of *adverse drug reactions* that occur as fixed or exanthematous drug eruption.

BURSA OF FABRICIUS

In birds, *B cells* originate from a special organ called the bursa of Fabricius. It is a lymphoepithelial organ found at the junction of the hind gut and cloaca. In mammals, *B cell differentiation* occurs in the *bone marrow*.

*C

C3a

(See *complement factor 3a*.)

C4a

(See *complement factor 4a*.)

C5a

(See *complement factor 5a*.)

CALCINEURIN

Calcineurin is a heterodimeric serine-threonine *phosphatase*, also called phosphatase 2B. It is an important molecule in *T cell antigen-receptor*-mediated *cytokine gene activation*. Activation of calcineurin occurs distal to *phospholipase C* stimulation and *calcium mobilization*.

> *Cyclosporin A* (CsA) and *tacrolimus* (FK506) block the phosphatase activity of calcineurin.

CALCITONIN-GENE-RELATED PEPTIDE (CGRP)

A 37-*amino acid peptide* found in small autonomic nerves (see *nervous system*), co-localized with *substance P* and *neurokinin A*. CGRP has a relaxant effect on *smooth muscle* cells mediated through a rise in intracellular *cAMP*. (*β2-agonists* also increase cAMP.) CGRP also dilates blood vessels, but has no effect on vascular permeability.

CALCIUM IONOPHORE

A calcium ionophore is a compound that bypasses *receptor*-mediated early *signal transduction* events, resulting in direct intracellular *calcium mobilization*. Several compounds are known and used, alone or together with a *phorbol ester*, to nonspecifically activate cells.

CALCIUM MOBILIZATION

> Activation of cells via many cell surface *receptors* results in stimulation of *phospholipase C* (PLC) and consequent increases in intracellular calcium levels (Table 15), a process that involves *tyrosine kinases* and/or *G proteins*.

PLC activation leads to the hydrolysis of *phosphatidylinositol-4,5-bisphosphate* (PIP_2) to *inositol-1,4,5-trisphosphate* (IP_3) and *diacylglycerol* (DAG). IP_3 generation induces the increase in $[Ca^{2+}]_i$, while DAG promotes the activation of *protein kinase C* (PKC) (see Figure 13).

The rapid and transient increase in intracellular calcium ion concentration $[Ca^{2+}]_i$ is associated with many different cell functions which are important in *allergic inflammation*. These calcium-dependent functions can be subdivided into two subgroups: (1) immediate cell responses, such as *degranulation* or *chemotaxis*, that do not require changes of the transcriptional activity; (2) other cell functions that depend on the activation of *genes* which control diverse functions such as adhesion (see *adhesion molecules*), *apoptosis*, or proliferation (see

TABLE 15
Examples of Cell *Surface Molecules* that Increase Intracellular Calcium Levels upon Activation

Via PLCβ	Via PLCγ
A1-*adrenergic receptor*	*T cell antigen receptor*
Muscarinic receptors	*B cell antigen receptor*
VIP receptor	*High-affinity IgE receptor*
Tachykinin receptor	
Bradykinin receptor	
PAF receptor	
Thromboxane receptors	
Chemokine receptors	
C5a receptor	
Serotonin receptor	
Histamine 1 receptor	
Angiotensin II receptor	

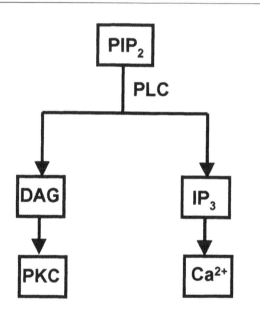

FIGURE 13   The immediate intracellular consequences of PLC activation.

T cell proliferation). In the latter subgroup, there is evidence that the size and duration of the calcium peak determine, at least partially, the activity of *transcription factors*. For instance, *nuclear factor-κB* (NF-κB) and c-*Jun-N-terminal kinase* (JNK) are selectively activated by large calcium fluxes, whereas *nuclear factor of activated T cells* (NF-AT) is more likely to translocate to the nucleus following lower amplitude calcium spikes. These mechanisms demonstrate a level of discriminatory control of gene activation that is achieved by the qualitative and quantitative levels of $[Ca^{2+}]_i$ generated following receptor ligation.

cAMP

(See *cyclic adenosine monophosphate*.)

CANDIDA

Common *fungus* associated with *immediate* and *delayed hypersensitivity* (see *molds*).

CANDIDATE GENE

This is a *gene* that, due to its function, is suspected to be responsible for a genetically determined disease or a putative genetic factor for disease susceptibility (see *genetic predisposition*). Since *allergic diseases* are complex and multifactorial diseases in which genetic and environmental factors interact to produce the ultimate disease *phenotype* (see *gene environmental interactions*), many genes might influence allergic susceptibility (see Tables 16 and 17). Candidate genes reflect our current understanding regarding the pathophysiology of a certain disease.

TABLE 16
Candidate Genes for Preferential *Th2* Activation

Role in Pathophysiology	Genes
Antigen recognition	*MHC, T cell antigen receptor*
Signal transduction	*STATs*, STAT5, STAT6
Cytokines	*Th2 cytokine gene cluster, IFN-γ*
Cytokine receptors	*IL-4/IL-13Rα, IL-2Rβ, IL-5R*
Transcription factors	*NF-AT, c-maf, GATA-3, AP*-1

TABLE 17
Candidate Genes for *Allergic Inflammation* and *Airway Hyperresponsiveness*

Role in Pathophysiology	Genes
Immunoglobulin receptor	*High-affinity IgE receptor*
Hormone receptors	*β2-adrenergic receptor*
	Corticosteroid receptor
	Muscarinic receptors
Adhesion molecules	*VLA-4, VCAM-1, ICAM-1, LFA-1*
Cytokines and receptors	*IL-1, IL-6, IL-10, TNF, TGF-β*
Chemokines and receptors	*RANTES, Eotaxin, MCP-1, MCP-3*
Mediator production/degradation	Inducible *nitric oxide synthase*
	Leukotriene C₄ synthase
	PAF acetylhydrolase

CAPSAICIN

Capsaicin is the active ingredient in red pepper. Capsaicin has been used as a tool for the study of *neurogenic inflammation*. It acts on unmyelinated C fibers. Capsaicin may stimulate primary sensory neurones to release *neuropeptides* such as *substance P, neurokinins*, and *calcitonin-gene-related peptide* (CGRP). At low concentrations, it causes excitation of these neuropeptides. At higher concentrations or upon repeated exposure, the neurons are depleted of their *peptide* content, and *desensitization* is achieved. When administered in the nasal cavity, capsaicin stimulates sensory nerves and produces cholinergic reflex-mediated glandular secretion. Intranasal capsaicin treatment is clinically effective in *vasomotoric rhinitis*.

CAP-SYSTEM

The CAP-system is an automatic test system that is widely used to measure *allergen*-specific *IgE antibodies* and autoantibodies (see *autoimmunity*). The principle of this assay is that of a nonradioactive *immunoassay*. To measure antibodies, allergen or *antigen* is bound to cellulose, which provides a large surface for binding resulting in high sensitivity of the test. The system is also used to measure cell-specific proteins such as *tryptase* and *eosinophil cationic protein* (ECP). Increased tryptase levels indicate *mast cell activation* (e.g., during *anaphylaxis*), whereas increased ECP levels suggest *eosinophil activation* (e.g., in *asthma*).

CARBACHOL

Carbachol is used as an alternative to *histamine* in *bronchial provocation tests* of *airway hyperresponsiveness*. It is also used to diagnose cholinergic *urticaria*.

CARBON MONOXIDE (CO)

The major effect of CO in the context of *environmental pollution* is exacerbation of cardiac disease due to blunting of oxygen-carrying capacity due to CO binding to hemoglobin. In occupational and domestic settings, exposure to increased levels of CO can cause severe neurotoxicity and death, again due to binding of hemoglobin by CO and the resultant inability of blood to carry oxygen (see *hypoxia*). This occurs when there is incomplete combustion or venting of natural gas or fossil fuels in a confined space, as is observed with poorly operating space heaters and poorly ventilated garages.

CARBOXYPEPTIDASE A

Carboxypeptidase A is a monomeric 34.5-kDa *metalloprotease* which removes the carboxyl terminal *amino acid* residues from a range of *peptides*, including *angiotensin*. It is a *neutral protease* localized in secretory granules of *mast cells*. Skin *fibroblasts* and *basophils* are also sources of this enzyme. Based on the cDNA-predicted amino acid sequence of the catalytic portion of the enzyme, the human enzyme is 86% identical to mouse carboxypeptidase A. When mast cells are activated, carboxypeptidase, *chymase*, and *cathepsin G* are released together in a 400–500 kDa complex to degrade proteins.

CARBOXYPEPTIDASE N

Carboxypeptidase N is, in addition to other *proteases*, important in degrading *bradykinin* in the circulation.

CARRIER

A carrier is an individual who is heterozygote for a certain *allele* (see also *mutation*) that causes disease in a homozygous state only.

CASEIN

Caseins and β-lactoglobulin are the most frequently involved *allergens* in *cow's milk allergy*. Since casein is also found in goat's and sheep's milk, patients allergic to cow's milk may not tolerate milk of other mammalian species (see *cross-reacting allergens*).

CASPASES

Caspases represent a family of at least 10 intracellular cysteine-containing, aspartate-specific *proteases* (<u>c</u>ysteine <u>aspartases</u>) which are involved in *apoptosis* and/or procytokine activation. Caspases exist as inactive proenzymes that are activated by proteolytic cleavage (Figure 14).

Caspases can activate other caspases, leading to an activation cascade.

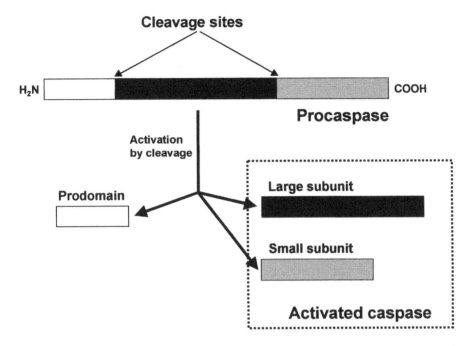

FIGURE 14 Proteolytic cleavage of a processed caspase. The active form of a caspase consists of large (black) and small chains (gray) released from the proenzyme by proteolysis. A linker segment and the prodomain (open box) are also released. The two chains form the catalytic site of the mature caspase. Both chains contain essential components of the catalytic machinery. Initiator procaspase aggregation is mediated by the binding of adapter molecules to the prodomain. Effector caspases have only short prodomains that may not allow interaction with adapter proteins.

The initial caspase activation occurs by aggregation of so-called initiator caspases (caspases 8 and 9). This occurs by adapter molecules allowing self-cleavage of the initiator caspase. For instance, caspase 8 is activated following *cross-linking* of *Fas* or *TNF receptors* in the described way. Effector caspases (caspases 3, 6, and 7) are activated by initiator caspases and then cleave a number of cellular substrates, leading to the morphological hallmarks of apoptosis including *DNA fragmentation* and condensation of cellular organelles. This final stage of apoptosis is also called execution. In contrast to other caspases, which promote apoptosis, *caspase 1* activates the precursors of *IL-1* and *IL-18*, and is therefore involved in the activation of proinflammatory *cytokines*. Its role in apoptosis is uncertain. Caspase 4 and 5 may also play a role in procytokine activation.

Caspases may represent suitable targets for therapeutic intervention.

For example, caspase 1 blockers may decrease inflammatory responses. Moreover, activation of caspases might be beneficial in cancer and in chronic *inflammation*. In contrast, patients with *acquired immunodeficiency syndrome* (AIDS), neurodegenerative disorders, or ischemic injury may benefit from caspase inhibition to prevent death. However, such drugs would have to be delivered to specific cells in order to prevent major side effects.

CASPASE 1

(See *interleukin-1-converting enzyme*.)

CATALASE

Catalase is a ubiquitous heme protein that catalyzes the dismutation of *hydrogen peroxide* (H_2O_2) into water and molecular oxygen.

$$H_2O_2 + H_2O_2 \rightarrow 2\ H_2O + O_2$$

CAT ALLERGEN (FELIS DOMESTICUS; Fel d 1)

Fel d 1 is the *major allergen* in cat extracts. It can be found in pelt, saliva, and lacrimal fluid. It is one of the best-characterized *allergens* (see also *animal dander*). It consists of two polypeptide chains with known *amino acid* sequences. *B cell epitopes* as well as *T cell epitopes* were found on both chains. The biologic function of the protein Fel d 1 is not known. For aerodynamic properties see *aeroallergens*.

CATECHOLAMINE

This term describes both *adrenaline* and *noradrenaline*.

CATHEPSIN G

Cathepsin G is a *neutral protease* normally associated with *neutrophils*. However, it has also been found in *mast cells* and *lymphocytes*. While neutrophils and lymphocytes transcribe cathepsin G without *chymase genes*, the genes of these two neutral *proteases* are cotranscribed in mast cells. When mast cells are activated, cathepsin G, chymase, and *carboxypeptidase A* are released together in a 400- to 500-kDa complex to degrade proteins.

CC10

CC10 is the abbreviation for Clara cell 10-kDa protein, and is produced by *Clara cells*. It inhibits *phospholipase A_2* (PLA_2), suggesting that CC10 may be an antiinflammatory molecule in the lung. The human CC10 *gene* has been localized to chromosome 11, p12-q13, a region occupied by other genes involved in the regulation of *allergic inflammation* (e.g., the gene for the β-chain of the *high-affinity IgE receptor*). Although CC10 *knockout mice* develop normally to adulthood, their response to lung injury is compromised in keeping with the hypothesis that CC10 regulates *inflammation* in the lung. No abnormalities in the *primary structure* of the CC10 gene have been identified in patients with *asthma* (see *genetic predisposition*).

CCAAT BOX

Promoters of inducible *genes* often contain the so-called CCAAT box or Y box motif (reversed CCAAT box). This element is found about 70 to 80 bp upstream of the initiation site of *transcription* and plays an important role in the efficient regulation of immunologically relevant molecules and in the cellular stress reaction. Further recognition motifs for the rapidly inducible *transcription factors NF-AT, AP-1, NF-κB*, and CREB have been found in multiple genes at variant locations and with different distances to the CCAAT box.

CC CHEMOKINES

Chemokine subfamily. In contrast to *CXC chemokines*, the structure of the CC chemokines is characterized by the position of the first two cysteine residues, which are not separated from each other. CC chemokines predominantly activate *monocytes*, *lymphocytes*, *eosinophils*, and *basophils*, suggesting that they play an important role in chronic inflammatory responses as seen in *asthma* and other *allergic diseases*. CC chemokines share 25 to 71% sequence identity and are encoded by *genes* on the human *chromosome* 17. Important members of this family are *eotaxin, RANTES, MCP-1, MCP-2, MCP-3*, MCP-4, and *MIP-1*. Different chemokines can often activate the same CC *chemokine receptor* (CCR), and one chemokine can often stimulate several *receptors* (see Table 18).

TABLE 18
CC Chemokines and Their Receptors (CCR)

	CCR1	CCR2	CCR3	CCR4	CCR5
MIP-1α	+	–	–	+	+
MIP-1β	–	–	–	–	+
RANTES	+	–	+	+	+
MCP-1	–	+	–	+	–
MCP-2	+	+	+	–	–
MCP-3	+	+	+	+	–
MCP-4	–	+	+	–	–
Eotaxin	–	–	+	–	–

CD ANTIGENS

CD (cluster of differentiation) antigens are cell *surface molecules* of *leukocytes* and *platelets* that are recognized and distinguished by *monoclonal antibodies* (mAbs). Such mAbs are used for the differentiation of leukocyte populations and subsets (see Table 19).

CD1

Nonclassical *major histocompatibility complex* (MHC)-like molecule expressed on the surface of several *antigen-presenting cells* (APCs). *Allergens* might be presented using CD1 to *gamma/delta* (γ/δ) *T cells*. These interactions are independent from *MHC class II molecules*. CD1 appears to be overexpressed by alveolar *macrophages* of patients with *asthma*.

CD2

CD2 is a *surface molecule* expressed on *T cells* throughout their entire development, as well as on some *NK cells* and a subset of *B cells*. CD2 ligation modulates *T cell antigen receptor* (TCR) activation.

CD3

CD3 is a cell surface *antigen* associated with the *T cell antigen receptor* (TCR). It is a complex of five different polypeptides (γ, δ, ε, and the dimeric ζ chains) with a co-stimulatory role in *signal transduction* during the process of *antigen recognition*.

CD4

CD4 is a *surface molecule* expressed on a subset of *T cells* known as *T helper (Th) cells*. CD4 is a co-receptor molecule (see *co-stimulation*) expressed in association with the *T cell antigen receptor* (TCR) complex and binds specifically to *MHC class II molecules* of *antigen-presenting cells* (APCs), which in these cells is essential for signaling via the TCR.

CD4+ T cells are central to the pathogenesis of many *allergic diseases*.

For instance, CD4+ T cells help *B cells* to generate large amounts of *allergen*-specific *IgE*. Moreover, they are central in the development of *delayed hypersensitivity* reactions.

TABLE 19
Cellular Expression and Functions of CD Antigens

CD Antigen	Cellular Expression	Function
CD1	Cortical thymocytes, Langerhans cells, dendritic cells, B cells, intestinal epithelium, smooth muscle, blood vessels	MHC class I-like molecule, may have specialized role in the presentation of lipid antigens and allergens
CD2	T cells, NK cells, thymocytes	Adhesion molecule and co-receptor, receptor for CD58
CD3	T cells, thymocytes	Associated with the T cell antigen receptor (TCR), required for cell surface expression and signal transduction
CD4	T helper cells, monocytes, macrophages, thymocyte subsets	Co-receptor for MHC class II molecules, receptor for HIV
CD5	T cells, thymocytes, B cell subset	Interactions with CD72
CD6	T cells, B cells in CLL, thymocytes	Unknown
CD7	Hematopoietic precursor cells, T cells, thymocytes	Unknown
CD8	T effector cells, thymocyte subset	Co-receptor for MHC class I molecules
CD9	Monocytes, eosinophils, basophils, platelets, activated T cells, vascular smooth muscle, pre-B cells, neuronal cells	Platelet activation via FcγRIIa
CD10	Bone marrow stromal cells, B cell precursors, T cell precursors	Zinc metalloproteinase, marker for pre-B ALL
CD11a	Lymphocytes, granulocytes, monocytes, macrophages	Subunit of the integrin LFA-1, associated with CD18, interactions with CD54 (ICAM-1), ICAM-2, and ICAM-3
CD11b	Monocytes, macrophages, granulocytes, NK cells	Subunit of the integrin Mac-1 (CR3), associated with CD18, interactions with C3b, CD54, and matrix proteins
CD11c	Monocytes, macrophages, granulocytes	Subunit of the integrin CR4, associated with CD18, interactions with fibrinogen
CD12	Monocytes, granulocytes, platelets	Unknown
CD13	Monocytes, macrophages, granulocytes	Zinc metalloproteinase (aminopeptidase N)
CD14	Monocytes, macrophages	LPS receptor, interacts with apoptotic cells
CD15	Monocytes, neutrophils, eosinophils	Ligand for ELAM (CD62E)
CD16	Neutrophils, NK cells, monocyte subset	Low-affinity IgG receptor (FcγRIII), mediates phagocytosis and cytotoxicity
CD17	Neutrophils, monocytes, platelets	Unknown
CD18	Leukocytes	Integrin β2 subunit, associates with CD11a, CD11b, CD11c
CD19	B cells	Co-receptor, associated with CD21 (CR2) and CD81
CD20	B cells	Possible calcium channel, regulates B cell activation
CD21	Mature B cells, follicular dendritic cells	CR for C3d and EBV, co-receptor, associates with CD19 and CD81
CD22	Mature B cells	Adhesion molecule
CD23	Activated B cells, activated macrophages, activated eosinophils, follicular dendritic cells, platelets	Low-affinity IgE receptor, ligand for CD19/CD21/CD81 complex
CD24	B cells, granulocytes	Unknown
CD25	Activated T cells, B cells, monocytes, activated eosinophils	α-Chain of the IL-2 receptor

TABLE 19 (continued)
Cellular Expression and Functions of CD Antigens

CD Antigen	Cellular Expression	Function
CD26	Activated T cells, activated B cells, macrophages	Exopeptidase (dipeptidyl peptidase IV)
CD27	T cells, NK cells, B cell subset	Co-stimulator for T and B cells, interactions with CD70
CD28	T cell subsets, activated B cells	Activation of naive T cells, interactions with CD80 (B7.1) and CD86 (B7.2)
CD29	Leukocytes	Integrin β1 subunit, associates with CD49a in VLA-1 integrin
CD30	Activated T cells, activated B cells, activated NK cells, monocytes	Interactions with CD30 ligand, stimulates T and B cell proliferation
CD31	Monocytes, platelets, T cell subsets, endothelial cells, neutrophils, eosinophils	Adhesion molecule (PECAM-1)
CD32	Monocytes, neutrophils, B cells, eosinophils	Low-affinity IgG receptor (FcγRII)
CD33	Myeloid progenitors, monocytes	Unknown
CD34	Hematopoietic precursors, endothelial cells	Ligand for CD62L (L-selectin)
CD35	Erythrocytes, B cells, monocytes, neutrophils, eosinophils, follicular dendritic cells	CR1, mediates phagocytosis, interactions with C3b and C4b
CD36	Platelets, monocytes, endothelial cells	Recognition and phagocytosis of apoptotic cells
CD37	Mature B cells, mature T cells, monocytes, macrophages, granulocytes	Unknown
CD38	Immature B and T cells, activated T cells, germinal center B cells, plasma cells	NAD glycohydrolase, augments B cell proliferation
CD39	Activated B cells, activated NK cells, macrophages, dendritic cells	Unknown
CD40	B cells, macrophages, dendritic cells, epithelial cells (basal)	Receptor for CD40L
CD41	Platelets, megakaryocytes	α-Integrin, associates with CD61 to form GPIIb, interactions with fibrinogen, fibronectin, von Willebrand factor, and thrombospondin
CD42	Platelets, megakaryocytes	Essential for platelet adhesion at sites of injury, interactions with thrombin and von Willebrand factor
CD43	Leukocytes, except resting B cells	Interactions with CD54 (ICAM-1)
CD44	Leukocytes, erythrocytes	Adhesion molecule, interactions with hyaluronic acid
CD45	Hematopoietic cells	Tyrosine phosphatase, essential for signaling via T cell antigen receptor and B cell antigen receptor
CD45RO	Memory T cells, B cell subset, monocytes, macrophages	Isoform of CD45, results from alternative splicing
CD45RA	Naive T cells, B cells, monocytes	Isoform of CD45, results from alternative splicing
CD45RB	T cell subsets, B cells, monocytes, macrophages, granulocytes	Isoform of CD45, results from alternative splicing
CD46	Nucleated cells	Receptor for C3b and C4b
CD47	All cells	Unknown
CD48	Leukocytes	Unknown
CD49a	Activated T cells, monocytes, neuronal cells, smooth muscle	α1-Integrin, associates with CD29 (VLA-1), interactions with collagen and laminin-1

TABLE 19 (continued)
Cellular Expression and Functions of CD Antigens

CD Antigen	Cellular Expression	Function
CD49b	B cells, monocytes, platelets, megakaryocytes, neuronal cells, endothelial cells, epithelial cells, osteoclasts	α2-Integrin, associates with CD29 (VLA-2), interactions with collagen and laminin
CD49c	B cells, monocytes, macrophages, granulocytes	α3-Integrin, associates with CD29 (VLA-3), interactions with laminin-5, fibronectin, collagen, entactin, invasin
CD49d	B cells, thymocytes, monocytes, granulocytes, dendritic cells	α4-Integrin, associates with CD29 (VLA-4), interactions with fibronectin, MAdCAM-1, VCAM-1
CD49e	Memory T cells, monocytes, platelets	α5-Integrin, associates with CD29 (VLA-5), interactions with fibronectin and invasin
CD49f	T cells, monocytes, platelets, megakaryocytes, trophoblasts	α6-Integrin, associates with CD29 (VLA-6), interactions with laminin, invasin, and merosin
CD50	T cells, B cells, monocytes, granulocytes, thymocytes	Interactions with CD11a/CD18 (ICAM-3)
CD51	Platelets, megakaryocytes	αv-Integrin, associates with CD61 (vitronectin receptor), interactions with vitronectin, von Willebrand factor, fibrinogen, and thrombospondin; involved in the recognition process of apoptotic cells
CD52	T cells, B cells, monocytes, granulocytes	Unknown
CD53	Leukocytes	Unknown
CD54	Hematopoietic and non-hematopoietic cells	ICAM-1, receptor for rhinovirus, interactions with LFA-1 and Mac-1
CD55	Hematopoietic and non-hematopoietic cells	Interactions with C3b, disassembles C3/C5 convertase
CD56	NK cells	Adhesion molecule
CD57	T cell subsets, B cells, monocytes, NK cells	Unknown
CD58	Hematopoietic and non-hematopoietic cells	Adhesion molecule, LFA-3, interactions with CD2
CD59	Hematopoietic and non-hematopoietic cells	Interactions with C8 and C9
CD60	T cell subsets, platelets, monocytes	Unknown
CD61	Macrophages, platelets, megakaryocytes	Subunit of β3-integrin, associates with CD41 or CD51
CD62E	Endothelial cells	Adhesion molecule (ELAM), important for rolling of neutrophils
CD62L	T cells, *B cells*, NK cells, monocytes	Adhesion molecule (LAM), important for rolling interactions
CD62P	Endothelial cells, platelets, megakaryocytes	Adhesions molecule, important for rolling interactions between endothelial cells and leukocytes or platelets
CD63	Monocytes, macrophages, activated platelets	Unknown
CD64	Monocytes, macrophages	High-affinity IgG receptor (FcγRI), mediates phagocytosis, antigen capture, and ADCC
CD65	Monocytes, macrophages, granulocytes	Unknown
CD66a	Neutrophils	Unknown
CD66b	Granulocytes	Unknown (former CD67)
CD66c	Neutrophils, colon cancer cells	Unknown
CD66d	Neutrophils	Unknown
CD66e	Colon cancer cells	Unknown, CEA
CD66f	Unknown	Unknown

TABLE 19 (continued)
Cellular Expression and Functions of CD Antigens

CD Antigen	Cellular Expression	Function
CD67	See CD66b	
CD68	Monocytes, macrophages, neutrophils, basophils, large lymphocytes	Unknown
CD69	Activated T cells, activated B cells, activated macrophages, activated NK cells, activated eosinophils	Unknown, early activation antigen
CD70	Activated T cells, activated B cells, activated macrophages	Co-stimulator of T and B cells, interactions with CD27
CD71	Activated leukocytes, proliferating cells	Transferrin receptor
CD72	B cells	Unknown, ligand for CD5
CD73	B cell subsets, T cell subsets	Ecto-5′-nucleotidase
CD74	B cells, monocytes, macrophages, dendritic cells, Langerhans cells	MHC class II molecule-associated invariant chain
CD75	Mature B cells, T cell subsets	Ligand for CD22, mediates B cell/B cell adhesion
CD76	Mature B cells, T cell subsets	Unknown
CD77	Germinal center B cells	Cross-linking induces apoptosis
CD78	B cells	Unknown
CD79α,β	B cells	Igα, Igβ, co-receptors of the B cell antigen receptor, required for surface expression and signal transduction
CD80	Monocytes, activated B cells, dendritic cells, macrophages	Co-stimulator (B7.1), ligand for CD28 and CTLA-4
CD81	Lymphocytes	Associates with CD19 and CD21 to form B cell co-receptor
CD82	Leukocytes	Unknown
CD83	Not yet assigned	
CD84	Monocytes, platelets, B cells	Unknown
CD85	Monocytes, B cells	Unknown
CD86	Monocytes, activated B cells, dendritic cells, macrophages	Co-stimulator (B7.2), ligand for CD28 and CTLA-4
CD87	Granulocytes, monocytes, macrophages, T cells, NK cells, many non-hematopoietic cells	Receptor for urokinase plasminogen activator
CD88	Neutrophils, eosinophils, basophils, macrophages, mast cells	Receptor for C5a
CD89	Neutrophils, eosinophils, monocytes, macrophages, T cell subsets, B cell subsets	IgA receptor
CD90	Thymocytes	Unknown
CD91	Monocytes, many non-hematopoietic cells	α2-Macroglobulin receptor
CD92	Neutrophils, monocytes, platelets, endothelial cells	Unknown
CD93	Neutrophils, monocytes, endothelial cells	Unknown
CD94	T cell subsets, NK cells	Unknown
CD95	Many hematopoietic and non-hematopoietic cells, including eosinophils, mast cells, and activated T cells	Death receptor (Fas receptor, APO-1), induces apoptosis in susceptible cells
CD96	Activated T cells, NK cells	Unknown
CD97	Activated T cells, activated B cells, monocytes, granulocytes	Interactions with CD55, G protein-coupled receptor
CD98	T cells, B cells, NK cells, granulocytes	Unknown

TABLE 19 (continued)
Cellular Expression and Functions of CD Antigens

CD Antigen	Cellular Expression	Function
CD99	Lymphocytes, thymocytes	Unknown
CD100	Hematopoietic cells	Unknown
CD101	Activated T cells, granulocytes, monocytes, dendritic cells	Unknown
CD102	Resting T cells, monocytes, endothelial cells	Interactions with LFA-1, but not Mac-1
CD103	T cell subsets	α-Integrin (HML-1)
CD104	Thymocyte subset; neuronal, endothelial, and epithelial cells; trophoblasts	β4-Integrin, associates with CD49f, interactions with laminins
CD105	Activated monocytes, activated macrophages, endothelial cells, bone-marrow subsets	Interactions with TGF-β
CD106	Activated endothelial cells	Adhesion molecule (VCAM-1), ligand for VLA-4
CD107a	Activated T cells, activated neutrophils, activated endothelial cells, activated platelets	Unknown (LAMP-1)
CD107b	Activated T cells, activated neutrophils, activated endothelial cells, activated platelets	Unknown (LAMP-2)
CD108	Lymphocytes, erythrocytes	Unknown
CD109	Activated T cells, activated platelets, endothelial cells	Unknown
CD110	Not yet assigned	
CD111	Not yet assigned	
CD112	Not yet assigned	
CD113	Not yet assigned	
CD114	Neutrophils, monocytes	Receptor for G-CSF
CD115	Monocytes, macrophages	Receptor for M-CSF
CD116	Monocytes, neutrophils, eosinophils, basophils, endothelial cells	α-Chain of the GM-CSF receptor
CD117	Hematopoietic progenitors, mast cells	Receptor for SCF (c-kit)
CD118	Broad cellular expression, including eosinophils	IFN-α,β receptor
CD119	Monocytes, macrophages, neutrophils, eosinophils, B cells, T cell subsets, endothelial cells	IFN-γ receptor
CD120a	Hematopoietic and non-hematopoietic cells, including eosinophils and neutrophils	TNF receptor I, belongs to death receptors
CD120b	Hematopoietic and non-hematopoietic cells	TNF receptor II, no death receptor
CD121a	T cells, thymocytes	IL-1 receptor I
CD121b	B cells, monocytes, macrophages, neutrophils, eosinophils	IL-1 receptor II
CD122	T cell subsets, NK cells, neutrophils, eosinophils	β-Chain of the IL-2 receptor
CD123	Neutrophils, eosinophils, basophils, monocytes, bone marrow stem cells, megakaryocytes	α-Chain of the IL-3 receptor
CD124	T cells, B cells, eosinophils, hematopoietic precursor cells	IL-4 receptor
CD125	Eosinophils, basophils	α-Chain of the IL-5 receptor
CD126	Activated B cells, plasma cells, most leukocytes	α-Chain of the IL-6 receptor

TABLE 19 (continued)
Cellular Expression and Functions of CD Antigens

CD Antigen	Cellular Expression	Function
CD127	Bone marrow lymphoid precursors, pro-B cells, mature T cells, monocytes	IL-7 receptor
CD128	Neutrophils, T cell subsets	IL-8 receptor, chemokine receptor, G protein-coupled receptor
CD129	Not yet assigned	
CD130	B cells, plasma cells, most leukocytes	Common β-chain of IL-6, IL-11, oncostatin-M, and LIF receptors
CD131	Neutrophils, eosinophils, basophils, myeloid progenitors	Common β-chain of IL-3, IL-5, and GM-CSF receptors
CD132	T cells, B cells, NK cells, neutrophils, eosinophils, mast cells	Common γ-chain of the IL-2, IL-4, IL-7, IL-9, and IL-15 receptors
CD133	Not yet assigned	
CD134	Activated T cells	Belongs to the TNF receptor superfamily (no death receptor)
CD135	Hematopoietic precursor cells	Growth factor receptor with tyrosine kinase activity
CD136	Monocytes, neuronal cells, epithelial cells	Receptor with tyrosine kinase activity
CD137	T cells, B cells, monocytes, some epithelial cells, activated eosinophils, neutrophils	Co-stimulator of T cell proliferation (ILA), belongs to the TNF receptor superfamily (no death receptor)
CD138	B cells	Interactions with collagen I
CD139	B cells	Unknown
CD140a,b	Stromal cells, some endothelial cells	α- and β-chains of the PDGF receptor
CD141	Endothelial cells	Anticoagulant
CD142	Keratinocytes, epithelial cells, astrocytes	Major initiating factor of clotting (thromboplastin)
CD143	Endothelial cells, epithelial cells, neuronal cells, activated macrophages, T cell subsets	Angiotensin-converting enzyme (ACE), also cleaves bradykinin
CD144	Not yet assigned	
CD145	Endothelial cells, some stromal cells	Unknown
CD146	Endothelial cells	Unknown
CD147	Leukocytes, erythrocytes, platelets, endothelial cells	Unknown
CD148	Granulocytes, monocytes, T cells, dendritic cells, fibroblasts, nerve cells	Contact inhibition of cell growth
CD149	Not yet assigned	
CD150	Not yet assigned	
CD151	Endothelial cells, epithelial cells, platelets, megakaryocytes	Associates with β1-integrins
CD152	Activated T cells	Ligand for CD80 and CD86, negative regulator of T cell activation (CTLA-4)
CD153	Activated T cells, activated macrophages, neutrophils, B cells	Ligand for CD30
CD154	Activated CD4+ T cells	CD40 ligand (TRAP, gp39)
CD155	Monocytes, macrophages, thymocytes, CNS neurons	Unknown normal function, receptor for poliovirus
CD156	Neutrophils, monocytes	Unknown
CD157	Granulocytes, monocytes, bone marrow stromal cells, endothelial cells, follicular dendritic cells	ADP-ribosyl cyclase

TABLE 19 (continued)
Cellular Expression and Functions of CD Antigens

CD Antigen	Cellular Expression	Function
CD158a	NK cell subsets	Inhibits NK cell cytotoxicity
CD158b	NK cell subsets	Inhibits NK cell cytotoxicity
CD159	Not yet assigned	
CD160	Not yet assigned	
CD161	T cells, NK cells	Regulates NK cell cytotoxicity
CD162	Not yet assigned	
CD163	Monocytes, macrophages	Unknown
CD164	Not yet assigned	
CD165	Not yet assigned	
CD166	Activated T cells, thymic epithelial cells, fibroblasts, neurons	Ligand for CD6

CD8

CD8 is a *surface molecule* expressed on a subset of *T cells* known as *T suppressor/cytotoxic cells*. CD8 is a co-receptor molecule expressed in association with the *T cell antigen receptor* (TCR) complex, and binds specifically to *MHC class I molecules* of *antigen-presenting cells* (APCs). *Allergens*, viral *antigens*, and autoantigens might be presented to CD8$^+$ T cells causing *delayed hypersensitivity* reactions.

CD8$^+$ T cells are involved in the pathogenesis of several diseases such as *asthma*, *atopic dermatitis*, *contact dermatitis*, and *autoimmunity*.

CD8 exists in two forms, CD8a (synonymous with Ly-2 or Lyt-2) and CD8b (Ly-3 or Lyt-3). CD8a is a heterodimer consisting of an α and β chain, CD8b a homodimer of two α chains. The expression and distribution of the two *isoforms* is thought to depend on whether the T cells matured in a thymic (see *thymus*) or extrathymic environment. Function distinctions at this level are not clear.

CD14

CD14 acts as a *receptor* expressed on *monocytes* and *macrophages* that binds bacterial lipopolysaccharide (LPS), triggering *inflammation*. Overstimulation of CD14 by LPS can cause the often fatal toxic-shock syndrome. Moreover, CD14 mediates recognition and *phagocytosis* of apoptotic cells (see *apoptosis*). However, apoptotic cells, unlike LPS, do not provoke the release of *cytokines* from macrophages.

CD16

CD16 is a low-affinity *IgG receptor* (FcγRIII) expressed by *NK cells*, *mast cells*, and *neutrophils*. Since *eosinophils* do not express CD16, this *surface molecule* is used to identify and/or purify eosinophils from mixed *granulocyte* populations. In contrast to mast cells, which express all three receptor α, β, γ subunits, NK cells express functional CD16 without the β-chain. The CD16 molecule of neutrophils, but not NK cells, is GPI-anchored.

CD23

(See *low-affinity IgE receptor*.)

CD25

α-Chain of the *IL-2 receptor*. CD25 is a marker of *T cell activation*. Anti-CD25 *antibodies* are used as *immunosuppressive drugs* (see *antibody therapy*).

CD28

Co-stimulatory molecule (see *co-stimulation*) expressed on the surface of *T cells*. Its ligand is *CD80* or *CD86*. Ligation of CD28 initiates a *signal transduction* pathway that supports *T cell antigen receptor* (TCR) signaling. CD28 signal transduction is blocked by *IL-10*. Lack of CD28-mediated *signaling* appears to be one major mechanism responsible for the induction of *anergy*. CD28 shares homology with the inhibitory *CTLA-4* molecule.

CD30

Surface marker of lymphoma cells. However, *allergens* can also induce expression of CD30 on *T cells* of atopic asthmatics (see *allergic asthma*). Therefore, CD30 may differentiate *CD4+* T cells between *Th1* (CD30-) and *Th2* (CD30+) functional phenotypes (see *Th1/Th2 markers*). However, the distinction does not appear to be absolute. CD30 is also expressed on *CD8+* T cells, which produce *Th2 cytokines* (see *Tc2 cells*).

CD40

CD40 is a 50-kDa transmembrane glycoprotein, and a member of the *TNF receptor super-family*. It is expressed on *B cells* at most stages of differentiation (with the exception of *plasma cells*), malignant B cells such as lymphomas and leukemias, and virally transformed B cells. CD40 is also expressed on interdigitating cells (= *dendritic cells* in *lymph nodes*), follicular dendritic cells, thymic epithelial cells, and on *monocytes* following treatment with *GM-CSF*, *IL-3*, or *IFN-γ*. The *gene* for CD40 has been mapped to *chromosome* 20 in humans and is located on chromosome 2 in the mouse.

> CD40/CD40 ligand (see *CD154*) molecular interactions and concurrent *IL-4* or *IL-13* stimulation induce *immunoglobulin class switching* to generate large amounts of *IgE* in B cells.

Moreover, such stimulation upregulates the expression of B cell *surface molecules* (e.g., *ICAM-1*, *CD23*, *Fas receptor*) as well as *B cell proliferation*. CD40 also plays a role in the regulation of *B cell apoptosis*. For instance, ligation of CD40 with anti-CD40 *monoclonal antibodies* (mAbs) delivers an anti-apoptotic signal to immature B cells, and rescues mature B cells from anti-IgM-induced *apoptosis*.

The biochemical events associated with CD40 *signal transduction* are beginning to emerge. Inhibitors of *tyrosine kinases* and *protein kinase C* (PKC) inhibit CD40-mediated B cell proliferation and IgE synthesis, suggesting a critical role of these signaling molecules. Indeed, CD40 activation leads not only to the activation of *Jak*3 and *STAT*3, but also *TRAF* proteins. Tyrosine *phosphorylation* of any of the other known STAT proteins in response to CD40 ligation has not been observed so far. Moreover, CD40 does not appear to be only a *receptor*, since it also supplies obligatory co-stimulatory signals (see *co-stimulation*) for *cytokine* production of CD40 ligand-expressing *T cells*.

CD40 LIGAND

(See *CD154*.)

CD44

CD44 has been implicated in *lymphocyte homing*. At least 20 different *isoforms* of CD44, arising from *differential splicing* of up to 10 alternative *exons* (v1–v10), have been identified to date. Variant forms of CD44 may play an important role in tumor metastasis. Moreover, CD44 appears to contribute to the molecular recognition process of apoptotic *neutrophils* (see *apoptosis*), but not *T cells*, by *macrophages*.

CD45

CD45 is a cell surface glycoprotein (gp) with four major *isoforms* of 180, 190, 205, and 220 (240) kDa. It is also known as the leukocyte common antigen (LCA) (synonyms T200 and B220).

> CD45 is present on all human *leukocytes* including *lymphocytes*, *monocytes*, *neutrophils*, *eosinophils*, and *mast cells*.

CD45 is absent from circulating erythrocytes, *platelets*, or mature erythroid cells of either the *bone marrow* or non-hematopoietic tissues. It has a cytoplasmic *tyrosine phosphatase* activity, and is, therefore, involved in *signal transduction*. The different isoforms of CD45 result from *alternative splicing*. The CD45RA (gp 205-220) isoform is found on approximately 50% of *CD4+* and *CD8+ T cells*, as well as some *B cells* and monocytes. This isoform is often referred to as *naive T cells*. CD45RB (gp 205-220) is expressed on B cells, T cells, monocytes, *macrophages*, and some *granulocytes*. Memory T cells (CD4+CD45RA−) exhibit differential expression of CD45RB. CD45RB bright staining cells are associated with proliferation (see *T cell proliferation*) and expression of *IFN-γ*. The CD45RO isoform (gp180) is found on activated T cells (see *T cell antigen receptor*) and *memory T cells*, but not on resting T cells. The numbers of CD4+CD45RO+ T cells is usually low, but is increased in allergic patients (see *allergic diseases*) following prolonged exposure to *allergen*. These CD45RO+ T cells are preferentially attracted to sites of *allergic inflammation* by the *chemokine RANTES*.

CD54

(See *intercellular adhesion molecule-1*.)

CD80

CD80 (=B7.1) is a cell *surface molecule* on several *antigen-presenting cells* (APCs). The expression appears to be regulated. For instance, *IFN-γ* upregulates surface expression on these cells.

> CD80 is the ligand for *CD28* and stimulates *T cell activation* and *Th1* differentiation.

On the other hand, CD80 may inhibit functional T cell responses when it binds to *CTLA-4*.

CD86

CD86 (=B7.2) is a cell *surface molecule* on several *antigen-presenting cells* (APCs). As *CD80*, CD86 is a ligand for both *CD28* and *CTLA-4*.

> Interestingly, blocking anti-CD86 (but not anti-CD80) *monoclonal antibodies* decreased *IL-5* production in *allergen*-specific *T cells* in patients with *asthma*.

Therefore, agents which block CD86-mediated *co-stimulation* may have therapeutic potential in *allergic diseases* associated with high *Th2* activity.

CD88

CD88 is a *G protein-coupled receptor* for *C5a*, which is an important *chemotactic factor* and activator molecule for *degranulation* in *allergic inflammation*. CD88 is expressed on most inflammatory cells (see *CD antigens*).

CD95

(See *Fas receptor*.)

CD117

Receptor for *stem cell factor* (SCF).

CD119

Receptor for *interferon-γ* (IFN-γ).

CD120

Receptor for *tumor necrosis factor* (TNF). See also *TNF receptor* and *TNF receptor superfamily*.

CD125

α-Chain of the *interleukin-5* (IL-5) *receptor*. In humans, CD125 is only expressed on *eosinophils* and *basophils*.

CD131

Common β-chain of *IL-3*, *IL-5*, and *GM-CSF receptors*.

CD137

CD137 is a member of the *TNF receptor superfamily*. It is expressed by *T cells* and may act as a co-stimulatory molecule to increase *T cell proliferation* (see *co-stimulation*).

> Interestingly, CD137 is selectively expressed on *eosinophils* derived from patients with *atopic dermatitis*, but not normal individuals.

Functional studies on *granulocytes* have shown that activation of CD137 may disrupt *signal transduction* pathways initiated by *survival factors* and may, therefore, limit granulocyte expansion in *inflammation* (see *immunosuppressive mechanisms*).

CD154

CD154 (CD40 ligand, CD40L) is a 33-kDa type II membrane glycoprotein belonging to the *TNF superfamily* of proteins. It is expressed on the surface of activated *CD4+ T cells*. The CD40L *gene* was mapped to the X *chromosome*. The critical role of CD40–CD40L interactions in immune function is highlighted by observations in special human diseases.

> Patients with a genetic defect in CD40L are unable to undergo *immunoglobulin class switching*. Such patients consequently develop a *hyper-IgM syndrome*.

In addition, mice with targeted disruption of their CD40L or CD40 genes fail to undergo immunoglobulin *isotype* switching and to form germinal centers in response to T-cell-dependent *antigens*. CD40L expression by *eosinophils* and *mast cells* has also been described under *IgE*-mediated allergic inflammatory conditions (see *allergic diseases*).

cDNA

(See *complementary DNA*.)

CELERY

Celery might be a food *allergen* (see *food allergy*), causing *oral allergy syndrome* (OAS), generalized *urticaria*, or even *anaphylactic reactions*. Celery contains *profilin* and is therefore a *cross-reacting allergen*.

CELL CYCLE

The cell cycle is a complex process that occurs during cell division (see *T cell proliferation*), which includes duplication of *DNA*.

CELL-MEDIATED HYPERSENSITIVITY

(See *delayed hypersensitivity.*)

CENTI-MORGAN (cM)

This is a definition of genetic distance. The unit 1 cM is defined by a recombination chance of 1% between two *gene* loci in a given meiotic event (see *meiosis*). One cM roughly corresponds to 1000 kb.

CENTROMERE

This is the central constriction of the *chromosome*.

CERAMIDE

Ceramide is a signaling molecule, generated from *sphingomyelin* by activated *sphingomyelinase*. The sphingomyelin–ceramide *signal transduction* pathway is initiated by *cross-linking* of *death receptors* and *IL-1*. Ceramide can directly or indirectly activate many target proteins, including *nuclear factor-κB* (NF-κB), *phospholipase D*, the *ζ-isoform* of *protein kinase C* (PKC), and *caspases*.

C1 ESTERASE-INHIBITOR

(See *C1 inhibitor.*)

CETIRIZINE

This is a second-generation H_1 antagonist (see *antihistamines*). Moreover, cetirizine has been shown to block *mediator* release from *mast cells* and *basophils*. It is the active carboxylic acid metabolite of *hydroxyzine*.

CFC PROPELLANTS

Chlorofluorocarbon (CFC) propellants have traditionally been used in a wide range of *aerosol* applications, including *metered dose inhalers* (and refrigeration units). Unfortunately, CFCs cause damage to the *ozone* layer, and are therefore being phased out under the Montreal Accord.

cGMP

(See *cyclic guanosine monophosphate.*)

CHARCOT–LEYDEN CRYSTALS

Granular debris from *eosinophils*, identified by microscopic examination of the *sputum* of patients with *asthma*.

CHEMOATTRACTANT

(See *chemotactic factors.*)

CHEMOKINES

Chemokines are traditionally defined as a subgroup of *cytokines* that share a common role in the inflammatory response, the chemoattraction (see *chemotaxis*) of specific *leukocytes* to the site of *inflammation*. The members of the chemokine family are structurally related, which means that they share variable degrees of sequence identity of at least 20%, suggesting that may have arisen by *gene* duplication. They are produced in response to inflammatory stimuli by a variety of cells, including *endothelial cells, T cells, monocytes, eosinophils, neutrophils,* and *mast cells*.

> Chemokines can be divided into two subfamilies according to the position of the first two cysteine residues, which are either separated by one *amino acid* (see *CXC chemokines*) or adjacent (see *CC chemokines*).

Most chemokines act on one cell or a selected panel of cells that depends on the expression of *chemokine receptors* by the target cell (see Table 20). Besides chemotaxis, chemokines may also activate *effector cells*. For instance, it has been shown that chemokines may stimulate *mediator* release and the generation of reactive *oxygen metabolites* in *eosinophils* and *basophils*.

TABLE 20
Chemotactic Activity of Selected Chemokines on *Granulocytes*

	Eosinophils	*Basophils*	*Neutrophils*
IL-8	(+)	(+)	+++
Eotaxin	+++	+++	–
RANTES	+++	+++	–
MCP-1	–	+	–
MCP-2	++	++	–
MCP-3	+++	+++	–
MCP-4	+++	+++	–
MIP-1α	+	+	–
MIP-1β	–	–	–

CHEMOKINE RECEPTORS

The *receptors* of *CC chemokines* and *CXC chemokines* are *G protein-coupled receptors*. Besides chemokine expression, the expression of chemokine receptors by the different inflammatory cells (see Tables 21 and 22) also determines which cells are attracted into inflammatory tissue. The receptor expression in specific cells can be determined by intracellular calcium measurements, since all G protein-coupled receptors are linked to *phospholipase C* (PLC) activation and consequent rapid increases in $[Ca^{2+}]_i$ (see *calcium mobilization*). When the same receptor is stimulated twice with the same chemokine, no increases of $[Ca^{2+}]_i$ are observed as a consequence of receptor *desensitization*.

> Desensitization after repeated stimulation is a sensitive test to determine functional chemokine receptor expression.

Interestingly, *Th1* and *Th2 cells* differ in their expression of chemokine receptors (see Tables 21 and 22). CC and CXC chemokines act on different chemokine receptors. In addition, other *chemotactic factors* such as *PAF, C5a, C3a,* FMLP, and *leukotrienes* have their own G protein-coupled receptors.

CHEMOTACTIC FACTORS

Mediators that attract and activate inflammatory cells in inflammatory processes, e.g., in *allergic inflammation* (see *chemotaxis, chemokines, IL-16, leukotrienes, PAF,* and *complement factors*).

TABLE 21
CC Chemokine Receptor (CCR) Expression by Inflammatory Cells

	CCR1	CCR2	CCR3	CCR4	CCR5	CCR6	CCR7
Eosinophils	(+)	–	+	–	–	–	–
Basophils	+	+	+	+	–	–	–
Neutrophils	(+)	–	–	–	–	–	–
Monocytes	+	+	–	–	+	–	–
Naive T cells	–	–	–	–	–	–	+
Th1 cells	(+)	+	–	–	+	–	–
Th2 cells	–	+	+*	+	–	–	–
B cells	–	–	–	–	–	–	+

* There are controversial findings regarding the expression of CCR3 on Th2 cells.

TABLE 22
CXC Chemokine Receptor (CXCR) Expression by Inflammatory Cells

	CXCR1	CXCR2	CXCR3	CXCR4	CXCR5
Eosinophils	–	–	–	–	–
Basophils	–	–	–	–	–
Neutrophils	+	+	–	–	–
Monocytes	–	–	–	+	–
Naive T cells	–	–	–	+	–
Th1 cells	–	–	+	–	(+)
Th2 cells	–	–	–	–	(+)
B cells	–	–	(+)	+	+

CHEMOTAXIS

Chemotaxis can be defined as the directional *migration* of cells toward a source of a *chemotactic factor*, following the increasing concentration gradient form of that source. Chemotactic responses are important in cell recruitment and migration to sites of *inflammation*. Chemotaxis in the *immune system* is mediated by specialized *cytokines* (see *chemokines* and *IL-16*), *lipid mediators* (see *leukotrienes* and *PAF*), and *complement factors* (see *C3a* and *C5a*).

CHESTNUT

Chestnut may generate *IgE*-mediated allergic reaction in patients with *latex allergy* (see *latex–fruit syndrome*).

CHILDHOOD ASTHMA

Approximately 80% of early-onset *asthma* is associated with allergic *sensitization* to indoor *aeroallergens*. Most frequently associated with the development of asthma are *house-dust mite*, *cockroach*, *cat,* and *alternaria allergens*. Moreover, *respiratory syncytial virus* (RSV) infection can cause childhood wheezing (see *wheeze*) and may lead to asthma. In addition, *rhinovirus* infection is associated with the majority of *asthma exacerbations* in children by upregulating *inflammation* in the lung. Males are more likely to develop early-onset asthma (gender ratio 2:1), whereas there is no gender difference in asthma onset in adulthood. Numerous studies indicate that approximately 50 to 60% of persons with asthma in childhood do not have clinical symptoms of asthma in adulthood. *Breast feeding*, while associated with protection against wheezing in early infancy, has not been associated with decreased incidence of asthma (see *risk factors*).

CHINESE RESTAURANT SYNDROME

Food *intolerance* reaction due to monosodium glutamate, which is often used to enhance flavor in Chinese food (see *adverse food reactions*).

CHOLINERGIC NERVES

Nerves whose transmitter is *acetylcholine*. Cholinergic nerves form the principal autonomic innervation of the airways (see *nervous system*). The fibers travel with the vagus nerve and maintain *airway tone*. The action of cholinergic nerves may be antagonized by *anticholinergic drugs*.

CHOLINERGIC RECEPTORS

(See *muscarinic receptors*.)

CHONDROITIN SULFATE A

Important *proteoglycan* produced by *basophils* (see *chondroitin sulfate E*).

CHONDROITIN SULFATE E

Important *proteoglycan* produced by *mast cells* and *monocytes*. It stabilizes mast cell *neutral proteases* and alters the biological activity of many enzymes (see *chondroitin sulfate A*).

CHROMATIN

This term describes nucleic acids and associated proteins of *chromosomes*. The *DNA* of eukaryotic cells is wrapped around *histones* to form *nucleosomes* with about 200 base pairs of DNA that are probably not accessible for the *transcription factor* proteins (see *DNase hypersensitivity*). Chromatin can be further compacted by folding of nucleosomes into higher-order structures, including the highly condensed metaphase chromosomes of cells undergoing *mitosis*.

CHROMOSOME

Eukaryotic *DNA* is present in the nucleus as linear DNA molecules that are visible in their transport form in the highly condensed metaphase chromosomes by light microscopy. The human *genome* is distributed among 24 chromosomes (22 *autosomes* and the 2 sex chromosomes), each containing between 5×10^4 and 26×10^4 kb of DNA.

CHROMOSOME WALKING

This is a method for consecutive isolation and characterization of *DNA* fragments overlapping with the starting *clone*. It is used for positional cloning to isolate the *gene* of interest located by linked markers (see *DNA cloning*).

CHRONIC BRONCHITIS

Chronic *bronchitis* is defined as the production of purulent *sputum* for at least 3 months during each of 2 consecutive years. This definition excludes those who have pneumonia or other acute respiratory illness and remain affected for several months with a productive *cough*. This definition has been useful for epidemiological purposes but is not always practical in clinical use. Patients with chronic bronchitis show *mucus* hyperplasia in their large airways (see *airway anatomy*) and produce increased volumes of mucus and sputum. Chronic bronchitis can therefore be identified histologically as well as epidemiologically. Chronic bronchitis commonly coexists with *emphysema* and is associated with a variable degree of *airway obstruction* (see *COPD*).

CHRONIC EOSINOPHILIC PNEUMONIA

(See *eosinophilic pneumonia*.)

CHRONIC INTERMITTANT URTICARIA

Any form of *urticaria* lasting for longer than 6 weeks, including symptom-free periods lasting for longer than 2 days.

CHRONIC OBSTRUCTIVE PULMONARY DISEASE (COPD)

COPD, also known as chronic obstructive lung disease or chronic obstructive airways disease, is a relatively new label applied to patients who have *airway obstruction*, *chronic bronchitis*, and/or *emphysema*. The air flow obstruction is usually more persistent and less reversible than in *asthma*. In extreme cases, the airway obstruction may be completely irreversible. Cigarette *smoking* is the major single risk factor for COPD, but exposure to cooking smoke, coal dust, and other respiratory *irritants* can also induce it. A minority of patients have deficiencies of α1-anti-protease, which can lead to premature emphysema, especially in those who have smoked. Table 23 compares known features of *inflammation* in asthma and COPD.

TABLE 23
Inflammatory Findings in Asthma and COPD

Feature	Asthma	COPD
Eosinophilia	Yes	No
Activated *T cells*	*CD4*+	*CD8*+
IL-4	Yes	Yes
IL-5	Yes	No
Eotaxin	Yes	No
IL-8	Yes	Yes
IgE	Yes	No
Mucus cell hyperplasia	Yes	Yes
Remodeling	*Subepithelial fibrosis*	*Fibrosis* and alveolar destruction

CHRONIC PERSISTANT URTICARIA

Any form of *urticaria* lasting for longer than 6 weeks lacking symptom-free periods.

CHURG–STRAUSS SYNDROME

A rare inflammatory condition characterized by eosinophilic *inflammation* (see *eosinophils*) of small blood vessels (vasculitis), pulmonary infiltrates, and *asthma*. Patients with Churg–Strauss syndrome usually respond well to oral *corticosteroids* with or without *cyclophosphamide*. Churg–Strauss syndrome forms part of a clinical spectrum, which includes polyarteritis nodosa. Patients usually have *intrinsic asthma* and go on to show signs of systemic *eosinophilia* and vasculitis after a few months or years. Churg–Strauss syndrome should be suspected in patients whose asthma is difficult to control except by oral steroids, and who show high blood eosinophil counts.

CHYMASE

In contrast to *tryptase*, chymase is only present in a subset of *mast cells* (MC_{TC}) found predominantly in the skin. It is a monomeric 30-kDa *neutral protease* and is stored in the same secretory *granules* as tryptase, but is independently (without tryptase) released in a macromolecular complex together with *carboxypeptidase* and *cathepsin G* to degrade proteins (see Table 24). The stored chymase needs no further processing before release. Of special interest in respect to *allergic inflammation* is that chymase contributes to the activation of *IL-1* (independent from *angiotensin-converting enzyme*) and degrades *IL-4*. Besides *angiotensin* I and *cytokines, bradykinin, kallikrein, substance P, vasointestinal peptide* (VIP), and matrix *metalloproteinases* (MMP 1 and MMP 3) represent targets of chymase, resulting in multiple biological functions (see Table 24).

TABLE 24
Biological Processes that Are Influenced by the Proteolytic Activity of Chymase

Activation of precursor IL-1
Angiotensin II generation
Basement membrane degradation
Cleavage of cytokines and *neuropeptides*
Leukocyte migration (see also *adhesion molecules* and *chemotaxis*)
Mast cell *degranulation*
Mucus secretion
Tissue degradation (see *extracellular matrix*)
Vascular exudation

CIGARETTE SMOKING

(See *smoking*.)

CILIA

Cilia are hair-like structures on the surface of *epithelial cells*, consisting of one pair of central microtubules surrounded by nine tubulin doublets. Each ciliated cell contains approximately 200 cilia. The airways (see *airway anatomy*) are ciliated from the nose to the *bronchioles*, with the exception of the larynx and parts of the pharynx. The ciliary beat cycle with its recovery stroke followed by an effective stroke results in continuous *mucus* transport.

In *asthma, epithelial damage* leads to an impairment of *mucociliary clearance*.

C1 INHIBITOR

C1 inhibitor is a member of a family of proteins called serine protease inhibitors (= serpins), which also include α1-antitrypsin and antithrombin III. It is mainly synthesized in the liver.

In case of C1 inhibitor deficiency, the first component of *complement system*, C1, is unrestrictedly activated in response to injury, stress, exercise, or other triggering factors. This results in activation of the complement cascade with the generation of *complement factors*.

C1 inhibitor is coded by two *genes*. In type I hereditary *angioedema*, there is a defect in one of these genes, resulting in a quantitative deficiency. In the rarer type II disease, one gene generates a normal C1 inhibitor at a reduced level, and the other gene produces a functionally incompetent protein. Moreover, an acquired deficiency of C1 inhibitor may occur in association with lymphoproliferative malignancies or autoimmune connective-tissue diseases, or due to autoantibodies directed against C1 inhibitor (see *autoimmunity*).

cis-ACTING PROTEIN

This is a transcriptional modulator (see *transcription*) acting on the same molecule of *DNA* (*chromosome*) in which it was expressed.

CLADOSPORIUM

(See *fungal allergens.*)

CLARA CELLS

Clara cells are nonciliated secretory *epithelial cells* lining the pulmonary airways (see *airway anatomy*), distinct from *mucus* secretory cells in morphology and their secretory products. In experimentally induced *epithelial damage* as it occurs in *asthma*, Clara cells lead to the recovery of epithelium, indicating a role in repair mechanisms (see *remodeling*). Moreover, Clara cells specifically produce the so-called Clara cell 10-kDa protein (*CC10*). CC10 is an inhibitor of *phospholipase A$_2$* (PLA$_2$), suggesting an antiinflammatory role of this protein in the lung.

CLIMATE THERAPY

Stays at the seaside or in the mountains may be beneficial for patients with *atopic dermatitis* and *asthma*. Intensive UV radiation (see *UV therapy*), absence of *air pollution*, air humidity (see *humidifiers*), temperature, marginal *pollen* concentrations, and absence of *house-dust mite allergens* are the main factors responsible for the dramatic relief of symptoms. High-altitude climate therapy has been associated with reduced *T cell activation*, *cytokine gene* expression, and eosinophilic *inflammation* (see *eosinophils*).

CLINICAL ECOLOGY

A branch of *alternative medicine* in which a wide range of symptoms are attributed to sensitivity to trace amounts of foreign chemicals including pesticides, *pollutants*, dental amalgam, etc. Several different diagnostic strategies are used including vega testing, reflexology, auriculocardiac tests, and applied kinesiology. Different treatment strategies are applied with varying levels of success, but no scientific evidence exists to support these techniques.

CLONE

A cell or an organism derived from a single parent cell or organism. A clone carries the same *genotype* and *phenotype* as the parent (see *monoclonal antibody, T cell clone*). *DNA cloning* is the process of isolating a particular *gene*, or gene fragment, and introducing the gene into a *vector* or *plasmid*.

CLONING OF ALLERGENS

By the mid-1980s a large number of *allergens* had been purified using biochemical techniques, but in general the yields were poor and, apart from physicochemical properties, the molecular structures of these proteins were poorly defined. With the advent of molecular cloning techniques (see *DNA cloning*), the *primary structures* of many *common allergens* were rapidly established and, by screening *cDNA* expression libraries with *IgE antibodies*, new allergens were identified and sequenced. More than 200 allergen sequences are now listed in protein databanks (e.g., GenBank), and a partial listing of *major allergens* is shown in Table 25.

> The aim of cloning and sequencing is to obtain the primary structure of the allergen and to produce *recombinant allergens*.

For many major allergens, *N*-terminal or internal *amino acid* sequences and monospecific antibodies were available to confirm the identity of cDNA *clones*. In some cases, e.g., *cat allergen*, Fel d 1, or *aspergillus* allergen, Asp f 1, the *nucleotide* sequences were obtained by *polymerase chain reaction* (PCR) using *primers* derived from *amino acid* sequences. However, the usual approach has been to isolate *mRNA* from allergen source material (e.g., *pollen, house-dust mite, cockroach*, or *fungal allergens*) and to use reverse transcriptase to generate double-stranded cDNA, which is then packaged into λGT11 or similar expression *vectors*. The cDNA libraries are screened with pooled IgE antibodies from six to eight allergic patients, or with high titer monospecific polyclonal antibodies, to identify cDNA clones expressing allergen. Increasingly, allergens are being identified solely based on screening cDNA libraries.

> Sequence similarity searches have enabled the protein families to which allergens belong to be ascertained and their biologic function to be identified.

The major *tree pollen* allergens (e.g., Bet v 1) are related to pathogenesis resistance proteins. Many mite allergens are proteolytic enzyme (cysteine and serine proteases, trypsin and chymotrypsin). Muscle proteins such as tropomyosin and troponin have been identified as allergens in mites, insects, and shellfish (see Table 25). Moreover, a family of proteins has been identified that causes IgE antibody responses — ligand binding proteins or calycins. These proteins bind small hydrophobic molecules such as pigments and pheromones. Calycins were first identified as a result of cloning cockroach allergens. However, the family also includes the major rodent urinary proteins, milk allergen β-lactoglobulin, as well as dog, bovine, and equine allergens (Figure 15).

It has been postulated that because many allergens, particularly from dust mites, are proteolytic enzymes, that this facilitates penetration through mucosal surfaces and induction of *allergen-induced immune responses*. There is evidence that Der p 1 may upregulate IgE synthesis through its ability to cleave *CD23*, the low-affinity receptor for IgE. However, several clinically important allergens have no enzymatic activity, and there are other allergens, that show no sequence homology to known proteins and whose function is as yet unknown (e.g., mite Group 5 allergens) (Table 25).

> It is quite common for a single allergen to show sequence polymorphisms, and variants with limited amino acid substitutions are termed *isoforms*.

In some cases, e.g., birch pollen allergen, Bet v 1, the isoforms may have altered IgE antibody binding properties (see *conformational epitopes*), which make them attractive candidates for *immunotherapy*.

CLONING VECTOR

(See *vector*.)

CLUSTER OF DIFFERENTIATION

(See *CD antigens*.)

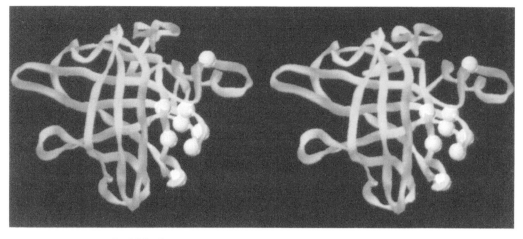

bgl2A-1   **bgl2A-2**

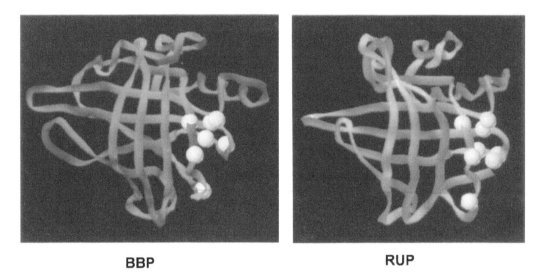

BBP   **RUP**

FIGURE 15   Molecular modeling of the cockroach calycin allergen, Bla g 4. The Cα backbone structures for two models of Bla g 4 (originally identified as clone bgl2A; upper panel) were modeled on the X-ray crystal coordinates for butterfly bilin binding protein (BBP; lower panel left) and are compared with rat urinary protein allergen (RUP, lower panel right), for which the X-ray crystal structure has also been determined. The spheres are conserved amino acid residues that form motifs, which define the ligand binding proteins, or calycins. (From Arruda, L.K., Vailes, L.D., Hayden, M.L., Benjamin, D.C., and Chapman, M.D., Cloning of cockroach allergen, Bla g 4, identifies ligand binding proteins (or calycins) as a cause of IgE antibody responses, *J. Biol. Chem.,* 270, 52, 1995. With permission.)

c-MAF

First identified as proto-*oncogene*, it is now clear that c-Maf is a *transcription factor* of the *activator protein 1* (AP-1) family, which binds the consensus recognition site called MARE. In mouse *Th2 clones*, c-Maf appears to be selectively expressed. Similarly, c-Maf expression was inducible in Th2, but not *Th1* development from naive mouse *T cells*. Mice lacking c-Maf (c-Maf[-/-]) were markedly deficient in *IL-4* synthesis but expressed normal levels of *IL-13* and *IgE*. Moreover, c-Maf does not transactivate *IL-5* or *IL-10 promoters*. In contrast, human *Th1*

TABLE 25
Molecular Properties of Common Allergens

Source	Allergen	MW (kDa)	Homology/Function
		Inhalants	
Indoor			
House-dust mite	Der p 1	25	Cysteine protease[b]
(Dermatophagoides pteronyssinus	Der p 2	14	Epididymal or molting protein[b]
	Der p 3	30	Serine protease
	Der p 5	14	Unknown
Cat (Felis domesticus)	Fel d 1	36	Uteroglobin[a]
Dog (Canis familiaris)	Can f 1	25	Cysteine protease inhibitor
Mouse (Mus musculus)	Mus m 1	21	Pheromone binding protein (calycin)[b]
Rat (Rattus norvegicus)	Rat n 1	21	Pheromone binding (calycin)[b]
Cockroach (Blattella germanica)	Bla g 2	36	Aspartic protease
Outdoor			
Pollens — Grasses			
Rye (Lolium perenne)	Lol p 1	28	Unknown
Timothy (Phleum pratense)	Phl p 5	32	Unknown
Bermuda (Cynodon dactylon)	Cyn d 1	32	Unknown
Pollens — Weeds			
Ragweed (Artemisia artemisifolia)	Amb a 1	38	Pectate lyase[a,b]
	Amb a 5	5	Neurophysins[b]
Pollens — Trees			
Birch (Betula verucosa)	Bet v 1	17	Pathogenesis-related protein[b]
		Foods	
Milk	β-Lactoglobulin	36	Retinol-binding protein (calycin)[a,b]
Egg	Ovomucoid	29	Trypsin inhibitor
Codfish (Gadus callarias)	Gad c 1	12	Ca-binding protein (muscle parvalbumin)
Peanut (Arachis hypogea)	Ara h 1	63	Vicilin (seed-storage protein)
		Venoms	
Bee (Apis melifera)	Api m 1	19.5	Phospholipase A_2
Wasp (Polestes annularis)	Pol a 5	23	Mammalian testis proteins
Hornet (Vespa crabro)	Ves c 5	23	Mammalian testis proteins
Fire ant (Solenopsis invicta)	Sol i 2	13	Unknown
		Fungi	
Aspergillus fumigatus	Asp f 1	18	Cytotoxin (mitogillin)
Alternaria alternata	Alt a 1	29	Unknown
		Latex	
Hevea brasiliensis	Hev b 1	58	Elongation factor unknown
	Hev b 5	16	

[a] Most allergens have a single polypeptide chain; dimers are indicated.

[b] Allergens of known three-dimensional structure are also indicated.

and Th2 cells did not differ in their c-Maf levels as assessed by quantitative *polymerase chain reaction* (PCR) analyses. It is possible that c-Maf needs additional *transcription* factors for efficient IL-4 *gene* activation in human cells. It is postulated that c-Maf and *nuclear factor of activated T cells* (NF-AT) synergize in transactivating the minimal IL-4 promoter.

CO

(See *carbon monoxide*.)

COCKROACH ALLERGENS

The two principal allergenic cockroach (CR) species, *Blattella germanica* and *Periplaneta americana*, both produce multiple *aeroallergens*. The first CR *allergens* to be identified were Bla g 1 and Bla g 2, which elicit *IgE antibody* responses in 30 to 50% and 60 to 80% of CR allergic patients, respectively. *DNA cloning* techniques determined the *amino acid* sequence of Bla g 2 and established that it is a 36-kDa aspartic protease. Other allergens identified by screening B. germanica *cDNA* expression libraries with IgE antibodies include Bla g 4, a lipocalin; Bla g 5, glutathione transferase; and Bla g 6, troponin. Bla g 1 has an unusual structure consisting of a series of up to seven tandem repeats, each ~100 amino acid residues in length. Bla g 1 is also the only B. germanica allergen that has a structural homologue in P. americana (Per a 1).

Several allergens have been cloned from P. americana, including Per a 1; Per a 3, an insect storage protein related to arylphorin; and tropomyosin (see Table 26). More than 90% of CR allergic patients living in Taiwan make IgE responses to Per a 3. CR tropomyosin is homologous to shrimp and dust mite tropomyosins, which are also important allergens (Pen a 1 and Der p 10).

Expression systems have been developed for producing recombinant CR allergens in either E. coli (pGEX or pET systems, see *plasmid*) or in the yeast, *Pichia pastoris* (pPIC9 system). The *recombinant allergens* produced in these systems are biologically active and can induce positive *immediate hypersensitivity* reactions in *skin tests* in CR allergic patients at concentrations as low as 10^{-5} µg/ml. Recombinant CR allergens can also be used for in vitro diagnostic tests. Using a cocktail of Bla g 1, Bla g 2, Bla g 4, and Bla g 5, it is possible to demonstrate *sensitization* to CR in >95% of CR allergic patients.

TABLE 26
Cloned P. americana Allergens

Allergen	MW	Function
Per a 1	24 kDa	Unknown
(CR-PII)	26–31 kDa	Unknown
Per a 3	72–78 kDa	Arylphorin
Tropomyosin	31 kDa	Muscle protein

CODOMINANCE

This means that both *alleles* of a pair are being expressed in the *heterozygote*.

CODON

A triplet of three bases in a *DNA* or *RNA* molecule specifying a single *amino acid*.

COELIAC DISEASE

(See *gluten-sensitive enteropathy*.)

COGNATE/NONCOGNATE INTERACTIONS

> Cognate interactions between *T cells* and other cell types (or between T cells and other T cells) require the specific recognition between the T cell and the target cell.

Examples of cognate interactions include *antigen* presentation and *antigen recognition* between *antigen-presenting cells* (APC) and T cells, T cell interactions with *B cells*, which provide help for *immunoglobulin* production, and direct cytotoxicity mediated by *CD8⁺* T cells on cells expressing viral, bacterial, or tumor antigens. Implicit in cognate interactions is the adherence of cells and effective *signal transduction*, mediated by *adhesion molecules* and co-stimulatory molecules (see *co-stimulation*), respectively.

> Noncognate interactions are cell interactions that occur over variable distances with no specific recognition.

Examples of noncognate interactions include the production by T cells of, and reaction by target cells to, *cytokines* and other *mediators*. In some instances intimate contact between the T cells and target cells is necessary so that concentration-dependent mechanisms of *receptor* engagement and activation may occur, for example in intercellular spaces bounded by tight junctions between cells. In other instances, hormonal interaction allows local production of messenger molecules to be effective over large distances on one or more target cell types bearing specific receptors.

COLD AIR CHALLENGE

The major trigger to exercise-induced *airway obstruction* is the cooling of the airways by mouth breathing. The response can be exaggerated by inhaling cold air, and this forms the basis of a simple *bronchial provocation test* to evaluate *exercise-induced asthma* and non-specific *airway hyperresponsiveness*.

COLLAGEN

Fibrils of collagen are deposited by the activity of *myofibroblasts* both as repair processes and as part of the process of scarring. In *asthma*, type 3 and type 5 collagen are deposited beneath the basement membrane (see *subepithelial fibrosis*) and may contribute to *airway remodeling*.

COLLAGENASE

This is a *metalloprotease* that degrades *collagen*.

COMMON ALLERGENS

Among the most common *aeroallergens* are *pollens*, *house-dust mite*, insect components (see *hymenoptera allergy*), and *animal dander*. Common food *allergens* (see *food allergy*) include nuts, shellfish, milk, and eggs, but also fruit, chocolate, food colorings, and many others. Occupational *allergies* (see *occupational asthma*) are often caused by small molecules (see *haptens*) that occur in industrial chemicals, flour, and animal body fluids. Other allergens include natural rubber latex (see *latex allergy*), seminal fluid, platinum, and *nickel* salts (see *metallic salts*). All allergens are characterized by the existence of allergenic *epitopes* that are recognized, after processing by *antigen-presenting cells* (APC), by *Th2 cells* and are capable of evoking an *IgE*-mediated response (see *immediate hypersensitivity*). Many allergens have intrinsic or inducible enzymatic activity (see *cloning of allergens*) that may be important in *T cell sensitization*.

COMPLEMENTARY

DNA consists of four different *nucleotides*, with either purine (*adenine* = A and *guanine* = G) or pyrimidine (*cytosine* = C and *thymine* = T) bases. The geometry of the double helix is provided by purine–pyrimidine base interactions (see *base pairs*) in nucleic acids through hydrogen-bonding (adenine with thymine and guanine with cytosine).

COMPLEMENTARY-DETERMINING REGIONS (CDRs)

These are the segments of *T cell antigen receptors* or *antibodies* that bind to soluble *antigen* or the *antigenic peptide–major histocompatibility complex* (MHC) presented by *antigen-presenting cells* (APCs).

COMPLEMENTARY DNA (cDNA)

cDNA is the *DNA* copy of an *RNA* molecule, typically 0.1 to 10 kb long. cDNA is generated in vivo by retroviruses during the replication of the viral RNA genome. The polymerase known as reverse transcriptase uses RNA as a template to synthesize the complementary DNA strand. In vitro, reverse transcriptase is used to generate cDNA from *messenger RNA* (mRNA) molecules in the process known as cDNA cloning (see *DNA cloning*). Thus a cDNA *clone* represents a *gene* that was transcribed from mRNA, and cDNA cloning is a method of "capturing" the genes encoding proteins. cDNA is also often used for mRNA expression studies by semiquantitative or quantitative reverse transcription *polymerase chain reaction* (RT-PCR).

COMPLEMENTARY PROCEDURES

Unconventional approaches to the diagnosis and treatment of *allergic diseases* are very popular among patients. Although case reports using homeopathy, hypnosis, and acupuncture have shown to be beneficial, these results have yet to be confirmed by controlled clinical trials. The effects of bioresonance, which had been claimed to neutralize *allergies*, was disproved. Alternative diagnostic tests such as leukocytotoxic test, hair analysis, kinesiology, and electroacupuncture do not appear to provide significant results.

COMPLEMENT FACTORS

Different effector functions are mediated by proteolytic fragments, which are generated during activation of the *complement system*. Such proteolytic fragments are called complement factors.

> *Inflammation*, consisting of recruitment (see *chemotaxis*) and *leukocyte* activation, is mediated by cleavage products of the complement proteins C3, C4, and C5, called *complement factor 3a* (C3a), *complement factor 4a* (C4a), and *complement factor 5a* (C5a), respectively (see Figure 16).

The activation of inflammatory cells by these complement factors is mediated via specific *G protein-coupled receptors*. Complement activation is central in the pathogenesis of many forms of *urticaria* and *angioedema*. Moreover, *opsonization* is largely due to a fragment called C3b.

COMPLEMENT FACTOR 3a (C3a)

C3a is a 9-kDa *peptide* fragment derived from proteolytic cleavage of the complement component C3 (see *complement system*). C3a *receptors* are *G protein-coupled receptors* and are expressed on cutaneous (but not lung or gut) *mast cells* (see *mast cell heterogeneity*), *basophils*, *eosinophils*, *neutrophils*, *lymphocytes*, and *smooth muscle* cells. C3a mediates *histamine* release from basophils and sensitive mast cells and increases vascular permeability, and belongs therefore to the *anaphylatoxins*. *Mediator* release is also triggered from eosinophils and neutrophils, resulting in *inflammation*. This also includes the generation of *leukotrienes* (LTs) and *prostaglandins* (PGs). C3a is also a *chemotactic factor* for *granulocytes*. In smooth muscle cells, C3a causes contraction. C3a is 20-fold less potent than *C5a*.

COMPLEMENT FACTOR 4a (C4a)

C4a is a 8.7-kDa *peptide* fragment derived from proteolytic cleavage of the complement component C4 (see *complement system*). C4a *receptors* are *G protein-coupled receptors* and are expressed on cutaneous (but not lung or gut) *mast cells* (see *mast cell heterogeneity*), *basophils, eosinophils, neutrophils, lymphocytes*, and *smooth muscle* cells. C4a mediates *histamine* release from basophils and sensitive mast cells and increases vascular permeability, and belongs therefore to the *anaphylatoxins*. C4a is 2500-fold less potent than *C5a*.

COMPLEMENT FACTOR 5a (C5a)

C5a is an 11-kDa *peptide* fragment derived from proteolytic cleavage of the complement component C5 (see *complement system*).

C5a is the most potent *complement factor*.

C5a *receptors* (CD88, see *CD antigens*) are *G protein-coupled receptors* and are expressed on cutaneous (but not lung or gut) *mast cells* (see *mast cell heterogeneity*), *basophils, eosinophils, neutrophils, monocytes, macrophages, endothelial cells, smooth muscle* cells, *epithelial cells*, and hepatocytes. C5a mediates *histamine* release from basophils and sensitive mast cells and increases vascular permeability, and belongs therefore to the *anaphylatoxins*. *Mediator* release is also triggered from eosinophils and neutrophils, resulting in *inflammation*. This also includes the generation of *leukotrienes* (LTs) and *prostaglandins* (PGs). Moreover, C5a generates reactive *oxygen metabolites* in these inflammatory effector cells. In addition, C5a is a *chemotactic factor* for *granulocytes*. In smooth muscle cells, C5a causes contraction. C5a-mediated effects are central in the pathogenesis of *allergic inflammation* as well as in many forms of *urticaria* and *angioedema*.

COMPLEMENT SYSTEM

The complement system comprises a group of more than 20 plasma proteins.

The proteins of the complement system provide many of the effector functions in *inflammation*.

The principal functions of the complement system are shown in Table 27.

TABLE 27
Biological Functions of the Complement System

Function	Description
1. Cytolysis	Following complement activation, components of the system form pores into membranes of bacteria.
2. *Opsonization*	Complement proteins bind to the surface of foreign organisms or particles. *Phagocytes* have *receptors* for the bound complement proteins, resulting in enhanced *phagocytosis*.
3. Inflammation	*Complement factors* (= *anaphylatoxins*) act on several inflammatory cells, causing *chemotaxis* and *mediator* release.
4. Antiinflammation	*Immune complexes* are bound by complement proteins and removed by phagocytosis.

The activation of the complement system occurs by limited proteolysis.

> This means that many proteins of the system are *proteases,* which cleave and thereby activate other proteases, resulting in a protease cascade.

Similar proteolytic cascades are seen in the coagulation, *kinin,* and *caspase* systems. The components of the complement system are controlled by inhibitors (see *C1 inhibitor*) and therefore are inactive in blood (or low level of spontaneous activation).

> *Immunoglobulins* that bond *antigen* can activate complement.

The sequence of events initiated by *antibody*–antigen complexes (= immune complexes) is called the classical pathway (see Figure 16). This pathway serves as a major effector mechanism of specific humoral immunity. In addition, the complement system can also be activated as a consequence of complement protein binding to bacterial surfaces. The sequence of events in the absence of antibody is called the alternative pathway. Both pathways result in the formation of pores in microbial surfaces and consequent killing by osmotic lysis.

> During complement activation, a number of proteolytic fragments are created which mediate inflammation.

These *peptides* are called *complement factors* (see Figure 16).

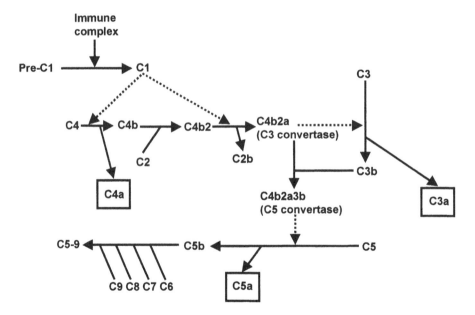

FIGURE 16 Overview of the classical complement activation pathway. The complement factors C3a, C4a, and C5a are generated in the process of complement activation.

COMPLIANCE

Compliance with therapy (doing what the doctor/nurse says) or *adherence* to therapy (strictly following the plan agreed upon between the patient and the doctor/nurse) is a complex area that can generate much heated discussion.

> Several studies demonstrate that patients with *asthma* do not follow medical advice.

In particular, few patients are willing to increase their maintenance doses of *inhaled corticosteroids* (ICS) to the extent that they abolish their need for *β2-agonists*. In practice, most patients taking ICS and short-acting β2-agonists for moderate asthma will titrate their dose of ICS so that they need around six puffs per day of salbutamol or equivalent. Patients are willing to increase their ICS if they need more than eight puffs of salbutamol per day but generally do not seem interested in abolishing the need for β2-agonist. The advent of long-acting β2-agonists has altered the situation somewhat, and a significant proportion of hospital clinic patients are now managed on ICS and long-acting β2-agonist with only occasional recourse to short-acting β2-agonists. The wide range of inhaler devices (see *metered dose inhaler*) available has made it easier to find a device that the patient prefers, and that may help compliance, but the most successful means of achieving better compliance is through cooperation and education. It has been difficult to perform properly controlled trials of asthma education, but patients who understand their disease are generally more committed to following the recommended treatment. Some doctors find patient education threatening, as it implies sharing medical knowledge, but doctors and nurses are now more willing to surrender their position as guardians of knowledge and are moving toward sharing that knowledge for the benefit of their patients.

COMPOSITAE

Artemisia (wormwoods, mugworts), Ambrosia (ragweeds), and Parthenium (feverfews) belong to the Compositae family of plants. Several species of Artemisia occur as widespread weeds. Their *pollens* may cause *allergic rhinoconjunctivitis* with a seasonal peak in July and August. Compositae are a common cause of airborne *contact dermatitis*, hand *dermatitis*, and light sensitivity. Sesquiterpene lactones are the main contact *allergens*.

COMPOUND 48/80

This polycationic molecule is one of the most potent *mast cell* activators, acting as a non-*IgE*-dependent stimulus (see *mast cell activation*) to activate specifically *connective tissue mast cells* (CTMC) but not *mucosal mast cells* (MMC) (see *rat mast cells*). The activation of the cells is the consequence of direct *G protein* activation. Compound-48/80-mediated release of *histamine* and *serotonin* occurs in faster kinetics compared to *high-affinity IgE-receptor*-mediated activation. Compound 48/80 stimulates histamine release from human skin mast cells, but not lung, adenoid, tonsil, or large intestine mast cells. Interestingly, this reactivity does not parallel protease phenotyping (see *mast cell heterogeneity*), since both intestine and tonsil mast cell populations contain large numbers of *tryptase*- and *chymase*-positive mast cells.

CONCORDANT

This term is used when both members of a twin pair (see *twin studies*) show the same phenotype or *trait*.

CONFORMATIONAL EPITOPES

T cell epitopes are generally linear *peptide* sequences presented in the *antigen* combining groove of either *MHC class I* or *MHC class II molecules* on the surface of *antigen-presenting cells* (APCs) after *antigen processing*. This method of presentation is restricted by the size of the *major histocompatibility complex* (MHC), and does not permit many *antigenic peptides* with *tertiary structure* to bind to the MHC. *Immunoglobulins* (Igs) and *B cell antigen receptors* are able to recognize larger proteinaceous structures exhibiting considerable three-dimensional structural variability (see *B cell epitopes*). Recognition of conformational *epitopes* by Igs is essential in the process of *antibody affinity maturation* and in the potential for multivalent interactions that permit *receptor cross-linking* when antigen/*antibody* complexes bind to cell surfaces via Ig receptors (e.g., *high-affinity IgE receptor*).

CONJUNCTIVITIS

Conjunctivitis is an *inflammation* of the whites of the eye. This is commonly due to infection, but can also be caused by *allergy.* Seasonal allergic conjunctivitis forms part of the syndrome of *hay fever* (see *allergic rhinoconjunctivitis*). Features of all types of allergic conjunctivitis are redness, itching, and swelling of the conjunctiva. The redness occurs as a result of dilation of the vascular bed, itching from sensory nerve stimulation, and *edema* from altered post-capillary venule permeability. In histological sections, a major finding is an increase in the number of *mast cells* (see also *mast cell numbers*).

CONNECTIVE TISSUE MAST CELLS (CTMC)

CTMC are *mast cells* within connective tissues with special functional characteristics that differ from those of *mucosal mast cells* (MMC) (see *rat mast cells*).

CONSTITUTIVE CYTOKINE PRODUCTION

In addition to *cytokines* whose production is induced (see *induced cytokine production*), some cytokines may exist in preformed stores or may be constitutively produced and released. As an example, examination of *TNF-α* and *TGF-β* production by *mast cells* and *T cells* has demonstrated differential mechanisms of expression for these cytokines. TNF-α was produced only after stimulation of the cells (see *cytokine gene activation*), and its production was suppressed by inhibition of *protein kinase C* (PKC) and calcium ion influx (see *calcium mobilization*). TGF-β, on the other hand, was constitutively expressed and released, but its production could be enhanced by cell activation, demonstrating an additional inducible component. Constitutive expression was found to be independent of PKC activation and resistant to suppression by *corticosteroids.*

CONTACT DERMATITIS

Allergic contact *dermatitis* is a unique skin reaction pattern of a sensitized individual toward a contact *allergen* due to a cell-mediated *delayed hypersensitivity* reaction (see *Coombs and Gell classification*, type IV). A *T cell sensitization* phase and an *elicitation* phase can be distinguished. However, in clinical dermatology, the sensitization phase (see *contact sensitization*) is not detectable. Based on the kinetics of the elicitation phase, an acute allergic contact dermatitis or a chronic allergic contact *eczema* is diagnosed.

Acute allergic contact dermatitis

This form of contact dermatitis takes a regular sequential course. In the *erythema* stage (stadium erythematosum), marked reddening and edematous swelling is witness for the onset of the dermatitis. During the following vesicular stage (stadium vesiculosum), small or large vesicules erupt from the erythematous skin. The eroded and oozing areas of the exudative stage (stadium exsudativum) become easily superinfected. In the crusted stage (stadium crustosum), the surface dries up, and this leads to formation of yellowish *crusts.* The scaling stage (stadium squamosum) marks the endpoint of the acute skin changes, but a residual erythema often persists in the previously affected location. Skin irritation and *pruritus* without fever and minimal systemic findings are the diagnostic hallmark of this disease. Acute irritant dermatitis, erysipelas, initial herpes zoster, and lupus erythematosus are the main differential diagnoses of acute allergic contact dermatitis and are made on clinical grounds. In contrast to *irritant contact dermatitis*, allergic contact dermatitis frequently shows satellite lesions and may even spread to distant locations.

Chronic allergic contact eczema

In this form of contact dermatitis, repeated contact with an allergen leads to the simultaneous occurrence of erythema, vesicles, oozing, crusts, and scaling. Chronic manipulation due to the itch sensation leads to *lichenification* of the affected areas. The differential diagnosis includes *lichen simplex chronicus* (lichen Vidal), *atopic dermatitis*, psoriasis vulgaris, and seborrheic dermatitis.

Diagnosis

For identification of the causative contact allergen, patch testing (see *patch test*) has to be performed. A carefully taken history and consideration of the distribution pattern of the lesions are mandatory for proper selection of the allergens to be tested. This is of particular importance, since the disease will heal only when the causative allergen is avoided. From the results of patch testing, a diagnosis of monovalent, oligovalent (two to five chemically unrelated contact allergens), or multivalent (at least six chemically unrelated contact allergens) contact sensitization is made.

Therapy

At present, there is no causative cure available for the sensitization against contact allergens. Therefore, therapy for *contact dermatitis* is always a combination of *allergen avoidance* and symptomatic therapy with antiinflammatory agents such as *corticosteroids* and *antibiotics* in cases of relevant superinfection.

CONTACT ECZEMA

(See *contact dermatitis*.)

CONTACT SENSITIZATION

Clinical manifestation of contact *hypersensitivity* is most often presented as allergic *contact dermatitis*. The signs and symptoms are brought on by contact with the *allergen* to which the subject has been sensitized and are commonly expressed as a form of *delayed hypersensitivity* (see *Coombs and Gell classification*, type IV). The result can be a prolonged and injurious eczematous type of pathology which, however, often resolves rapidly on removal of the agent to which the subject is sensitive.

Contact sensitivity differs from *sensitization* in the lungs or across the gut in that there is no induction of *IgE* and, therefore, there is no evidence of a *type I reaction*.

This might be due to different mechanisms of *antigen* presentation that occur in the skin after epicutaneous exposure to contact allergens (see also *T helper cell differentiation*). The skin possesses specialized *antigen-presenting cells* (APCs) known as *Langerhans cells,* which are able to take up allergens or protein-haptenated molecules, process them, and present them either in *MHC class I* or *class II molecules*. Langerhans cells have been shown to migrate to regional *lymph nodes*, where effective presentation to *T cells* can occur. At the same time, skin *keratinocytes* are activated by the contact allergen to secrete inflammatory *cytokines*, which further activate the migrating Langerhans cells. Langerhans cells, activated in this way (or directly by haptens), rapidly secrete *IL-1*. Production of this cytokine has been shown to correlate with the ability of a chemical to effect contact sensitization, but it is still unclear if the action of IL-1 on T cells is directly responsible for their sensitization. Many other cytokines are known to be upregulated during this process, including *IL-6, IL-12, TNF-α, GM-CSF*, and some *chemokines*. Although Langerhans cells are not obligatory for T cell activation (dermal *dendritic cells* can function in the same way), they probably contribute significantly to this process in vivo.

> In the lymph nodes, most contact allergens are *haptens* and presented by Langerhans (or dendritic) cells in the context of MHC class I molecules and evoke an oligoclonal *CD8⁺* T cell response.

The consequence of this is the production of *Th1*-like (*Tc1*) cytokines such as *IFN-γ*, and the expression of *adhesion molecules* and *chemokine receptors* by CD8⁺ T cells. The activated T cells migrate and are recruited to the epidermal layers of the skin where mild inflammatory reactions may occur locally. On re-exposure, the sensitized T cells release IFN-γ (which activates resident APCs) and other inflammatory cytokines such as TNF-α and chemokines which recruit inflammatory effector cells such as *neutrophils*.

> This inflammatory response can be downregulated by removing the hapten (sensitizing agent) or by hapten-specific *CD4⁺* T cells secreting antagonistic cytokines (e.g., *TGF-β*, *IL-10*).

This balance and the control mechanisms involved in this process are still poorly understood (see *immunosuppressive mechanisms*). However, the major difference between contact sensitization and other forms of delayed hypersensitivity might be the type of the participating T cells. Whereas in contact dermatitis, IFN-γ-producing CD8⁺ T cells are primarily involved, CD4⁺ T cells are central in classical delayed hypersensitivity reactions (see *allergic inflammation*).

CONTACT URTICARIA

Any type of *urticaria* induced by direct contact of an agent with the skin (e.g., *latex* contact urticaria).

COOMBS AND GELL CLASSIFICATION

This is a classification of *hypersensitivity* reactions that was established by Coombs and Gell in 1963. It has remained the most commonly used classification of allergic reactions. The new type V and type VI reactions were added later, but have not been accepted by all authors.

Type I reactions (immediate-type) are *immediate hypersensitivity* reactions that are mediated by *allergen*-specific *IgE* bound to *mast cells* and *basophils* via *high-affinity IgE receptors*. *Cross-linking* of the *receptor*-bound IgE molecules by allergens induces the release of *histamine* and other vasoactive *mediators* that cause acute allergic symptoms (e.g., *allergic rhinoconjunctivitis*).

Type II reactions (cytotoxic-type) are caused by cytotoxic *antibodies*, which bind to the cell membrane, activate the *complement system*, and thereby cause cytolysis (e.g., *thrombocytopenic purpura*, allergic agranulocytosis — see *drug allergy*).

Type III reactions (immune complex-type) are caused by soluble *immune complexes*, activating the complement system (e.g., *extrinsic allergic alveolitis*, *serum sickness*, and *allergic vasculitis*).

Type IV reactions (delayed-type) are *delayed hypersensitivity* reactions that are caused by antigen-specific *T cells* and their *cytokines*. Both predominant *Th1* (e.g., *contact dermatitis*) or *Th2* cytokine expression (chronic *allergic diseases* in association with *atopy*) can occur.

Type V reactions (granulomatous reactions) are defined as granulomatous reactions to a given *antigen* (e.g., injection granuloma).

Type VI reactions include all pathogenic effects caused by binding of an antibody to a biological structure (e.g., myasthenia gravis).

COOMBS TEST

This is a hemagglutination technique that allows the detection of Rh incompatibilities (*antibodies* against erythrocytes). A Rh– mother of a Rh+ fetus can become immunized to fetal erythrocytes that enter the maternal circulation at the time of delivery. In a subsequent pregnancy with a Rh+ fetus, anti-Rh *IgG* antibodies can cross the placenta and induce hemolytic disease in the fetus. The Coombs test detects anti-Rh antibodies in the mother's serum.

COPD

(See *chronic obstructive pulmonary disease*.)

CORD BLOOD IgE

IgE levels in cord blood have been measured in studies over many years. They have proved to be of low predictive value for the development of an *IgE*-mediated *allergic disease* later in life.

CORD BLOOD MAST CELLS

Human cord blood *mast cells* (HCMC) are considered to be a powerful tool for the investigation of *IgE*-mediated allergic reactions. These cells contain *histamine*, carry surface *high-affinity IgE receptors*, and express mast cell-specific *neutral proteases* such as *tryptase* and *chymase* resembling human skin mast cells. *SCF*, together with *IL-6*, promotes the growth of immature cord blood cells into mature mast cells with a phenotype similar to lung mast cells.

CORTICOSTEROIDS

Corticosteroids (also known as glucocorticoids or steroids) are complex molecules based on the 4-ring sterol structure and are manufactured in the adrenal cortex. Deficiency of corticosteroids leads to Addison's syndrome. Excess of corticosteroids causes *Cushing's syndrome*.

> Corticosteroids have several antiinflammatory properties. Therefore, they are useful in the treatment of *allergic inflammations*, especially in *asthma*.

Inhaled corticosteroids can control asthma in most patients. Oral corticosteroids retain a place in the management of *asthma exacerbations* and in other severe cases. Beneficial effects of corticosteroids in asthma include reduction of airway *inflammation*, improved airway function, reduced airway secretions, reduced *airway hyperresponsiveness*, and restoration of airway integrity. Commonly used corticosteroids include budesonide, *prednisolone*, *dexamethasone*, deflazacort, fluticasone, and beclomethasone diproprionate.

Upon binding of corticosteroids to the intracellular *corticosteroid receptor*, this protein complex migrates into the nucleus and acts as a *transcription factor*.

> One major molecular mechanism of action is the inhibition of the transcription factor *nuclear factor-κB* (NF-κB) by the induction of its inhibitor, the IκBα *gene*.

This leads to a downregulation of NF-κB-regulated genes (see Table 28). For instance, corticosteroids reduce *IL-5* gene expression in *T cells* and perhaps other cells such as *mast cells* and *eosinophils*, resulting in decreased production and accelerated *eosinophil apoptosis* and, therefore, in reduced eosinophil numbers.

> Thus, the mechanism of action of corticosteroids can be considered as a transcriptional inhibition of inflammatory gene products, resulting in the downregulation of T cell, as well as allergic effector cell, responses.

In contrast, immediate *IgE*-mediated allergic responses are relatively unaffected by corticosteroid treatment.

However, corticosteroids not only reduce *Th2 cytokine* expression, they also reduce gene expression of important components of the *immune system* needed for host defense mechanisms.

For instance, high doses of corticosteroids (see *corticosteroid-dependent asthma*) downregulate *IgG* subclasses, HLA-DR expression on *monocytes*, proliferative responses of *lymphocytes* in vitro (see *lymphocyte proliferation test*), and may even induce *apoptosis* in activated T cells. These immunosuppressive effects can lead to increased risk of viral and bacterial respiratory infections, both of which are major triggers of exacerbation of asthma and have clinical importance in the management of asthma.

TABLE 28
Corticosteroid-Mediated Reduction of Gene Expression

Cytokines (*IL-1*, *IL-2*, *IL-3*, *IL-4*, IL-5, *IL-6*, *IL-8*, IL-11, *IL-12*, *IL-13*, *IFN-γ*,
 TNF-α, *GM-CSF*, *RANTES*, *MIP-1α*, *SCF*)
Inducible nitric oxide synthetase (iNOS)
Inducible *cyclooxygenase* (COX-2)
Inducible *phospholipase* A_2 (cPLA$_2$)
Adhesion molecules (e.g., ICAM-1)

CORTICOSTEROID-DEPENDENT ASTHMA

Even with currently available *inhaled corticosteroids* (ICS) and other anti-asthmatic drugs (see *asthma treatment strategies*), there is still a significant number of *asthma* patients who require long-term oral *corticosteroids* or short courses of steroids for acute *asthma exacerbation*. Maintenance of oral steroids is only needed in asthmatic patients with the most severe asthma, which cannot be controlled with maximal doses of ICS (2000 μg daily) and additional *bronchodilators*. Oral steroids are usually given as a single morning dose, as this reduces the risk of side effects (see *Cushing's syndrome*), since it coincides with the peak diurnal concentrations. Administration in the afternoon may be optimal for some patients with severe *nocturnal asthma*. The side effects of oral corticosteroids taken for prolonged periods may be serious, in particular the effects on bones, muscles, and the *immune system*. Suppression of the normal adrenal production of *cortisol* occurs after 10 to 14 days of treatment.

CORTICOSTEROID RECEPTOR

Corticosteroids exert their effects via binding to an intracellular corticosteroid *receptor*. The nonstimulated receptor is associated with several inhibitory proteins (e.g., 90-kDa heat shock protein or 59-kDa immunophilin protein) that prevent receptor translocation from the cytoplasma into the nucleus. Only upon corticosteroid binding do the associated proteins dissociate, allowing nuclear localization of the ligand-activated corticosteroid receptor, which binds to a corticosteroid recognition sequence (see *corticosteroid responsive element*). Interestingly, reduced corticosteroid receptor binding affinity associated with decreased steroid responsiveness has been observed at night in patients with *nocturnal asthma*.

The immunosuppressive and antiinflammatory actions of corticosteroids have been shown to be mediated by the induction of *inhibitory κB* (IκB) synthesis (see also *nuclear factor-κB*).

CORTICOSTEROID-RESISTANT ASTHMA (CRA)

CRA is a subgroup of patients with *asthma* that does not respond to high-dose oral *corticosteroids*. These patients have reversible *airway obstruction* in that they show spontaneous variability in *lung function tests*, and will respond to inhaled *β2-agonists*. The mechanism of CRA has been intensively investigated. Patients with CRA have normal numbers of *corticosteroid receptors*, and seem to develop just as many side effects from oral corticosteroids as those with SRA.

> The patients' *monocytes* and *T cells* appear resistant to the effects of corticosteroids. Therefore, signs of immunosuppression are usually not present in CRA patients.

Current thoughts are that CRA patients may show impaired binding of corticosteroid receptors to the *corticosteroid response element* (CRE). Interestingly, corticosteroid resistance may vary over time. Therefore, it may be worthwhile to test CRA patients again after a certain time period. A minority of patients has pharmacokinetic handling problems and may respond better to betamethasone than to *prednisolone*. Recent data suggest that *IFN-α* therapy may abolish corticosteroid resistance.

CORTICOSTEROID RESPONSIVE ELEMENT (CRE)

CRE is a recognition sequence of the *corticosteroid/corticosteroid receptor* complex on the 5'-upstream *promoter* sequence of steroid-responsive *genes*. CRE may decrease or increase *transcription* (see Table 28), resulting in decreased or increased *mRNA* and protein production.

CORTISOL

Cortisol is a steroid hormone produced by the adrenal glands. Its secretion is regulated by the hypothalamic–pituitary–adrenal axis (HPA) and may be suppressed by systemic *corticosteroid* therapy. The degree of HPA suppression depends on dose, duration, frequency, and timing of corticosteroid administration. A prolonged adrenal suppression may lead to reduced adrenal response to stress. The adrenal cortisol secretion is estimated by measuring the morning plasma cortisol level, a 24-hour urinary cortisol, or a plasma cortisol profile over 24 hours. Several studies in asthmatic patients demonstrated that there are no significant suppressive effects of *inhaled corticosteroids* (ICS) on HPA axis function at doses of <1500 μg/day in adults and <400 μg/day in children.

CO-STIMULATION

In order to activate an *antigen*-specific *CD4+ T cell*, two fundamental requirements have to be met.

> First, the T cell must recognize the *antigen* presented by *MHC class II molecules* of an *antigen-presenting cell* (APC). Second, it must receive an additional activating signal from that APC (or possibly another APC) known as a co-stimulatory signal.

Failure of the *T cell antigen receptor* (TCR)/*major histocompatibility complex* (MHC) interaction (i.e., antigenic mismatch) will have no effect on the ability of a T cell to react to a subsequent and appropriate antigen/MHC configuration, but inadequate co-stimulation following TCR ligation can result in T cell *anergy* or activation-induced *apoptosis*. One of the most important co-stimulatory interactions is between *CD28* (expressed on the surface of T cells) and its ligands, *CD80* and *CD86*, which are expressed on APCs. CD80 (B7.1) is an inducible *surface molecule* primarily expressed by *B cells*, but also by *macrophages* and *dendritic cells*. CD86 (B7.2) is expressed on the surface of *monocytes* and activated B cells. Ligation of CD28 initiates a *signal transduction* pathway that is independent of the TCR.

It appears that CD28 stimulation lowers the *threshold* of antigen-stimulated TCRs needed for *T cell proliferation*.

CD28 expression is upregulated on *allergen*-specific T cells, but appears relatively unaffected by *immunotherapy*. CD28 shares homology with *CTLA-4*. *Cross-linking* of *IgG receptors* on APCs strongly inhibits CD80/CD86 expression and can induce T cell anergy when antigen is presented in the absence of CD28/CD80 co-stimulation. Both *Th1* and *Th2* responses are dependent on co-stimulation.

In contrast to CD80, CD86 appears to contribute to the preferential differentiation of *Th2 cells* in *IgE*-mediated *allergic inflammations*.

Similar to the TCR, the *B cell antigen receptor* also has co-receptors (see *B cell co-receptor*). The function of these co-receptors is similar to that of CD28. They enhance *signaling* of the *antigen receptor* by activating more *Src*-family *tyrosine kinases*. Thus, when the co-receptor is triggered at the same time as the B cell antigen receptor, a lower amount of antigen is needed to activate the B cell.

Another important interaction is that between *CD40* and *CD40 ligand* (CD40L, *CD154*), which are co-stimulatory molecules expressed on the surface of Th2 cells and *mast cells/basophils/eosinophils* (CD40L) and B cells (CD40). As well as supplying obligatory co-stimulation for *T cell cytokine* production, the interaction mediates adhesion between B cells and CD40L-expressing cells (see *cognate/noncognate interactions*). CD40 expression on B cells is upregulated in atopic asthmatics (see *allergic asthma*) when exposed to specific allergen.

COUGH

A reflex response involving rapid contraction of the diaphragm and expulsion of air from the lungs. Cough may be dry (without *sputum*) or productive (with sputum). Cough may be the dominant or indeed the only symptom in a minority of patients with *asthma* (see *cough variant asthma*).

COUGH SUPPRESSANT

Codeine and other opiate drugs suppress the *cough* reflex and may be useful in managing respiratory tract infections. Cough suppressants are not generally appropriate for treating cough associated with *asthma* since, in this case, the cough reflects poorly controlled airways *inflammation*, and treatment should be directed toward the underlying cause. Cough suppressants can also be dangerous in patients with respiratory failure, since they will tend to depress the respiratory center and can lead to *hypercapnia*.

COUGH VARIANT ASTHMA

A relatively rare variant of *asthma* in which *cough* is the only symptom. Most patients with asthma will report a *wheeze* as well as cough.

COW ALLERGENS

Allergen extracts of cow hairs and dander (see *animal dander*) contain three *allergens* (Bos d 1, Bos d 2, and Bos d 3). Cow *allergy* may occur in farmers and veterinarians.

COW'S MILK ALLERGY

Cow's milk *allergy* is a common *adverse food reaction* and occurs in 2 to 3% of children under 2 years of age and in approximately 1% of adults. The most important sensitizing proteins are bovine β-globulin, caseins, α-lactalbumin, and serum albumin (see *food allergy*).

COX

(See *cyclooxygenase.*)

COX-2 INHIBITORS

(See *cyclooxygenase-2 inhibitors.*)

CREOLA BODIES

(See *epithelial damage.*)

CROMOGLYCATE

Sodium cromoglycate was originally used as a *mast cell* stabilizer (see *cromones*), although it is now thought to have antiinflammatory properties. The related *nedocromil* sodium has potent effects on inflammatory cells. These compounds are particularly effective in the treatment of *asthma* in children (see *childhood asthma*) and young adults, as well as in *exercise-induced asthma*, but do not alleviate *airway obstruction* when administered acutely. Moreover, sodium cromoglycate nasal sprays can be used as an alternative to local *corticosteroid* sprays. Eye symptoms are particularly distressing symptoms of *hay fever* and are not always controlled by *antihistamines*. Sodium cromoglycate drops (2%) are often very effective in such cases of *allergic rhinoconjunctivitis*. Their mode of action is believed to be an inhibition of *G protein*-regulated chloride channels that regulate, besides other mechanisms, *calcium mobilization* upon *receptor*-mediated stimulation. Sodium cromoglycate has no effect on skin mast cells (see *mast cell heterogeneity*).

CROMOLYN

(See *cromoglycate.*)

CROMONES

Cromones represent a class of *anti-allergic/anti-asthmatic drugs* (see *asthma treatment strategies*) that contain chromium within an organic structure. Cromones were originally developed as *mast-cell*-stabilizing agents (they prevent mast cell *degranulation*), but their anti-*asthma* properties are probably related to their ability to block ion channels in mast cells and airway *epithelial cells*. Treatment with cromones blocks *early-* and *late-phase responses* in asthma (see *immediate* and *delayed hypersensitivity*).

> Cromones are effective in *exercise-induced* and in *childhood asthma*, but are less effective in adult asthma.

Sodium *cromoglycate* and *nedocromil* are the only cromones in current use. In *allergic asthma*, they are administrated by inhalation. In *allergic rhinoconjunctivitis*, they are applied locally using nasal sprays or eye drops.

CROSS-ALLERGY

(See *cross-reacting allergens.*)

CROSSING-OVER

Crossing-over is a reciprocal exchange of *DNA* between homologous *chromosomes* in meiotic prophase I (see *meiosis*) due to the breaking and rejoining of the DNA molecules, resulting in the exchange of chromosomal segments.

CROSS-LINKING

Signal transduction through *surface molecules* is usually initiated by ligand binding. Ligand binding brings the *receptors* in closer proximity to each other, resulting in dimerization (e.g., *cytokine receptors* and *antigen receptors*) or trimerization (e.g., *death receptors*) of receptor components. This ligand-mediated process is called cross-linking and can often be mimicked by specific *antibodies* against the receptor. Cross-linking provides the possibility for molecular interactions between the cytoplasmic regions of the receptors to initiate a downstream *signaling* cascade.

CROSS-REACTING ALLERGENS

There are well-known clinical observations whereby patients, who are allergic to a given *allergen,* have symptoms upon being exposed to apparently unrelated substance(s). A typical manifestation is the *oral allergy syndrome*, the best example of which occurs in *birch* or *grass-pollen*-allergic patients, who experience allergic symptoms after eating fruits, such as apples (see *apple allergen*) and pears (see *food allergy*). The symptoms may include itching at the back of the throat, swelling of the lips, and facial swelling. Likewise, ragweed (see *ragweed pollen*) allergic patients may have oral *allergy* symptoms after eating watermelon, and patients with *latex allergy* may also be sensitive to kiwifruit, avocado, banana, and chestnuts (*latex-fruit syndrome*).

> Such cross-allergies can be explained by the existence of the same or similar *epitopes* present in different allergens.

For instance, structural homologues of the birch pollen allergens, Bet v 1 and Bet v 2, occur in other trees (e.g., hazelnut) as well as in apples, pears, *celery*, carrots, *potato*, and buckwheat (see Table 29). The symptoms are caused by *IgE antibodies* against birch allergens that show partial cross-reactivity with the food-derived allergens. These cross-reactive IgE antibodies cause *mast cell degranulation* with the release of *histamine* and other inflammatory *mediators*. Similar cross-reactive IgE antibodies are produced by latex allergen (Hev b 5), which has 40% *amino acid* sequence *homology* (see *cloning of allergens*) with a kiwifruit protein (function unknown).

Tropomyosin is another potential source of allergenic cross-reactivity. Tropomyosin is the major allergen of shrimp (Pen a 1) and is also found in *house-dust mite* (Der p 10) and *cockroach allergens*. Therefore, consumption of seafood and other molluscs (shellfish and snails) can give rise to food allergic symptoms in mite-allergic patients. *Asthma* has also been reported in mite-allergic subjects who have eaten snails. The problem may be exacerbated in mite-allergic patients receiving *immunotherapy*, and it has been reported that mite-immunotherapy may be a risk factor for induction of food allergy in some patients.

Carbohydrate interactions with IgE can also give rise to apparent cross-reactivities. Some vegetable sources (e.g., peas) contain lectins, which bind to the sugar moieties on IgE itself, can give false positive results in serologic *immunoassays* for IgE antibody (see *RAST, Phadiatop*, and *CAP-system*). Conversely, some vegetable glycans can elicit IgE antibody responses (e.g., potato lectin), and these responses can then be cross-reactive with other food, insect (see *hymenoptera allergy*), or plant glycoproteins. Cross-reactive carbohydrate determinants (CCD) include *N*-linked mannose/xylose/fucose glycans as well as *O*-linked arabinose-containing glycans. CCD are found in almost all vegetable foods, in pollen extracts, purified pollen allergens, and in insect venoms.

TABLE 29

Cross-Reactivity between IgE Antibodies to Allergens and Foods ("Oral Allergy Syndrome")

Allergen	Food
Bet v 1	Hazelnut (Cor a 1), apple, pear, celery
Bet v 2 (profilin)	Carrot, celery, potato, buckwheat
Tropomyosin (mite, cockroach, shrimp)	Shrimp, shellfish, snails
Latex (Hev b 5)	Kiwifruit
Other latex allergens	Avocado, banana, chestnuts
CCD (N-linked plant glycans)	Vegetables, peanuts

Note: CCD — cross-reacting carbohydrate determinants (*N*- or *O*-linked plant glycans).

CRUDE ALLERGEN EXTRACTS

Crude *allergen extracts* are sometimes used to test for skin reactivity (see *skin tests*). In their simplest form, they can be applied as the entire suspected *allergen*, for example the juice of a fruit or the touch of a nut. Aqueous or solvent extracts have also been used. Crude allergen extracts, however, are usually proteinaceous mixtures derived from phenolic extraction procedures, often delipidated with ether, and then dialyzed. Initial standardization was attempted by lyophilizing crude extracts and presenting them in known weight/volume proportions. *Immunotherapy* attempts with crude extracts have failed due to low concentrations of suspected allergens (e.g., whole bee extracts for *hymenoptera allergy*) and high, sometimes sensitizing, amounts of irrelevant proteins swamping specific *T cell* responses.

CRUST

A basic skin lesion consisting of dried exudate, secretion, or hemorrhage.

CRUSTACEA

The crustacean family includes shrimp, prawns, crabs, lobster, and crayfish. They are common causes of *food allergy*.

CRUSTA LACTEA

Milk scurf, a unique type of skin lesion seen in young children, resembling the scurf of cooked milk. Frequently, this is the first clinical manifestation of an underlying atopic constitution (see *atopy* and *genetic predisposition*).

CRYPTOGENIC FIBROSING ALVEOLITIS

Cryptogenic fibrosing *alveolitis* is a progressive fibrotic condition that affects older people and causes respiratory failure. The *fibrosis* tends to start in the lower lobes and may be seen radiographically as a fine reticulo-nodular appearance. *Lung function tests* show a restrictive pattern, and the carbon monoxide *transfer factor* is always reduced. An acute form (Hamman–Rich syndrome) has been described, which can respond to systemic *corticosteroids*, but the more chronic forms tend to be progressive and lead to respiratory failure. Some benefit may be achieved with corticosteroids or cyclophosphamide, but it is difficult to reverse the condition, and the best hope is to arrest its progression. *IFN-γ* treatment has recently been demonstrated to be beneficial for these patients. In addition, *antioxidant* therapy might be useful.

CRYSTALLOGRAPHY

(See *X-ray crystallography.*)

C-TERMINAL TYROSINE KINASE (Csk)

Csk is a non-*receptor* protein *tyrosine kinase*. One of its major functions is to phosphorylate a specific conserved C-terminal tyrosine on the proto-oncogene *Src* and other Src family members (including Lck, *Lyn*, Fyn, Yes, etc.), and downregulate them by shutting off their *kinase* activity (compare downregulation by inhibitory *tyrosine phosphatases*). In this way, Csk plays a role in cell growth and differentiation in a variety of organs, including the *immune* and *nervous system* (see *immunosuppressive mechanisms*).

CTLA-4

(See *cytolytic T lymphocyte associated antigen-4.*)

CURSCHMANN SPIRALS

Inspissated *mucus* originally noted on microscopic examination of *sputum* samples from patients with *asthma*.

CUSHING'S SYNDROME

Patients with functioning tumors of the adrenal cortex produce excessive amounts of *cortisol*. This leads to muscle wasting, thinning of the skin, bruising, diabetes mellitus, fat deposition in the trunk, thinning of the bones, premature development of cataracts, and arterial hypertension. This is Cushing's disease. A similar constellation of symptoms occurs in patients who receive excessive amounts of exogenous *corticosteroids*. Cushing's syndrome can develop within a few years of starting oral corticosteroids, and is almost universal in patients who have received oral corticosteroids for more than 15 years.

> The risk of Cushing's syndrome can be reduced by keeping the dose of steroids as low as possible, ideally by giving the necessary dose by inhalation rather than by tablet (see *inhaled corticosteroids*).

CUTANEOUS-LYMPHOCYTE ANTIGEN (CLA)

CLA is considered to be a *homing receptor* for skin *T cells*. The majority of skin T cells in skin inflammatory disorders (e.g., *atopic dermatitis*, *contact dermatitis*, psoriasis) express CLA. CLA binds to E-selectin (CD62E, see *adhesion molecules*), which is expressed on inflamed superficial dermal postcapillary venules and *endothelial cells*. CLA is induced by *TGF-β* and *IL-12*.

> CLA$^+$ T cells represent CD45RO$^+$ memory/effector T cells that are in an activated state in patients with atopic dermatitis.

They express large amounts of *IL-5* and *IL-13*, but only little *IL-4*, contributing to delayed *eosinophil apoptosis* and elevated *IgE* production. Therefore, CLA$^+$ T cells play an important role in the initiation, maintenance, and exacerbation of atopic dermatitis.

CXC CHEMOKINES

Chemokine subfamily. In contrast to *CC chemokines*, the structure of the CXC chemokines is characterized by the position of the first two cysteine residues, which are separated by one *amino acid*.

> CXC chemokines predominantly activate *neutrophils*, suggesting that they play an important role in acute inflammatory responses as seen in tissue injury and bacterial infections.

CXC chemokines share 20 to 40% sequence identity and are encoded by *genes* on the human chromosome 4. Important members of this family are *IL-8*, NAP-2, ENA-78, PF4, Gro, and GCP-2. Different chemokines can often activate the same *chemokine receptor* (especially CXCR2), and IL-8 can use two different receptors (see Table 30).

TABLE 30
CXC Chemokines and Their Receptors (CXCR)

	CXCR1	CXCR2	CXCR3
IL-8	+	+	–
GCP-2	+	+	–
NAP-2	–	+	–
Gro	–	+	–
ENA-78	–	+	–
IP-10	–	–	+

CYCLIC ADENOSINE MONOPHOSPHATE (cAMP)

cAMP is a ubiquitous intracellular second messenger that transduces signals (see *signal transduction*) initiated by several hormones, *neuropeptides*, autocoids, and drugs. cAMP is formed from adenosine triphosphate (ATP) by the catalytic action of *adenylate cyclase*. This enzyme can be directly activated by forskolin. Indirect activation of adenylate cyclase is achieved through ligand binding of many cell surface *receptors* (e.g., *β2-agonists*). cAMP activates *protein kinase A* (PKA), which phosphorylates target proteins (Figure 17). *Phosphorylation* results in an alteration in the activity of these substrates. Consequently, cell functions are modulated.

> Increased cAMP levels induce *bronchodilation*. Therefore, β2-agonists and *phosphodiesterase inhibitors*, which prevent cAMP degradation, are effective in the treatment of *asthma*.

Moreover, increases in cAMP levels suppress the activity of inflammatory cells, since PKA can uncouple heterologous receptors from *phospholipase C* (PLC). For instance, increased intracellular cAMP levels are associated with decreased release of *mediators* from *mast cells* and *basophils*, decreased *degranulation* and reduced reactive *oxygen metabolites* formation in *neutrophils* and *eosinophils*, decreased *T cell cytokine* expression and *T cell proliferation* (see *immunosuppressive mechanisms*). The levels of *gene* expression are influenced by binding of PKA to so-called cAMP responsive elements in the *promoter* region of various genes.

CYCLIC GUANOSINE MONOPHOSPHATE (cGMP)

cGMP is a ubiquitous intracellular second messenger that transduces signals (see *signal transduction*) initiated by several hormones, *neuropeptides*, autocoids, and drugs. cGMP is

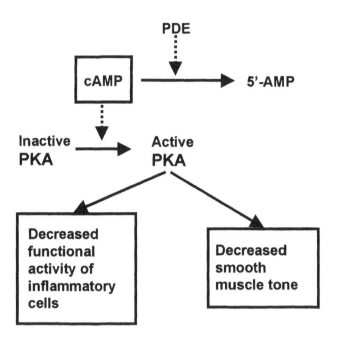

FIGURE 17 Protein kinase A (PKA) is activated by cAMP. Phosphodiesterase (PDE) decreases cAMP levels by catalyzing the synthesis of 5′-AMP, which is blocked by PDE inhibitors (e.g., theophylline). Activated PKA mediates bronchodilation and antiinflammation.

formed from guanosine triphosphate (GTP) by the catalytic action of guanylyl cyclase. This enzyme can be directly activated by *nitric oxide* (NO). Indirect activation of guanylyl cyclase is achieved through ligand binding of many cell surface receptors. cGMP activates *protein kinase G* (PKG), which phosphorylates target proteins. Phosphorylation results in an alteration in the activity of these substrates. Consequently, cell functions are modulated. For instance, PKG induces bronchorelaxation (like PKA). In contrast to the role of cAMP, only little evidence supports an important role in inflammatory cells. However, a recent report suggests a role in blocking of *Fas-receptor*-mediated *caspases* activation in *eosinophils*.

CYCLOOXYGENASE (COX)

Cyclooxygenase, also called prostaglandin H synthase, metabolizes *arachidonic acid* (AA) to form *prostaglandins* (PGs) and *thromboxane*.

In contrast to *5-lipoxygenase* (5-LO), COX is found in almost all cells. However, the further distal enzymatic activities that are responsible for the generation of specific COX pathway products (see Figure 18) vary between cells. For instance, *mast cells* preferentially generate PGD_2, *platelets* make TXA_2, *endothelial cells* synthesize PGI_2, *epithelial cells* are producers of PGE_2, and *macrophages* generate PGF_2, PGE_2, and TXA_2. In contrast, *eosinophils*, *neutrophils*, and *basophils* do not produce significant amounts of COX pathway products. Several isoforms of COX have been identified, including COX-1, constitutively expressed, and COX-2, induced at sites of *inflammation. Nonsteroidal antiinflammatory drugs* (NSAIDs) (e.g., *aspirin*) inhibit both molecules. COX-1 inhibition leads to side effects of the drug, while COX-2 inhibition results in clinical efficacy (see *cyclooxygenase-2 inhibitors*).

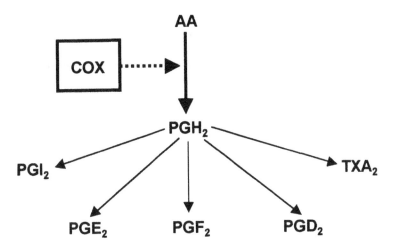

FIGURE 18   The cyclooxygenase (COX) pathway. All products are originally generated from arachidonic acid (AA).

CYCLOOXYGENASE-2 (COX-2) INHIBITORS

Prostaglandins (PGs) have important functions which are not always associated with *inflammation* (e.g., protection of the gastric mucosa). Such PGs are produced by *cyclooxygenase*-1 (COX-1). Therefore, nonspecific inhibition of cyclooxygenases (e.g., treatment with *aspirin*) may result in significant side effects.

Selective COX-2 inhibitors have been developed which only act as antiinflammatory drugs.

Whether these new drugs can be used in patients with aspirin *intolerance* (see *adverse drug reactions* and *aspirin-sensitive asthma*) remains to be determined.

CYCLOPHILIN

Cyclophilin is an intracellular *cyclosporin A* (CsA) *receptor*.

CYCLOSPORIN A (CsA)

CsA is an *immunosuppressive drug* of fungal origin that selectively targets activated *T cells* and is widely used in transplantation surgery to prevent rejection of allografts, such as kidney or heart transplants. CsA has been used to treat patients with *corticosteroid-resistant asthma* and provides modest benefit in this group of patients.

The mechanism of action is the downregulation of *cytokine gene* expression (and many other genes) by inhibiting *transcription*.

Thus, the efficacy of CsA in *asthma* probably lies in its ability to inhibit *Th2* cytokine formation, notably that of *IL-5*. By reduction of *survival factors* for inflammatory cells, the numbers of *eosinophils* and *mast cells* are reduced as a consequence of CsA therapy (see *apoptosis*). Moreover, CsA can inhibit all *immunoglobulin* isotype production. Thus, it does not reduce *IgE* levels in a specific manner. However, CsA is a potent inhibitor of *high-affinity IgE receptor*-mediated *histamine* and PGD_2 (see *prostaglandins*) release from mast cells, suggesting that CsA not only downregulates chronic inflammatory processes, but may also reduce *immediate hypersensitivity* reactions. However, there are contrasting reports regarding the in vivo relevance of the latter effect.

> CsA (as *tacrolimus*) binds to an intracellular *cyclophilin* (intracellular CsA receptor), forming a complex that inhibits the Ca^{2+}-calmodulin-dependent (see *calcium mobilization*) *phosphatase*, *calcineurin*.

Calcineurin-mediated *dephosphorylation* of *nuclear factor of activated T cells* (NF-AT) is essential for the translocation of this *transcription factor* into the nucleus. Since CsA blocks the phosphatase activity of calcineurin, the translocation of NF-AT cannot occur (Figure 19). However, NF-AT translocation is important for the transcription of cytokine and many other genes. CsA also inhibits the activity of the *nuclear factor-κB* (NF-κB), but not *activator protein 1* (AP-1).

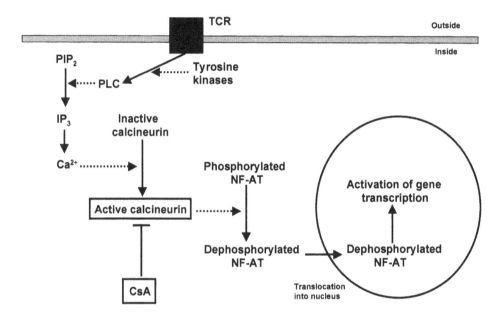

FIGURE 19   Simplified scheme of T cell antigen receptor (TCR)-mediated signal transduction. CsA blocks the phosphatase activity of calcineurin, thereby preventing the translocation of NF-AT into the nucleus.

CYSTEINYL LEUKOTRIENES

Collective term for the *leukotrienes* LTC_4, LTD_4, and LTE_4, because of the presence of a peptide linked to the *eicosanoid* backbone through a thioether link at C-6. Due to their biological activity, these three leukotrienes were formerly called *slow-reacting substance of anaphylaxis* (SRS-A). It has been shown that there are increased levels of cysteinyl leukotrienes in biological fluids from patients with *asthma*, especially *aspirin-sensitive asthma*, but also from those with *allergic rhinoconjunctivitis*. The physiological role of cysteinyl leukotrienes may include a role as modulators of central nervous system activity (see *leukotriene C_4 synthase*).

CYSTIC FIBROSIS (CF)

CF is the most common inherited disease, which affects approximately 1 in 2000 children. The protein product of the *gene* that causes the disease is a *cAMP*-regulated chloride channel.

Many different mutations of the CF gene have been identified that may explain the heterogeneity in the severity of the disease among patients. The recessive disorder is mainly characterized by lung disease, especially after chronic Pseudomonas aeruginosa infection, which is acquired in more than 90% of the patients.

> *Bronchoalveolar lavage* (BAL) fluid studies revealed that CF patients develop a strong neutrophilic *inflammation*.

The expansion of *neutrophils* appears to be, at least partially, due to delayed *neutrophil apoptosis*. *GM-CSF* and *G-CSF* are important neutrophil *survival factors* expressed in the inflamed lung tissue. Respiratory failure due to inflammation-mediated chronic *mucus* obstruction and lung destruction is often responsible for the premature death of CF patients. CF has to be considered as a differential diagnosis in children with *wheeze*. Up to 15% of the patients develop *allergic bronchopulmonary aspergillosis* (ABPA) due to colonization of the airways with *Aspergillus* fumigatus. Moreover, CF is a multisystem disorder and is also characterized by malabsorption due to exocrine pancreatic insufficiency, increased salt loss in sweat (used as a diagnostic mean), and male infertility. Interestingly, CF ΔF508 heterozygosity is overrepresented among patients with *asthma* (see *genetic predisposition*).

CYTOCHROME OXIDASE

(See *NADPH oxidase*.)

CYTOKINES

Cytokines are polypeptides (6 to 30 kDa) made by cells that affect the function of other cells by noncognate interactions (see *cognate/noncognate interactions*). Cytokines are released from cells and stimulate cells that express the appropriate surface *cytokine receptor*. They mediate proinflammatory, proliferative, or antiinflammatory mechanisms. Cytokines are divided into subgroups such as *interleukins* (ILs), *chemokines*, *growth factors*, *interferons* (IFNs), *tumor necrosis factor* (*TNF*) *superfamily*, and colony-stimulating factors (CSFs). As indicated by the several existing subgroups, cytokines are a diverse group of proteins. However, there are a number of properties shared by these molecules (see Table 31).

In the pathogenesis of *allergic diseases*, *T cell cytokines* are of particular importance, since they orchestrate *allergic inflammation* (see Table 32).

CYTOKINE CONTROL MECHANISMS

Inhibition of *cytokine* production/secretion can occur at three levels, pre- or post-transcriptional or post-translational. Pre-transcriptional inhibition prevents *cytokine gene activation* following *receptor* activation (see *transcription*); post-transcriptional inhibition prevents *translation* of the *gene* product. Post-translational control inhibits the release of translated gene product (cytokine).

> Considerable evidence suggests that cytokines are primarily controlled by pre-transcriptional mechanisms.

On the other hand, *mast cells* can produce cytokines, which remain stored in intracellular vesicles (see *constitutive cytokine expression*) and are only released upon activation. For ex vivo experiments, inhibition of cytokine secretion using monensin or brefeldin A can be useful in measuring intracellular cytokine production of in vivo activated inflammatory cells by *flow cytometry* or *immunohistochemistry*.

TABLE 31
Ten Properties Shared by Cytokines

1. Cytokines serve to mediate and regulate immune and inflammatory responses.
2. With a few exceptions (see *constitutive cytokine expression*), cytokines are usually not stored as preformed *mediators*. Their synthesis is the consequence of new *gene transcription*.
3. Without stimulation, cytokine synthesis is rapidly downregulated. Therefore, cytokine production is a transient event.
4. A cytokine can be synthesized by many different cells. Therefore, the terms *lymphokines* or *monokines* are used less frequently in current terminology.
5. Cytokines act on many different cells. This property is called *pleiotropism*.
6. Cytokines often have several different effects on the same target cell.
7. Many cytokines share the same function. This property is called *redundancy*.
8. Cytokines often influence the synthesis and/or function of other cytokines. This may include positive (cytokine cascade) or negative regulatory mechanisms.
9. Cytokines act via specific cytokine receptors.
10. Most cytokine-mediated cellular responses require newly synthesized *mRNA* and protein.

TABLE 32
T Cell Cytokines with Major Activity in the Manifestation of Allergic Diseases

Cytokine	Major Functional Role in Allergic Diseases	T Helper Functional Phenotype	Molecular Weight (kDa)	Receptor* and (Expression)
IL-1	Initiation of inflammation	Th0/Th1?	18(α) 17(β)	CD121a (T, Thy, F, Endo), CD121b (M, B, Mø)
IL-2	T cell proliferation	Th1	15	CD122 (NK, T, B, Mø)
IL-3	Priming	Th0	15	CDw123 (My p) CD123 (B, T, Endo, p)
IL-4	IgE production, Th2 differentiation	Th2	14	CD124 (B, T, Endo, Hem p)
IL-5	Eosinophilic inflammation	Th2	28–31	CDw125 (My p)
IL-6	B cell differentiation	Th2	20.5	CD126 (B, Epi)
IL-8	Neutrophil chemotaxis	Th0?	8	CDw128 (N, Ba, T, Mø, K)
IL-10	Limitation and resolution of inflammation	Tr1	18.5	NA
IL-12	Downregulation of Th2 cells	Th1	35, 40, 70	NA
IL-13	IgE production	Th2	13	CD124 (B, T, Endo, Hem p)
IFN-γ	Downregulation of Th2 cells	Th1	35	CDw119 (M, Mø, B, NK)
TNF-α/β	Initiation of inflammation	Th1	17.5(α) 19(β)	CD134, CDw136 (T, Broad)
RANTES	T cell chemotaxis	Th0?	8	CD4, CD45RO+ T

Notes: B: B cell, Ba: basophil, Endo: endothelial cell, Epi: epithelial cell, F: fibroblast, Hem: hematopoietic, K: keratinocyte, M: macrophage, Mø: monocyte, My: myeloid cell, N: neutrophil, NK: natural killer cell, p: precursor cell, T: T cell. NA: Not assigned as of 6th HLDA workshop, Kobe, Japan, 1996.

* Many receptors share common chains. Only the major identifying CD numbers are given.

CYTOKINE DETECTION METHODS

Several methods are now available to measure and determine the cell source of *cytokines*, including *in situ hybridization* and *immunohistochemistry*, as well as reverse transcription-*polymerase chain reaction* (RT-PCR) and measurement of secreted products by *immunoassays* (mostly *ELISA*) from purified cell populations. Using these techniques, it has been possible to show that coordinate *transcription* and expression of primarily *Th2* cytokines occurs in *IgE*-mediated *allergic inflammations*.

CYTOKINE GENE ACTIVATION

The study of *T cell genes* has led to an abundant literature on activation of *cytokine* genes, many of which are related to *allergic diseases*. As an example, the sequence of events from *T cell antigen receptor* (TCR) engagement to secretion of *IL-2* is illustrated here. IL-2 is a growth factor secreted by T cells following activation with *antigen*. In resting *CD4⁺* T cells, *mRNA* for IL-2 cannot be detected, but appears within 30 minutes of *T cell activation*.

Following TCR binding, a series of *phosphorylation* events causes intracellular *calcium mobilization* and activation of cytosolic *transcription factors*, which translocate to the nucleus where they bind to regulatory elements on the *DNA* and initiate *transcription*.

The IL-2 *promoter* has four known transcription factors: *nuclear factor of activated T cells* (NF-AT), octamer protein (Oct), *activator protein 1* (AP-1), and *nuclear factor-κB* (NF-κB) (see Figure 20). NF-AT has two binding regions on the IL-2 promoter and binds cooperatively with Fos and Jun (= AP-1). Various other transcription factors (e.g., Ets-1) can also bind the NF-AT motif and may have regulatory potential on the IL-2 gene. The Oct proteins act as transactivating factors, facilitating AP-1 binding and also functionally cooperating with Fos and Jun. The NF-κB element binds Rel family proteins and may not contribute greatly to enhancing activity, but a p50 homodimer of RelB may be important in repressing IL-2 gene transcription in *Th2 cells* or in states of *anergy*. Fos and Jun have to bind as a dimer, and dominant binding of Jun to other promotor regions can inhibit its function. NF-AT, NF-κB, and certain Oct family protein activity is blocked by *cyclosporin A* (CsA) or *tacrolimus* (FK506), which illustrates the dependence of these transcription factors on the calcium-dependent *phosphatase calcineurin*. Factors affecting the duration of IL-2 mRNA persistence are not fully understood but could be linked to removal of the stimulating *antigen* (thus, no further transcription factor activation via the TCR). Other possible mechanisms include the production of inhibitory factors to transcription, which either compete with or block activating transcription factor function or degrade the mRNA (see also *immunosuppressive mechanisms*).

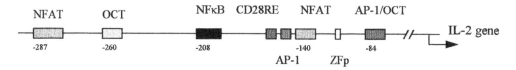

FIGURE 20 Simplified diagram showing the IL-2 promoter with transcription factor binding sites. Each position is shown with the numbers in base pairs upstream of start of the major transcription site for IL-2. CD28RE is a *CD28* response element, ZFp is a zinc finger protein.

CYTOKINE GENE CLUSTER

(See *T helper 2 cytokine gene cluster*.)

CYTOKINE mRNA EXPRESSION

Cytokine effects are transient. Cytokine *mRNA* expression is rapidly up- and downregulated. To understand pathogenic mechanisms in *allergic diseases*, it is important to study cytokine mRNA expression. Several methods have been developed, e.g., reverse transcription-*polymerase chain reaction* (RT-PCR) and *in situ hybridization*. These powerful techniques have been used to detect cytokine mRNA in tissues as well as in purified blood and tissue cells. A major finding using such techniques was the direct demonstration of *Th2 cell* infiltration into the lungs of patients with *asthma*.

CYTOKINE RECEPTORS

Cytokine receptors have been grouped into five large families based on the presence of conserved folding motifs or sequence homologies (see Table 33). The cellular expression and CD numbers of cytokine receptors are given in Table 34. The major function of cytokine receptors is the transduction of the signal that has been initiated following cytokine binding into the cell (see *cytokine receptor signal transduction*).

TABLE 33
Cytokine Receptor (R) Families and Their Members

Cytokine Receptor Family	Members
1. *Immunoglobulin superfamily* domain-containing receptors	*IL-1*R, PDGFR, *SCF*R, M-CSFR
2. Type I family containing a WSxWS motif just proximal to the transmembrane region	*IL-2*R, *IL-3*R, *IL-4*R, *IL-5*R, *IL-6*R, IL-7R, IL-11R, *IL-13*R, *GM-CSF*R, G-CSFR
3. Type II family (defined at sequence level)	*IFN-α/β*R, *IFN-γ*R
4. *TNF receptor superfamily* (also called Type III family)	*TNF*RI, *TNF*RII, *NGF*R, *Fas*R, TRAILR, *CD40*, and many others
5. Seven transmembrane domain receptors (see *G protein-coupled receptors*)	*IL-8*R, *chemokine* receptors

---

TABLE 34
CD Classification and Cellular Distribution of Cytokine Receptors

CD Number	Receptor	Main Distribution
CD25	IL-2Rα	Thymocytes, activated *T cells*, pre-*B cells*
CD114	G-CSFR	*Granulocytes, monocytes, platelets*
CD116	GM-CSFRα	Monocytes, granulocytes
CD117	SCFR	Hematopoietic progenitors, *mast cells*
CD121a	IL-1RI	Thymocytes, T cells, *fibroblasts, endothelial cells*
CD122	IL-2β	T cells, *NK cells,* granulocytes
CD123	IL-3Rα	Granulocytes, hematopoietic progenitors
CD124	IL-4Rα IL-13Rα	T cells, B cells, hematopoietic progenitors, fibroblasts
CD125	IL-5Rα	*Eosinophils, basophils*
CD126	IL-6Rα	Activated B cells, plasma cells, T cells, monocytes, epithelial cells, fibroblasts, neural cells
CD127	IL-7Rα	Immature thymocytes, hepatocytes, pre-B cells, T cells
CD129	IL-9R	T cells, B cells, *macrophages,* megakaryoblasts
CD131	IL-3Rβ IL-5Rβ GM-CSFRβ	Hematopoietic progenitors, granulocytes, monocytes
CD132	IL-2Rγ IL-4Rγ IL-7Rγ IL-9Rγ IL-15Rγ	T cells, B cells, hematopoietic progenitors, granulocytes, fibroblasts

CYTOKINE RECEPTOR SIGNAL TRANSDUCTION

The first step in *signaling* processes of *cytokines* is ligand-induced dimerization of *receptor* components (see *cross-linking*), resulting in molecular interactions among cytoplasmic regions of these components to initiate a downstream signaling cascade.

> Many of the *cytokine receptors* have a specific recognition domain but share common subunits, which serve as signal transducers.

For example, *IL-3, IL-5,* and *GM-CSF* receptors share a common β-subunit. *IL-6* and IL-11 receptors share the signal transducer gp130, and *IL-2, IL-4,* IL-7, and *IL-15* receptors a common γ-subunit. All these signal transducers lack an enzymatic motif in their cytoplasmic structure.

> Receptor dimerization forms contact surfaces, which allow molecular interactions with cytoplasmic *tyrosine kinases*, resulting in tyrosine *phosphorylation* of intracellular proteins.

The tyrosine kinases, which interact with cytokine receptor components, belong mostly to the families of *Src* and *Janus kinases*. Important downstream molecules activated by cytokine receptors are *Ras, Raf-1,* and *mitogen-activated protein kinases* (MAPK) as well as *signal transducers and activators of transcription* (STAT). During *inflammation*, cytokines elicit the production of new proteins. This means that the *signal transduction* cascade initiated by cytokine receptors often activates *transcription factors* (see Figure 21). However, there are many unresolved questions, especially how specific responses can be achieved when many cytokines share common signaling pathways. One current hypothesis to explain this phenomenon is that the signaling pathways are modified by other stimuli. For more specific information on cytokine receptor signaling, see *interleukin-4 receptor* and *interleukin-5 receptor.*

CYTOKINE THERAPY

Besides indirect modulation of *cytokine* expression during *immunotherapy* or *corticosteroid* therapy, there are other options to influence the pathologic immune response in *allergic diseases*. For instance, *cytokines* can selectively be blocked by *monoclonal antibodies* or directly given as a recombinant protein.

> In the future, cytokines might be applied using *gene therapy* methods.

In *allergic inflammation* associated with a *Th2*-driven immune response, therapeutically applied cytokines such as *IL-12, IL-18,* or *IFN-γ* may favor *Th1* and block Th2 differentiation. Also, natural *IL-1* as well as created *IL-4, IL-5,* or *IL-13 receptor* antagonists might be beneficial in these diseases. In addition, *IL-10* and *TGF-β* are also possible candidates to downregulate inflammatory responses. However, note that TGF-β can also induce *fibrosis.*

CYTOLYTIC T LYMPHOCYTE ASSOCIATED ANTIGEN-4 (CTLA-4)

CTLA-4 is co-expressed or transiently expressed with *CD28⁺ T cells*. CTLA-4 and CD28 share considerable homology, and both react with *CD80/CD86* (B7.1/B7.2) expressed on the surface of *antigen-presenting cells* (APCs).

> Whereas CD28 positively regulates *T cell activation*, CTLA-4 is considered to be a negative regulator for these cells.

CTLA-4 contains a *tyrosine-based inhibitory motif* (ITIM) within the cytoplasmic tail that is phosphorylated by the *tyrosine kinase* Lck. The inhibitory *tyrosine phosphatase* SHP-2 is recruited to the tyrosine-phosphorylated ITIM. SHP-2 dephosphorylates *T cell antigen receptor* (TCR)-mediated *signaling* events by *dephosphorylation* (Figure 22).

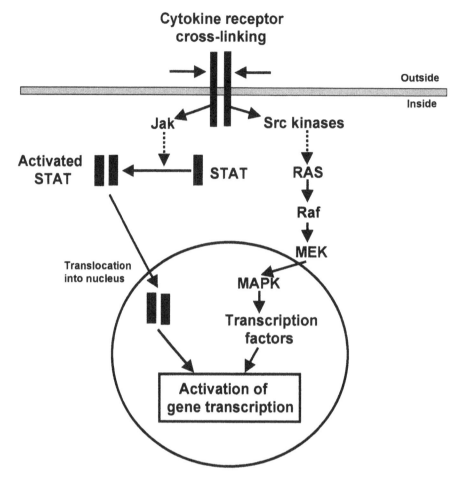

FIGURE 21   A model for cytokine signaling pathways from cytokine receptor binding to activation of transcription.

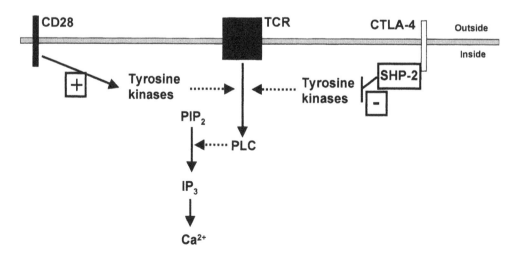

FIGURE 22   Inhibition of TCR signal transduction by CTLA-4.

CYTOPENIA

Cytopenia is a term to describe decreased cell numbers within one or more cell populations. For instance, *lymphopenia* is often observed during systemic therapy with *corticosteroids* or other *immunosuppressive drugs*. Moreover, agranulocytosis, anemia, and thrombocytopenia are sometimes the consequence of *drug allergies*.

CYTOSINE

A pyrimidine base that is an essential component of *DNA*.

CYTOSOLIC PHOSPHOLIPASE A$_2$ (cPLA$_2$)

Important *isoform* of *phospholipase A$_2$* (PLA$_2$) that initiates *leukotriene* synthesis.

CYTOTOXICITY OF ALLERGENS

Food *allergens* (see *food allergy*) and *haptens*, such as *nickel* or platinum salts, can form complexes with inherent cytotoxicity. Moreover, *bee venom phospholipase A$_2$* (PLA$_2$) is cytotoxic by hydrolyzing membrane phospholipids. It is this characteristic evident or latent cytotoxic capacity that may be responsible for primary *T cell sensitization* in these cases.

Interaction of *allergens* with cell membranes of *mast cells* in mucosal surfaces and *mucosa-associated lymphoid tissue* (MALT) or in the skin (e.g., *contact sensitization*) may lead to the disruption of mast cell membranes and release of preformed *IL-4*.

Allergen-specific *T cells* recruited to an IL-4-rich environment develop into *Th2 cells*, which drive *IgE* selection and synthesis (see *immunoglobulin class switching*) and chronic eosinophilic *inflammation*.

CYTOTOXIC THERAPY

Drugs such as azathioprine, cyclophosphamide, and *methotrexate,* which are often used to treat malignant disease, also have some immunosuppressive potential (see *immunosuppressive drugs*). Trials of cytotoxic therapy in severe *asthma* have provided mixed results. Methotrexate and *cyclosporin A* (CsA) are the only immunosuppressive agents in current use for *asthma*.

D

DANDER

(See *animal dander*.)

DEATH FACTORS

Death factors can be defined as soluble or membrane-bound proteins which induce *apoptosis*. For instance, *CD8⁺ T cell*-derived *mediators* induce apoptosis in virus-infected cells. *Fas ligand* and some other members of the *TNF superfamily* induce apoptosis via specific *receptors* (see *TNF receptor superfamily*). A common feature of death factors is the direct or indirect activation of *caspases*.

> Death factors regulate as *survival factors* the life span of cells and therefore cell numbers.

Resistance toward death factors can be associated with *delayed apoptosis* or even tumorigenesis.

DEATH FROM ASTHMA

Asthma causes a significant number of deaths each year, but the number of fatalities is relatively small compared to the number of people who have the condition. Death from asthma can occur in a number of different ways.

> The most common patterns recognized are acute death occurring within a few hours of onset of an attack and a more prolonged asphyxiating death occurring over several days.

In acute death from asthma, the patient's airways may be relatively clear. *Neutrophils* may be present in the airways, and there may be marked *smooth muscle bronchospasm*, but there is rarely much to see in the way of *eosinophils* or *mucus*. These patients may die from acute *hypoxia*, causing cardiac rhythm disturbance.

More commonly, patients will present with a prolonged attack and deteriorate with a progressively worsening *ventilation–perfusion mismatch*, hypoxia, and eventually exhaustion. At post mortem, the airways are plugged with mucus and eosinophilic debris, demonstrating that the problem is asphyxia due to internal blockage of the airways.

> Prompt treatment of *asthma exacerbations* with nebulized *bronchodilators* and parenteral *corticosteroids* is recognized as the best way of reducing the risk of death from asthma.

A small minority of asthma deaths may be associated with pneumothorax, which requires treatment in its own right.

DEATH RECEPTORS

A subgroup of *surface molecules* of the *TNF receptor superfamily* contains in their cytoplasmic parts a motif (death domain) which allows the initiation of *apoptosis signaling* pathways. There are at least six *death receptors* known that are expressed on most cells, suggesting an important role for these molecules in the maintenance of correct cell numbers.

DECONGESTANTS

The topical or oral administration of nasal decongestants results in vasoconstriction of the nasal mucosa. They activate post-junctional *α-adrenergic receptors* of precapillary and post-capillary blood vessels.

> The effect of decongestants is temporary, and they do not relieve nasal *inflammation*.

However, decongestants can be used when a completely blocked nose (see *allergic rhinitis*) prevents penetration of *corticosteroid* nasal sprays. Because of the risk of inducing *rhinitis medicamentosa*, it is not recommended to use them for more than 7 to 10 days.

DEGRANULATION

(See *exocytosis*.)

DEHUMIDIFIERS

Dehumidifiers may reduce the *house-dust mite* growth in areas where outdoor humidity is high most of the year (see *allergen avoidance*).

DELAYED APOPTOSIS

Under normal conditions, inflammatory cells such as *eosinophils* or *neutrophils* rapidly die via *apoptosis*. However, under inflammatory conditions, these cells receive survival signals that prevent apoptosis (see *survival factors*).

> Delayed apoptosis is an important mechanism for the accumulation of inflammatory cells at inflammatory sites.

The most important survival factor for eosinophils in *allergic diseases* appears to be *IL-5* (see *eosinophilia*). In contrast, *G-CSF* and *GM-CSF* mediate delayed neutrophil apoptosis in diseases associated with bacterial infection (e.g., *cystic fibrosis*). In the resolution of *inflammation*, a downregulation of the survival factor expression is observed that is associated with the induction of *granulocyte* apoptosis.

> Besides overexpression of survival factors, the disruption of death *signaling* pathways (see *TNF receptor superfamily*) may represent another possibility to prevent apoptosis of inflammatory cells (Figure 23) (see *nitric oxide*).

In a subgroup of patients with the *hypereosinophilic syndrome*, an *intrinsic defect of apoptosis* has been observed.

DELAYED HYPERSENSITIVITY

Delayed *hypersensitivity* is a late allergic reaction (see *allergy*) to an *antigen* or *allergen*. It is also called *type IV reaction* (see *Coombs and Gell classification*). Sensitized *T cells* (see *T cell sensitization*) accumulate at the inflammatory site following antigen or allergen exposure.

> Delayed hypersensitivity reaction may lead either to a beneficial immunity (e.g., tuberculin, see *tuberculin test*) or *allergic disease*.

The classical delayed hypersensitivity reaction (type IVa1) involves *CD4+* T cells that produce *Th1 cytokines* (e.g., *contact dermatitis*). However, under different pathologic conditions,

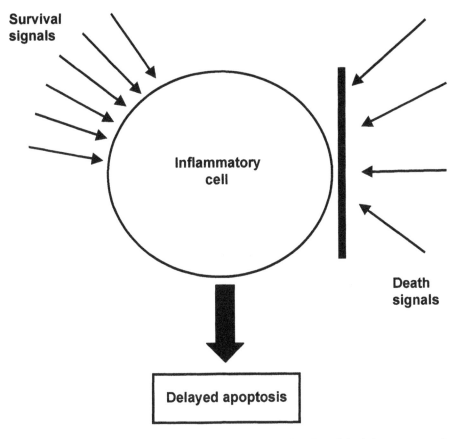

FIGURE 23   Increased expression of survival factors and/or inhibition of death factors are two important mechanisms that delay apoptosis in inflammatory cells.

cytotoxic *CD8⁺* T cells (type IVb) accumulate that kill target cells (e.g., diabetes mellitus). In *asthma*, specific *allergen challenge* causes not only an *immediate hypersensitivity* reaction, but also a *late-phase response* (LPR). Therefore, asthma usually demonstrates features of both *type I* and type IV reactions.

> *Bronchial provocation tests* with *antigenic peptides* representing *T cell epitopes* of allergens have demonstrated that delayed hypersensitivity reactions can occur without and independent of immediate hypersensitivity reactions in asthma.

Such an LPR demonstrates many features of the chronic *allergic inflammation* present in asthmatic patients. The delayed hypersensitivity reaction in asthma and other *allergic diseases* is associated with eosinophilic *inflammation* (see *eosinophils* and *eosinophilia*) and an accumulation of CD4⁺ as well as CD8⁺ T cells that express *Th2* cytokines (see also *Tc2 cells*). In addition to cytokines (including *chemokines*), many *mediators* are generated in this inflammatory response, such as *leukotrienes, prostaglandins, PAF,* and *complement factors*. Delayed hypersensitivity associated with abnormal Th2 activation is now called type IVa2 reaction (see Table 35).

DELETION

Deletion describes the loss of a *DNA* sequence or a *gene* whereby the neighboring regions are joined together.

TABLE 35
Forms of Delayed Hypersensitivity (Type IV Following the Coombs and Gell Classification)

Type	T Cell Subpopulation(s)	Cytokines	Description
IVa1	CD4+	Th1	Classical delayed hypersensitivity
IVa2	CD4+	Th2	Chronic allergic inflammation
	CD8+		
IVb	CD8+	Th1	Cytotoxic responses

DENATURATION

Process leading to single-stranded *DNA* or *RNA* molecules. The separation of two *complementary* strands or the opening of internal base interaction on the same strand is commonly achieved by increasing the temperature (melting). The term is also used in protein chemistry when denaturing agents are used.

DENDRITIC CELLS

Morphological aspects determined the name of these cells.

> Mature dendritic cells are the most efficient *antigen-presenting cells* (APCs) known at the moment. They are the only APCs able to induce a *primary immune response*.

Dendritic cells originate from a *bone marrow* progenitor, travel through the blood, and are seeded into non-lymphoid tissues. In most tissues, dendritic cells are present in a so-called immature state, with a low stimulatory capacity toward naive *T cells* (see *naive lymphocytes*). Following *antigen* uptake and *antigen processing*, the dendritic cells mature (see Table 36), express co-stimulatory molecules (see *co-stimulation*), and migrate to the draining *lymph nodes*.

> In the lymph nodes, they interact with naive T cells to facilitate *T cell sensitization*.

The process of dendritic cell maturation can be mimicked in vitro: immature cells incubated with *CD40 ligand*, LPS, or *TNF-α* develop into mature dendritic cells.

There are two subtypes of dendritic cells present in the human body. (1) Interdigitating dendritic cells are present in the interstitium of most organs and are abundant in lymph nodes and spleen. They are extremely efficient in the uptake and presentation of protein antigens

TABLE 36
Some Characteristics of Immature and Mature Dendritic Cells

Immature Dendritic Cells	Mature Dendritic Cells
High intracellular *MHC class II* content	High surface MHC class II expression
High *endocytosis* rate	Low endocytosis rate
High Ig-receptor expression	Low Ig-receptor expression
Low co-stimulatory molecule expression	High co-stimulatory molecule expression
Good processors, weak presenters of *antigenic peptides*	Weak processors, good presenters of antigenic peptides

to *CD4*+ helper T cells. They originate from *monocytes* following interactions with *endothelial cells*, the subendothelial *extracellular matrix*, and *cytokine* activation (*IL-4* and *GM-CSF*). Epidermal *Langerhans cells* are well-investigated organ-specific dendritic cells of this subtype. (2) Follicular dendritic cells are present in the germinal centers of the lymphoid follicles in the lymph nodes, spleen, and *mucosa-associated lymphoid tissues*. They may trap antigens bound to soluble *antibodies* or complement via *Fc receptors* or *complement factor* receptors and are able to directly activate *B cells*.

DENNIE–MORGAN INFRAORBITAL FOLD

A doubled infraorbital fold, which is one of the most important *atopy stigmata*.

DEOXYRIBONUCLEIC ACID

(See *DNA*.)

DEPHOSPHORYLATION

Dephosphorylation is an enzymatic reaction mediated by *phosphatases*. Several proteins have phosphate groups on tyrosine, serine, or threonine residues (see *amino acids*). To activate these molecules (e.g., some *Src kinases*), dephosphorylation has to occur. *CD45* is a *tyrosine phosphatase* that is essential for *antigen receptor signaling*. *Calcineurin* is a serine-threonine phosphatase important in *T cell antigen receptor*-mediated *cytokine gene activation*. Other phosphatases are needed to terminate or to have inhibitory functions on *signal transduction* pathways.

DERMATITIS

Any acute skin *inflammation* with metachronic polymorphism. Lesions follow the sequential pattern of *erythema*, vesiculation, oozing, *crusts*, and desquamation (e.g., sunburn dermatitis).

DERMATITIS EXFOLIATIVA

A morphologically defined group of exfoliative skin diseases, leading to an intraepidermal or subepidermal blister formation, including the following diseases: (1) staphylococcal scalded skin syndrome; an exfoliative *dermatitis* with an intraepidermal split level due to a toxin from a group II Staphylococcus aureus (phage type 71); (2) *toxic epidermal necrosis*, an exfoliative dermatitis with subepidermal split level due to a drug *intolerance* reaction.

DERMATOPHAGOIDES

Genus of *house-dust mite* (order Acarina, class Arachnida, family Pyroglyphidae). House-dust mites of the genus Dermatophagoides are the most common indoor mites of North America and Europe. Their primary food source is human skin scales (thus their name "skin eating"), and they are found in carpets, upholstered furniture, and bedding. Epidemiologic studies have demonstrated a strong correlation between *sensitization* to mite *aeroallergens* and *allergic diseases*. The most common species of Dermatophagoides are D. pteronyssinus and D. farinae. There are several possibilities to reduce mite exposure (see *allergen avoidance* and *climate therapy*).

DERMIS

The dermis is the second layer of the skin (see *epidermis*).

DERMOGRAPHISM

The skin reaction induced by a localized short-term pressure, resembling writing on the skin. While normal subjects show red dermographism, atopic subjects (see *atopy*) tend to exhibit a white dermographism. Urticarial dermographism (see *urticaria*) is a third, less common pattern of reaction.

DESENSITIZATION

Desensitization describes a condition of unresponsiveness of a cell following ligand stimulation. In contrast to *anergy* or *tolerance*, this term usually describes unresponsiveness of *granulocytes* and *monocytes*, but not *lymphocytes*. Also, the ligands are inflammatory *mediators*, but not *antigens*.

> The phenomenon of desensitization is frequently used to determine the *receptor* specificity of *CC chemokines* and *CXC chemokines* using *calcium mobilization* experiments.

Desensitization might be due to the mechanisms shown in Table 37.

TABLE 37
Possible Mechanisms of Desensitization

1. Occupation of the receptor by ligand.
2. Receptor inactivation by *signaling* mechanisms.
3. Internalization of the receptor–ligand complex.
4. Inability of the cell to carry out a specific function (e.g., no mediator content due to previous stimulations).

The term "desensitization" is also used to describe the situation of a patient following successful *immunotherapy*.

DEVELOPMENT OF T CELLS

(See *thymus*.)

DEXAMETHASONE

Dexamethasone is a highly active *corticosteroid*.

DEXTRAN

Dextran appears to release *histamine* from *mast cells* by *cross-linking* of glucose *receptors* on the cell membrane (see *idiosyncrasy*).

DIACYLGLYCEROL (DAG)

DAG is a lipid-soluble cleavage product generated by *phospholipase C* (PLC)-mediated hydrolysis of membrane phosphoinositides or *phospholipase D* (PLD)-mediated hydrolysis of phosphatidylcholine. DAG activates *protein kinase C* (PKC).

DIESEL EXHAUST

Important *dust* particle (see *PM-10*). Diesel exhaust has been associated with cell activation leading to *cytokine* production. In general, it appears that it enhances *inflammation* and *airway hyperresponsiveness* in *asthma*. Epidemiological studies in Japan supported this hypothesis, demonstrating a higher prevalence of *allergic rhinitis* among children in districts polluted by automobile exhaust than in nonpolluted districts (see *pollution*).

DIET

Once certain foods are suspected to provoke allergic symptoms, they should be completely excluded from the food uptake. The food *allergen* elimination diet might be helpful in diagnosing *food allergy*, but should be completed by blinded *food challenge* tests (see *allergen challenge* and *exposition test*).

DIET DIARY

For the diagnosis of *adverse food reactions*, a diet diary, in which patients record all ingested foods as well as the symptoms experienced, is useful. This method may help to identify a relationship between ingested food(s) and disease symptom(s) (see *food allergy* and *intolerance*).

DIPLOID

This term is used to describe the number of *chromosomes* in most somatic cells, which is double that in gametes (*haploid*); two sets of autosomal chromosomes (*autosomes*) and two sex chromosomes (gonosomes).

DISCOID ECZEMA

A clinically defined type of *eczema* with coin-shaped lesions, hence the name numular eczema (Lat.: numulus = coin). Subtypes include numular atopic eczema (see *atopic dermatitis*) and microbial eczema.

DISKHALER

This is a kind of *dry powder inhaler* (DPI). It can be loaded with a strip of up to 60 drug-containing packets. The diskhaler is breath-actuated and efficient at low inspiratory flow rates.

DISODIUM CROMOGLYCATE

(See *cromoglycate*.)

DISSEMINATED NEURODERMITIS

(See *atopic dermatitis*.)

DNA

Most organisms store their genetic information in deoxyribonucleic acid (DNA).

The genetic information of life is physically stored in the cellular nucleus by the polymer deoxyribonucleic acid, which is a double-helix structure with two antiparallel *complementary nucleotide* chains (strands). DNA consists of four different nucleotides linked by phosphodiester bonds. Thus the backbone of each strand consists of an invariant sugar–phosphate–sugar–phosphate polymer. In DNA the sugar is deoxyribose. Joined at the 1′ position of the sugar is one of four nitrogen-containing bases, either purine (*adenine* = A and *guanine* = G) or the less bulky pyrimidine (*cytosine* = C and *thymine* = T). The architecture of the DNA macromolecule was discovered by *X-ray crystallography*. The double helix is held together by hydrogen bonds that form between A and T bases and between G and C bases, called base pairs (Figure 24). The complementarity of the DNA leads to equimolar amounts of adenine and thymine and guanine and cytosine in a given double-stranded DNA molecule. This feature (that the genetic information is present on both strands) allows accurate replication of DNA during cell division in two identical copies that can then be equally distributed to the daughter cells.

DNA CLONING

Method to isolate and characterize single *genes*. Two basic varieties of this method have been undertaken, depending on the nature of the original *DNA*. For genomic DNA cloning, DNA

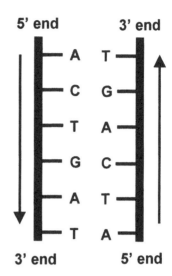

FIGURE 24   Structure of DNA.

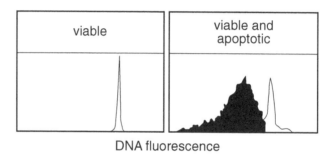

DNA fluorescence

FIGURE 25   Analysis of DNA fragmentation by flow cytometry. High-molecular-weight DNA is indicated by the narrow peak. DNA fragments are shown in black.

molecules are cleaved into pieces of manageable sizes and then cloned. For *cDNA* cloning, isolated *mRNA* is used to produce cDNA before cloning.

DNA FRAGMENTATION

Besides morphological changes, *DNA* fragmentation is another hallmark of cells undergoing *apoptosis*. In contrast to *necrosis*, where a random DNA fragmentation occurs, in apoptotic cells an internucleosomal fragmentation is present. There are many different techniques to analyze the apoptotic DNA fragmentation. The classical technique is DNA electrophoresis. This technique visualizes a ladder pattern in apoptotic, but not normal or necrotic cells. However, although this method is specific, it does not give quantitative information about the amount of apoptosis. Another way to analyze DNA fragmentation is based on the observation that cellular DNA of apoptotic cells is less stainable with fluorescent dyes. Measurements are performed by *flow cytometry*. The advantage of this technique is that apoptotic cells can be measured quantitatively as a hypodiploid cell population (see Figure 25). To detect apoptotic cells in tissues, DNA fragmentation is analyzed by the so-called *TUNEL technique*.

DNA IMMUNOTHERAPY

Immunization with *DNA* is a new approach in *allergen*-specific *immunotherapy*. It was found that *plasmid*-DNA encoding an *antigen* is taken up in vivo by *antigen-presenting cells* (APCs), but also other cells including muscle cells, *keratinocytes*, and *fibroblasts*. Interestingly, these cells then start to produce the protein, which is encoded within the plasmid. These "self-made" antigens induce a long-lasting *antigen*-specific cellular and humoral *immune response*. Antigen-stimulated *CD4⁺ T cells* from plasmid-DNA-immunized mice secrete *IFN-γ*, a potent inhibitor of *Th2 cells* and *IgE* production. At the moment, the safety and clinical efficacy of DNA vaccination for infectious diseases (e.g., influenza and mycobacterial antigens) is being tested in humans.

> It is likely that clinical trials will be performed to investigate the potential of DNA immunotherapy for the treatment of IgE-mediated *allergic diseases*.

Current problems include low efficiency of transfection, the limited time of immunity, and possible side effects.

DNA POLYMERASE

This enzyme synthesizes *DNA* after unwinding the double helix by adding one *nucleotide* after the other to the 3′ end of a *primer*, leading to the synthesis of a new *complementary* strand, thus faithfully copying the information in each strand. The DNA double helix in the daughter cells comprises a parental and a newly synthesized deoxyribonucleic strand (semi-conservative replication) (see also *DNA sequencing* and *polymerase chain reaction*).

DNase HYPERSENSITIVITY

Changes in the *chromatin* structure allow molecular interactions between *transcription factors* and *promoter* sequences of *genes* following activation of a cell. As a result of such chromatin configuration changes, the *DNA* becomes sensitive toward DNase (see *transcription*).

DNA SEQUENCING

The determination of the exact linear *nucleotide* sequence of a segment of *DNA*. The first DNA sequencing was performed by chemical degradation; treating the DNA fragment with chemicals that specifically destroyed one or two of the four bases. Sequencing based on the enzymatic activity of *DNA polymerase* is used today and has been automated. DNA polymerase uses deoxynucleotides (dNTP) to synthesize a *complementary DNA* (cDNA) strand from a single strand DNA template and an oligonucleotide *primer*. In the presence of a mixture of dNTP and dideoxynucleotides (ddNTP), the newly synthesized strand is terminated upon random incorporation of the ddNTP due to the lack of a 3′-hydroxyl group required for formation of the phosphodiester bond that links the nucleotides. Four separate reaction mixtures are prepared, each containing a percentage of the dideoxy derivative of one of the four bases. The fragments from a particular reaction mix correspond to pieces of DNA that terminate at that particular base. The fragments resulting from the four reactions are resolved by size using gel electrophoresis, and the DNA sequence is determined by the pattern of fragments.

DNA VACCINATION

(See *DNA immunotherapy*.)

DOG ALLERGEN (CANIS FAMILIARIS; Can f 1)

The dog *allergen* (Can f 1) is present in hair, dander, and saliva (see *animal danders*). For aerodynamic properties see *aeroallergens*.

DOMAIN

This is a segment of a *gene* or a protein with a certain function.

DOMINANT

A *trait* expressed in the *heterozygote*.

DPI

(See *dry powder inhalers*.)

DRUG ALLERGY

In allergic reactions, only high-molecular-weight drugs (e.g., insulin) may directly stimulate an *immune response* (see *allergen-induced immune responses*), whereas most drugs act as *haptens*. The risk of drug *sensitization* depends on the route of administration (oral < intravenous < subcutaneous < topical). The clinical manifestation varies and depends at least partially on the underlying immunological mechanisms, which are usually classified according to *Coombs and Gell* (see Table 38).

TABLE 38
Immunological Mechanisms of Drug *Allergy*

Immunologic Type	Clinical Manifestations	Drugs
IgE-mediated reactions (type I)	*Urticaria, asthma, anaphylaxis*	*Penicillin, allergen extracts*, muscle relaxants
Cytotoxic reactions (type II)	Agranulocytosis, anemia, thrombocytopenia, *vasculitis*	Penicillin, cephalosporin, metamizole, carbamazepine
Immune complex reactions (type III)	Vasculitis, *alveolitis*	Penicillin, sulphonamides, *dextrans*, allopurinol, thiouracils, phenytoin
T-cell-mediated reactions (type IV)	*Eczema, fixed drug eruption,* exanthema, *dermatitis exfoliativa*	*Antibiotics*, topical anesthetics, ethylenediamine, barbiturates, chinin, penicillin, β-blocker, *gold* salts, sulphonamides, *NSAID*, phenytoin, barbiturates, allopurinol

---

According to the clinical manifestation, drug allergies can also be classified as anaphylactic, cutaneous, hematological, pulmonary, hepatic, renal, or cardiac reactions.

> Skin symptoms, such as measles-like rashes, urticaria, and *purpura*, are seen most frequently.

However, severe and life-threatening reactions such as anaphylaxis, *dermatitis exfoliativa*, or erythrodermia may also occur. Pseudoallergic reactions such as direct *histamine* release induced by opionides and activation of the *complement system* induced by radiocontrast media may mimic immunologic reactions (see *idiosyncrasy*). The diagnosis of drug *allergy* is mainly based on the clinical history. *Skin tests* (patch, prick, scratch, and intracutaneous tests) and laboratory tests (specific *IgE, IgG*, IgM, *lymphocyte transformation test*) can be helpful and should be done before a rechallenge (see *allergen challenge* and *exposition test*) is considered.

> Avoidance of the drug in question may be the only treatment.

In diabetic patients with insulin allergy, *immunotherapy* can be tried.

DRUG ERUPTION

Drug eruptions are diagnosed if cutaneous reactions are likely to be related to the uptake of a drug (see *drug allergy*). The proper diagnosis includes the morphology (macular, maculopapular,

papular, urticarial, morbiliform, rubeoliform, multiform), the location (localized, generalized, genital, trunk, extremities), and the generic name of the accused drug.

> Exanthematous drug eruptions due to β-lactam-*antibiotics* and *fixed drug eruptions* due to *nonsteroidal antiinflammatory drugs* (NSAID) represent the most frequently observed cases.

A careful history usually leads to the correct working diagnosis. *Skin tests* should be performed, but are mostly negative. In less severe cases, oral *provocation tests* should be considered.

DRUG-INDUCED EOSINOPHILIA

A variety of drugs have been described that are able to induce *eosinophilia* or *hypereosinophilia* (see Table 39). The pathomechanism may involve hapten/carrier-protein-induced *Th2* activation (see *drug allergy*) with high *IL-5* expression.

TABLE 39
Drugs Associated with Eosinophilia or Hypereosinophilia

Amiodaron	Naproxen
Carbamazepin	Nitrofurantoin
DNCG (see *cromones*)	Rifampicin
Gold	Sulfasalazin
Heparin	L-Tryptophan
Mesalazin	

DRY POWDER INHALER (DPI)

A variety of devices are available that provide a measured amount of a dry powder containing respiratory drugs for the treatment of *asthma*. The powder is inhaled by the patient taking a deep breath in. Deposition is dependent on the size of the particles in the powder and is less dependent on timing and technique than in *metered dose inhalers* (MDI).

DRY SKIN

Dry skin is one of the stigmata of the atopic constitution (see *atopy stigmata*). Furthermore, the clinically uninvolved skin in *atopic dermatitis* patients has been shown to bear a minimal disease activity with a mild *T cell* infiltrate and increased numbers of *Langerhans cells*. Thus, the clinically uninvolved skin of atopic dermatitis patients seems to represent a minimal eczematous disease (see *eczema*).

DUST

Particles of air *pollution* are divided into coarse (>50 μm), medium (10 to 50 μm), fine (0.5 to 10 μm), and finest dust (<0.5 μm). About 80% of the floating dust consists of particles smaller than 10 μm (see *PM-10*), which may contain asbestos, heavy metals (lead, cadmium), acids (sulfur trioxide, sulfureous acid), and organic components (polycyclic aromatic hydrocarbons, *diesel exhaust*, halogen hydrocarbons). An increased concentration of these substances can provoke *airway obstruction*.

DYSHIDROSIS

The term dyshidrosis describes small (less than 2 mm in diameter), clear subcorneal blisters translucent through the thick stratum corneum of the palms and soles. The name reflects the historically proposed pathophysiological hypothesis of this disease entity. Frequently, a secondary type of dyshidrosis occurs in palmoplantar *eczema*, leading to the diagnosis of *dyshidrotic eczema*.

DYSHIDROTIC ECZEMA

A morphologically defined disease entity, dyshidrotic *eczema* of the palms and soles is diagnosed if there is an eruption of dyshidrosiform blisters in an otherwise typical palmar or plantar eczema. Oral uptake of contact *allergens* (e.g., *nickel*) by atopic individuals (see *atopy*) may be a relevant trigger factor for this type of eczema.

DYSHIDROTIC ECZEMATOUS DERMATITIS

(See *dyshidrotic eczema*.)

DYSPHONIA

Hoarseness of the voice is a local side effect of *inhaled corticosteroids* (ICS). Dysphonia is due to myopathy of laryngeal muscles. It is reversible following *corticosteroid* withdrawal.

DYSPNEA

The sensation of breathlessness caused by a pathological process (e.g., in *asthma*). Breathlessness due to psychological factors or *hyperventilation* is not usually included in the definition of dyspnea.

E

EAACI

European Academy of Allergology and Clinical Immunology.

EARLY ASTHMATIC REACTION

Airway obstruction occurring within 15 to 30 minutes of inhalation of an *allergen* as the consequence of an *immediate hypersensitivity* reaction. The early asthmatic reaction usually resolves within 90 to 120 minutes and may be followed by a *late-phase asthmatic reaction.*

ECZEMA

Eczema is defined as a chronic type of skin *inflammation* with isochronic polymorphism of the basic skin lesions seen in an acute *dermatitis*. Therefore, eczema lesions may show all stages of an acute dermatitis at the same time (i.e., *erythema*, vesicules, oozing, *crusts*, *scales*).

ECZEMA HERPETICUM

Any *eczema* with a herpes simplex virus (HSV) superinfection. However, more than 95% of the patients suffer from underlying *atopic dermatitis*. Patients usually feel sick, have high fever and disseminated, monomorphic vesicules in all regions affected by the eczema. The disease frequently requires hospitalization and antiviral therapy.

ECZEMA VACCINATUM

A severe complication of *atopic dermatitis*, caused by contact of an *eczema* patient with the vaccina virus. To avoid this disease, atopic dermatitis patients should not be vaccinated on a routine basis. Patients usually feel sick, have high fever, and have disseminated, monomorphic vesicules, which are larger than in *eczema herpeticum*. Since vaccination was stopped years ago, the disease is now limited to a few cases in occupational dermatology (see *occupational dermatitis*).

EDEMA

An accumulation of liquid in tissues, especially in the dermis and subcutis. Edema is a main symptom in *urticaria* (wheal), *angioedema*, and acute *contact dermatitis*. It can also be found in *allergic rhinoconjunctivitis*. Moreover, mucosal edema contributes to *airway obstruction* present in *asthma*. In response to *mediators* such as *histamine, prostaglandins, leukotrienes, bradykinin,* and *platelet-activating factor* (PAF), which act directly or via neural reflexes, contraction of *endothelial cells* in post-capillary venules leads to the formation of gaps that allow the outflow of plasma.

EDUCATION

Increasingly, *asthma* is managed by patients themselves rather than by their medical attendants. This requires that patients understand the nature of their disease and what to do when things go wrong. Successful education programs require the active engagement of patients, and it is not enough simply to hand out information leaflets. When properly conducted, asthma education programs can lead to a substantial improvement in disease management and to a reduction in the rate of hospital admission (see *asthma treatment strategies*).

EGG ALLERGY

Egg *allergy* is one of the most frequently implicated causes of *immediate hypersensitivity* reactions following food uptake. A number of egg-white proteins could be identified as *major allergens*, such as ovomucoid (Gal d 1), ovalbumin (Gal d 2), conalbumin (Gal d 3), and lysozyme (Gal d 4). Ovaflavoprotein can be found in both egg white and egg yolk. Egg yolk may also contain *allergens*, such as apovitellenin, phosvitin, and livetins. Hens' eggs and eggs from other birds may contain *cross-reacting allergens*.

EICOSANOIDS

Inflammatory *mediators* derived from *arachidonic acid*. These include *prostaglandins* (PGs) and *leukotrienes* (LTs).

ELASTIC RECOIL

In good health, the airways are held open by a combination of negative intrapleural pressure and connective tissue links to the substance of the lung. The elastic recoil mechanism may be damaged by destruction of the lung parenchyma in *emphysema* or by peribronchial *edema* in *asthma*.

ELECTROACUPUNCTURE

Electroacupuncture is a treatment method that belongs to the *complementary procedures*.

ELICITATION

In allergic *contact dermatitis*, two disease stages are differentiated. In the *T cell sensitization* phase, which takes a few days, the *immune system* of the individual is sensitized against a specific *hapten*. The immunological background of this sensitization phase is a *primary immune response* to the contact *allergen*. It is usual that neither the patient nor the physician is aware of the underlying sensitization. In the second stage, every contact the individual makes with the causative allergen starts an elicitation phase, leading to clinically visible skin lesions.

> The immunological background of the elicitation phase is a *secondary immune response* against the contact allergen.

In clinical dermatology, the manifestation of skin lesions leads to the diagnosis of allergic contact dermatitis. Patch testing (see *patch test*) is the method of choice to identify the causative allergen.

ELISA

(See *enzyme-linked immunosorbentassay.*)

EMESIS

Symptom that can occur in patients with *food allergy*, as well as during reactions to additives (see *intolerance reaction*) or contaminants (infectious organisms toxins).

EMPHYSEMA

> Emphysema is a destructive process in the parenchyma of the lung which affects the terminal *bronchioles,* leading to enlargement of the air spaces and loss of alveoli septae.

This leads to loss of *elastic recoil* and premature closure of the airways during expiration, which in turn causes *air trapping* and inequality of gas distribution within the lungs. This makes the process of gas transfer inefficient and leads to *ventilation-perfusion mismatch* and *hypoxia*. Typically, a patient with emphysema will have a normal p_aCO_2 and a reduced p_aO_2.

On exertion, both p_aO_2 and p_aCO_2 will fall. Severe emphysema can be seen on chest X-ray, but mild forms of the condition do not show any obvious radiographic abnormality. Emphysema forms part of the cluster of conditions now known as *chronic obstructive pulmonary disease* (COPD) and commonly coexists with *chronic bronchitis* and severe *asthma*. Although emphysema is primarily a pathological definition, it has characteristic pathophysiological consequences, which may be demonstrated by *lung function tests*.

ENCASING

Mattress covers of semipermeable material are efficient in reducing *house-dust mites* and mite *allergens*. Such *allergen avoidance* is followed by a decrease in symptoms of the *IgE*-mediated *allergic disease*.

ENDOCYTOSIS

Endocytosis is the process of uptake of extracellular proteins into a cell and their inclusion into vesicles (= *endosomes*). Endocytosis may occur without a *receptor*-mediated mechanism.

> Receptor-mediated endocytosis is much more efficient.

The receptors mediating endocytosis can be specific for a certain protein (e.g., LDL, transferrin, or insulin receptors) or nonspecific (*Fc receptors*). *Antigen–antibody* complexes can be bound via Fc receptors by *antigen-presenting cells* (APCs). In contrast to *phagocytosis*, all cells are able to perform endocytosis.

ENDOGENOUS ECZEMA

(See *atopic dermatitis*.)

ENDONUCLEASE

Endonucleases open phosphodiester bonds within nucleic acid molecules. Restriction endonucleases are enzymes isolated from bacteria, able to cleave the double-stranded nucleic acid chain at specific residues in a sequence-specific manner, thus resulting in distinct fragments unique to the *DNA* sequence. Each restriction enzyme is named by the bacteria species from which it was isolated and numbered accordingly (e.g., EcoRI, Escherichia coli RY13). These restriction enzymes are widely used for characterization of DNA segments (restriction mapping analyses) and for *DNA cloning* in biotechnology.

ENDOSOMES

Endosomes are membrane-coated vesicules filled with extracellular fluid and derived from the cell membrane following *pinocytosis*.

> During *antigen* uptake, the formation of endosomes is an essential part of the endocytotic pathway of *antigen-presenting cells* (APCs).

Early endosomes (freshly derived from the cell membrane) are distinguished from late endosomes. Late endosomes are filled with loaded *major histocompatibility complex* (MHC) molecules ready to be reexpressed on the cell surface.

ENDOTHELIAL ADHESION MOLECULES

> Members of the *immunoglobulin superfamily* and *selectin* family are *adhesion molecules* on the surface of *endothelial cells* that are important for the *recruitment of inflammatory cells*.

Various inflammatory *cytokines* upregulate these *surface molecules* on the endothelium of postcapillary venules. The ligands for *intercellular adhesion molecule-1* (ICAM-1) include the *integrins* CD11a/CD18 (expressed on *lymphocytes*) and CD11b/CD18 (expressed on *macrophages*, *monocytes*, and *granulocytes*) (see *LFA-1*). ICAM-2 is found on endothelial cells with the integrin CD11a/CD18 acting as its ligand. *Vascular adhesion molecule-1* (VCAM-1) is expressed on endothelial cells and *dendritic cells*. Its ligand is the integrin CD49d/CD29, also known as *very large antigen 4* (VLA-4), which is expressed by *eosinophils*. *IL-1*, *TNF*, LPS, and *IL-4* upregulate the expression of VCAM-1 on endothelial cells.

ENDOTHELIAL CELL

Endothelial cells form a barrier between the blood and tissues.

> Adherence of *leukocytes* to vascular endothelial cells is essential for *migration* from the circulation to sites of tissue *inflammation*.

This requires a coordinated series of events involving enhanced expression of *adhesion molecules* on the endothelium of postcapillary venules. Exposure of endothelial cells to various *cytokines* or inflammatory *mediators* such as *IL-1*, *TNF*, or lipopolysaccharides induces or upregulates the expression of several adhesion molecules including E-selectin (see *selectins*), P-selectin, *intercellular adhesion molecule-1* (ICAM-1), ICAM-2, and *vascular adhesion molecule-1* (VCAM-1) on these cells. Following adhesion, the movement of inflammatory cells through extravascular spaces is directed by *chemotactic factors* (see *recruitment of inflammatory cells*).

ENDOTHELIN

A potent *peptide* that mediates *airway obstruction*. It is secreted by airway *epithelial cells*.

ENDOTHELIUM NITRIC OXIDE SYNTHETASE

(See *nitric oxide synthetase*.)

ENHANCER

An enhancer is a *DNA* sequence that acts in cis to increase the *transcription* of a nearby *gene*. They are composed of multiple, different, specific DNA-binding sites, which are recognized by *transcription factors*. Enhancers can be present upstream, downstream, or within a *gene*. They act in either orientation and also over large distances.

ENHANSON

This is a region or composite *DNA*-binding site comprising different regulatory activities. In multiple *promoter* studies, cross-talk between several groups of *transcription factors* could be demonstrated. A regulatory network is formed by the action of different families of transcription factors creating different heterodimers in order to bind DNA elements with variant effects on the transcriptional level. DNA elements can be shared by different transcription factors and can be bound in a mutually exclusive fashion (e.g., *AP-1* and the *glucocorticoid receptor*).

ENZYME-LINKED IMMUNOSORBENT (ELISA)

ELISA is an *immunoassay* or binder-ligand assay. It allows accurate measurement of hormones, drugs, *antibodies*, tumor markers, infectious agents, and many molecules whenever a ligand or an antibody for detection is available.

> For the measurement of *allergen*-specific *IgE* concentrations, allergen-coated particles or plates are exposed to a patient's serum and the allergen-bound IgE is detected by means of an enzyme-labeled anti-IgE antibody.

The addition of substrate results in the development of a color reaction, which is analyzed. In all ligand assay systems, a calibration curve using different known quantities of the substance of interest must be established. The amount of unknown allergen-specific antibodies is interpolated according to the standard curve. *Phadiatop* and the *CAP-system* are based on this principle.

EOSINOPHIL

Eosinophils are terminally differentiated *leukocytes* with a bilobed nucleus. They contain prominent *granules* which can be stained by the acidic dye eosin. This is due to the highly basic nature of the *eosinophil granule proteins*. Eosinophil growth and survival (see *eosinophil apoptosis*) is regulated by *IL-5*, but also by *IL-3* and *GM-CSF*. Eosinophil recruitment is mediated through several *endothelial adhesion molecules* including *ICAM-1* and *VLA-4*, and a variety of *chemokines* including *eotaxin*.

> Eosinophils are associated with responses to parasitic infection (see *parasitic diseases*), as well as *IgE*- and non-IgE-mediated *allergic diseases* (see *eosinophilia*).

In *asthma*, both circulating and airway eosinophil numbers are upregulated (see *eosinophil apoptosis*) and correlate with the severity of the disease. The specific mechanisms by which eosinophils contribute to *airway obstruction*, *allergic inflammation*, and *airway hyperresponsiveness* are not completely understood, but certainly require *eosinophil activation*.

EOSINOPHIL ACTIVATION

> *Eosinophils* have to be activated in order to be able to release products that directly participate in inflammatory tissue damage (see *epithelial damage*). Nonactivated eosinophils do not cause *inflammation*.

Eosinophils generate several cationic proteins (see *eosinophil granule proteins*), *oxygen metabolites*, *leukotrienes*, *platelet-activating factor* (PAF), and *cytokines* (see *eosinophil cytokines*) (see Table 40). For the production of *mediators* that promote inflammation, eosinophils are activated via specific cell-surface *receptors* (see *eosinophil surface molecules*). Important stimuli include *immunoglobulins*, *complement factors*, PAF, *adenosine*, FMLP, and cytokines. The activation of *signal transduction* pathways responsible for *degranulation*, *chemotaxis*, and *respiratory burst* is often mediated via *G protein-coupled receptors* and involves *phospholipase C* activation and *calcium mobilization*. Eosinophil priming (see *granulocyte priming*) enhances functional responses.

EOSINOPHIL APOPTOSIS

Although *apoptosis* is a physiologic form of cell death, it can be dysregulated and may then contribute to a number of pathogenic processes. For instance, in both eosinophilic and neutrophilic *inflammations*, apoptosis of inflammatory cells appears to be delayed (see *neutrophil apoptosis*).

> *Delayed apoptosis* is an important mechanism for accumulating *eosinophils* in allergic tissues (see *eosinophilia*).

Inhibition of apoptosis can be achieved by at least two mechanisms: (1) increased expression of eosinophil *survival factors* (e.g., *IL-5*), and (2) disruption of *death receptor*-mediated signals (see *TNF receptor superfamily*) (see Figure 26). For instance, it has been shown that *nitric oxide* (NO) and its second messenger (*cGMP*) disrupt *signal transduction* pathways initiated via the *Fas receptor* (APO-1, CD95).

TABLE 40
Mediators Released Following Eosinophil Activation

1. Eosinophil granule proteins
   Eosinophilic cationic protein (ECP)
   Eosinophil-derived neurotoxin (EDN)
   Eosinophil *peroxidase* (EPO)
   Major basic protein (MBP)
2. Lipid mediators
   Prostaglandins D2, E2, F2
   Leukotrienes A4, B4, C4, D4, E4
   15-HPETE
   15-HETE
   Platelet-activating factor (PAF)
   Thromboxane B2
3. Cytokines
   IL-1, IL-2, IL-3, IL-4, IL-5, IL-6, IL-8, IL-10, IL-12, IL-13, IL-16, GM-CSF, TNF-α, TGF-α, TGF-β,
   IFN-γ, RANTES, MIP-1α, PDGF-B, MIF, *NGF, eotaxin*
4. Reactive oxygen metabolites
   Superoxide anion (O_2^-)
   Hydrogen peroxide (H_2O_2)
5. Enzymes
   Hexosaminidase
   Arylsulfatase B
   Collagenase
   Histaminase
   Catalase
   β-Glucuronidase
   Acid phosphatase
   Gelatinase (MMP-9) (see *metalloproteases*)

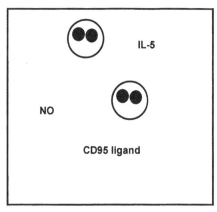

No inflammation

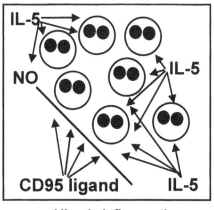

Allergic inflammation

FIGURE 26 Role of delayed apoptosis in eosinophilia. In normal tissues (left), only a few eosinophils are present. The expression of the eosinophil survival factor IL-5 and the death factor CD95 ligand is low. Concentrations of NO are also relatively low. Under these conditions, eosinophils rapidly die via apoptosis. In contrast, in allergic tissues (right), IL-5 is highly expressed and delays eosinophil apoptosis. This mechanism is important for the development of tissue eosinophilia. In spite of high CD95 ligand expression, eosinophils are often resistant toward CD95-mediated apoptosis because of high NO concentrations.

TABLE 41
A List of Agents Known to Induce or Inhibit
Granulocyte Apoptosis[a]

	Eosinophils	Neutrophils
Antiapoptotic signals		
IL-3	+	+
IL-5	+	−
GM-CSF	+	+
G-CSF	−	+
IFN-γ	+	+
Fibronectin	+	?
TNF-α[b]	+	−
TGF-β	−	+
Apoptotic signals		
Fas ligand	+	+
TNF-α[c]	−	+
TGF-β[c]	+	−
Survival factor withdrawal	+	+
Corticosteroids[d]	+	+
Theophylline[e]	+	?
CD69 ligand[b]	+	?
CD137 ligand[c]	+	+

[a] This list is not complete. *CD40 cross-linking* has been reported to inhibit eosinophil apoptosis. In contrast, *CD45 cross-linking* may induce apoptosis in eosinophils. Moreover, *IL-13* was reported to delay, whereas *IL-4* may induce eosinophil apoptosis. However, these are controversial findings. Therefore, the significance of these data is not completely clear at the moment, and they were excluded from the table.
[b] TNF-α indirectly delays eosinophil apoptosis in vitro via the induction of the GM-CSF *gene*.
[c] These signals may not directly activate apoptotic pathways; however, they may block survival signals.
[d] Corticosteroids inhibit survival factor synthesis, block *signal transduction* pathways, and directly induce eosinophil apoptosis. In neutrophils, they may block apoptosis at early time points, but at later time points it is clear that survival factor *signaling* is also blocked in these cells.
[e] Theophylline induces eosinophil apoptosis at low concentrations, but at higher concentrations it may block apoptosis.

Several *cytokines*, *mediators*, and drugs have been reported to influence *granulocyte* apoptosis in vitro. Table 41 summarizes some of the published data on this issue and compares the effects of these compounds on eosinophils and *neutrophils*.

EOSINOPHIL CATIONIC PROTEIN (ECP)

ECP is an important basic protein in the matrix of *eosinophil granules* (see *eosinophil granule proteins*).

> By installing small amounts of ECP into the airways of experimental animals, a pathology similar to human *asthma* has been observed.

This includes *epithelial damage* and basement membrane thickening (see *subepithelial fibrosis*). Indeed, it has been shown that ECP can stimulate *fibroblasts* (see *airway remodeling*). ECP can be released from eosinophils following *priming* with *cytokines* (*IL-3*, *IL-5*, *GM-CSF*) and stimulation via *complement factor* (e.g., *C5a*), lipid (e.g., *PAF*), and *immunoglobulin receptors* (IgA, *IgG*) (see *eosinophil activation*).

> ECP levels in serum, *sputum*, and in *nasal* or *bronchoalveolar lavage* (BAL) fluids have been measured (see *CAP-system*) to monitor eosinophilic *allergic inflammation*.

Using *immunohistochemistry*, *antibodies* against ECP are used to specifically detect eosinophils in tissues of patients with *allergic diseases*.

EOSINOPHIL CYTOKINES

It had been suggested that *eosinophils* have a limited capacity to transcribe (see *transcription*) and translate new proteins (see *translation*).

> It is now clear that the eosinophil is a transcriptionally active cell.

Among other *genes*, the eosinophils express important inflammatory and regulatory *cytokines* (see Table 40). However, in many cases, eosinophils express only marginal amounts of a certain cytokine. Moreover, in many studies the functional activity of the eosinophil-derived cytokines has not been demonstrated. Therefore, the in vivo significance of eosinophil cytokine generation for the inflammatory process in *asthma* and other *allergic diseases* is still not completely understood.

EOSINOPHIL CYTOLYSIS

In eosinophilic *inflammation* as seen in *nasal polyps* or skin of patients with *atopic dermatitis*, disrupted *eosinophils* might be observed.

> In contrast to *eosinophil apoptosis*, eosinophil cytolysis is a pathologic form of cell death, which demonstrates characteristic features of *necrosis*.

Eosinophil cytolysis is associated with the release of toxic *mediators* such as *eosinophil granule proteins* and reactive *oxygen metabolites*, and therefore causes additional inflammation. Eosinophil cytolysis might be the consequence of overactivation of eosinophils by inflammatory mediators.

EOSINOPHIL-DERIVED NEUROTOXIN (EDN)

(See *eosinophil granule proteins*.)

EOSINOPHIL GRANULE PROTEINS

Eosinophil granules contain several highly charged basic proteins including *major basic protein* (MBP), *eosinophil cationic protein* (ECP), eosinophil-derived neurotoxin (EDN), and eosinophil *peroxidase* (EPO). Other granule proteins are *β-glucuronidase*, acid phosphatase, and *arylsulfatase* B. MBP, ECP, EDN, and EPO are among the most basic proteins found in animals, due to their high content of the basic *amino acids* arginine and lysine.

> The eosinophil granule proteins are released upon *eosinophil activation* or due to *eosinophil cytolysis*, but not during *eosinophil apoptosis*.

The eosinophil granule proteins disrupt cell membranes. In this way, they cause the killing of parasites (see *parasitic diseases*), but also direct *epithelial damage* in human *asthma*.

EOSINOPHILIA

The term eosinophilia describes increased numbers of *eosinophils* in blood or tissue. Common causes of eosinophilia are parasitic infections (see *parasitic diseases*) and *allergic diseases*.

> Accumulation of eosinophils in tissues is at least partially due to inhibition of *eosinophil apoptosis*. In contrast, blood eosinophilia is mostly the consequence of increased eosinophil generation in the *bone marrow*.

Moreover, many authors suggest that a preferential recruitment of eosinophils would allow the specific accumulation of these cells in tissues (see *adhesion molecules*). In addition, some authors observed that the differentiation of *eosinophil progenitors* into mature eosinophils occurs at allergic inflammatory sites, and suggested that this mechanism may also contribute to the development of tissue eosinophilia.

High increases in blood eosinophil numbers (see *hypereosinophilia*) raise the possibility of complications such as *drug allergies* (see also *drug-induced eosinophilia*), *Churg–Strauss syndrome*, *T cell lymphoma*, or *allergic bronchopulmonary aspergillosis* (ABPA). Table 42 provides a more complete list of diseases that can be associated with eosinophilia.

TABLE 42
Diseases Associated with Eosinophilia

1. *Allergies*
   Rhinoconjunctivitis
   Asthma
   Atopic dermatitis
   Food allergy
   Drug allergy
2. *Parasitic diseases*
3. Vasculitis
   Churg–Strauss syndrome
   M. Wegener
   Panarteritis nodosa (see *allergic vasculitis*)
4. Pulmonary diseases
   Asthma
   Extrinsic allergic alveolitis
   Eosinophilic pneumonia
   Löffler syndrome
5. Gastrointestinal diseases
   Eosinophilic esophagitis
   Eosinophilic gastroenteritis
   Eosinophilic colitis
6. Cancer diseases
   T cell lymphoma
   Epithelial cancers
   Eosinophilic leukemia
   M. Hodgkin

EOSINOPHILIC GASTROENTERITIS

Eosinophilic *gastroenteritis* is characterized by *eosinophil* infiltration of the wall of the digestive tract (mainly the stomach and small intestine). The eosinophilic *inflammation* is followed by malabsorption, obstruction, and eosinophilic ascites. The disease is frequently associated with peripheral blood *eosinophilia*. The diagnosis is made by histologic examination. Since the eosinophilic infiltrates may be sporadic, multiple biopsies are often required. The differential diagnosis of the possible cause responsible for the eosinophilic inflammation of the gastrointestinal tract may include *food allergy, parasitic diseases, hypereosinophilic syndrome, T cell lymphoma*, and systemic *allergic vasculitis*. For treatment, *corticosteroids*, oral *cromoglycate*, and an *amino acid*-based elemental *diet* are recommended.

EOSINOPHILIC INFILTRATES

(See *Churg–Strauss syndrome*.)

EOSINOPHILIC INFILTRATION

The mechanisms of *eosinophil* infiltration and accumulation in tissues (see *eosinophilia*) include three important mechanisms: (1) increased production in the *bone marrow,* and perhaps at the inflammatory site (see *eosinophil progenitors*), (2) preferential recruitment (see *adhesion molecules*) and *chemotaxis* (see *eotaxin, RANTES*, and *IL-16*), and (3) delayed *eosinophil apoptosis*.

EOSINOPHILIC PNEUMONIA

Eosinophilic pneumonia is an *eosinophilic infiltration* and *edema* within the alveolar spaces, bronchial wall, and interstitium.

Depending on the clinical course of the disease, two forms can be distinguished: acute and chronic eosinophilic pneumonia. In both forms, strong *eosinophil activation* with subsequent *exocytosis* of *eosinophil granule proteins* is observed.

Acute eosinophilic pneumonia

Patients have severe hypoxia, high fever, pleuritic chest pain, and myalgia. The chest X-ray reveals intensive alveolar and interstitial infiltrates involving all lobes.

The *bronchoalveolar lavage* (BAL) fluid contains many *eosinophils* (>25%). In contrast, no blood *eosinophilia* is found.

The etiology of the disease is unknown. However, acute *hypersensitivity* reactions to an unidentified inhaled *aeroallergen* have been suggested. A similar rapid *granulocyte* influx is seen in the adult respiratory distress syndrome; however, in this case *neutrophil* infiltration is observed. Patients with acute eosinophilic pneumonia usually respond to high doses of *corticosteroids*.

Chronic eosinophilic pneumonia

Patients present with *cough*, fever, *dyspnea*, and weight loss; 50% of the patients have *intrinsic asthma*. Chest X-ray and computer tomography show a peripheral distribution of shadowing.

In contrast to the acute form of eosinophilic pneumonia, patients demonstrate *leukocytosis* and blood eosinophilia, suggesting increased eosinophil production in the *bone marrow.*

Most patients respond well to corticosteroid therapy, which should be continued for at least 6 months. In some patients, chronic eosinophilic pneumonia may progress into *Churg–Strauss syndrome*.

EOSINOPHIL PEROXIDASE (EPO)

(See *eosinophil granule proteins* and *peroxidase*.)

EOSINOPHIL PROGENITORS

Eosinophils and *basophils* share a common late-stage progenitor, which is called Eo/B-colony forming unit. Commitment to eosinophil and basophil lineages appears to be regulated by *IL-3, IL-5,* and *GM-CSF. Allergic inflammation* is often associated with high expression of IL-5, which may reach the *bone marrow,* where it stimulates production of eosinophils. In this process, it is possible that some eosinophil progenitors leave the bone marrow and are subsequently recruited to allergic inflammatory sites. For instance, eosinophil progenitors have been identified in *nasal polyps,* where the process of production of mature eosinophils continues. It has been suggested that this process contributes to the development of tissue *eosinophilia.*

EOSINOPHIL SURFACE MOLECULES

Eosinophils express a large number of known *surface molecules* (see Table 43). Many of them are listed within the *CD antigen* classification. *Cross-linking* of many *receptors* induces functional responses, such as *degranulation, respiratory burst, cytokine* or *leukotriene* generation, or *delayed apoptosis.* Whereas most of the surface molecules are shared with other cells, *IL-5* and *eotaxin* receptors are almost selectively found on eosinophils. Normal eosinophils do not express *CD16,* which is expressed on *neutrophils,* allowing purification of eosinophils by negative selection from mixed *granulocyte* populations.

EOTAXIN

Eotaxins 1, 2, and 3 represent a family of *CC chemokines* that specifically activate *eosinophils* and *basophils,* but not *neutrophils.*

All eotaxins bind to the same *chemokine receptor.* Eotaxin is expressed in allergic inflammatory tissues (see Table 44). Therefore, eotaxin represents an important *chemotactic factor* for eosinophils contributing to tissue *eosinophilia* in *allergic diseases.* After eosinophil priming (see *granulocyte priming*), eotaxin is also able to stimulate *exocytosis* (see *eosinophil activation*). Originally described as a specific eosinophil factor, the specificity of eotaxin appears to be broader. Besides eosinophils and basophils, embryogenic *mast cell* progenitors may also respond to eotaxin. There are controversial findings regarding the expression of eotaxin *receptors* on *Th2 cells.*

EPIDERMAL BARRIER

The epidermal barrier (see *epidermis*) of the stratum corneum may be thought of as a wall formed by brick and mortar, with protein-enriched corneocytes being the bricks and lipid-enriched intercellular material being the mortar. Artificial damage to this barrier (e.g., with repetitive Scotch tape stripping) leads to an increased transepidermal water loss and an increased uptake of *allergens* (also drugs) from the environment.

In *atopic dermatitis* patients, dry-looking skin (see *dry skin*) with an increased transepidermal water loss is present in predilection and nonpredilection sites.

EPIDERMIS

The epidermis is the first, uppermost layer of the skin. As shown by dermatohistopathology, there are four layers of the epidermis: a basal cell layer or "stratum basale," a prickle cell layer or "stratum spinosum," a granular layer or "stratum granulosum," and the uppermost horny layer or "stratum corneum." The *keratinocytes* originate from the basal cell layer and migrate upward while changing their morphology and keratin program within the respective layers.

TABLE 43
Eosinophil Surface Molecules[a]

Subgroup	Surface Molecule	Ligand
	Complement Receptors (CRs)	
	C3aR	*C3a*
	C5aR (CD88)	*C5a*
	CR1 (CD35)	C3b
	CR3 (CD11b/CD18)	C3bi, *ICAM-1*
	P150, 95 (CD11c/CD18)	C3bi
	CD46	C3b, C4b
	CD55	C3b
	CD59	C8, C9
	Cytokine Receptors	
	IL-1R (CD121b)	*IL-1*
	IL-2R (CD25[b], CD122, CD132)	*IL-2*
	IL-3R (CD123, CD131)	*IL-3*
	IL-4R (CD124, CD132)	*IL-4*
	IL-5R (CD125[c], CD131)	*IL-5*
	GM-CSFR (CD116, CD131)	*GM-CSF*
	IFN-α,βR (CD118)	*IFN-α*, IFN-β
	IFN-γR (CD119)	*IFN-γ*
	TNFR (CD120a, CD120b)	*TNF*
	FasR (CD95)	*Fas ligand*
	TRAILR	TRAIL
	CCR1[c]	*MIP-1α, RANTES MCP-2, MCP-3*
	CCR3[c]	*RANTES, Eotaxin*, MCP-2, MCP-3, MCP-4
	Adhesion Molecules	
	Immunoglobulin superfamily	
	ICAM-1 (CD54)[b]	CD11a/CD18 (*LFA-1*)
	ICAM-3 (CD50)	CD11a/CD18
	LFA-3 (CD58)	*CD2*
	PECAM-1 (CD31)	*Heparin* sulfate
	Integrins	
	LFA-1 (CD11a/CD18)	ICAM-1, ICAM-2, ICAM-3
	Mac-1 (CD11b/CD18)	ICAM-1, C3bi
	P150, 95 (CD11c/CD18)	C3bi
	αdβ2	ICAM-3
	α4β1, *VLA-4* (CD49d/CD29)[c]	*VCAM-1, fibronectin*
	α6β1, VLA-6 (CD49f/CD29)	*Laminin*
	α4β7	MAdCAM-1, VCAM-1, fibronectin
	Selectins	
	L-selectin	GlyCAM-1, CD34
	Others	
	PSGL-1	*P-selectin*
	Sialyl-Lewis[x] (CD15)	E-selectin, P-selectin
	Sialyl-dimeric Lewis[x]	E-selectin
	Leukosialin (CD43)	ICAM-1
	Pgp-1 (*CD44*)	Hyaluronic acid

TABLE 43 (continued)
Eosinophil Surface Molecules[a]

Subgroup	Surface Molecule	Ligand

Enzymes

	Tyrosine phosphatase (CD45)	
	P24 kinase (CD9)[c]	FcγRIIa
	Aminopeptidase N (CD13)	

Immunoglobulin Receptors

	FcαR (CD89)	IgA
	FcγRI (CD64)[b/c]	*IgG*
	FcγRII (CD32)	IgG
	FcγRIII (CD16)[b]	IgG
	εBP (Mac-2)	*IgE*

Lipid and Other Inflammatory Mediator Receptors

	PAFR	*PAF*
	LTB_4R	LTB_4 (see *leukotrienes*)
	$LTC_4/D_4/E_4R$	LTC_4, LTD_4, LTE_4
	PGER	PGE (see *prostaglandins*)
	Histamine receptor	*Histamine*
	fMLPR	fMLP

MHC Molecules

	MHC class I	*CD8*
	MHC class II[b]	*CD4*

Other Surface Molecules

	CD52	Unknown
	CD63	Unknown
	CD69[b]	Unknown
	β-Adrenergic receptors	*Adrenaline, noradrenaline*

[a] This list is not complete. *High-* and *low-affinity IgE receptors*, as well as functional *IL-8* receptors, have also been reported on eosinophils. However, these are controversial findings. Therefore, the significance of these data is not completely clear at the moment, and they were excluded from the table.

[b] These molecules are expressed upon activation only.

[c] These molecules are not expressed by neutrophils.

TABLE 44
Eotaxin-Producing Cells

Epithelial cells
Endothelial cells
Fibroblasts
Eosinophils
Th1 cells
Th2 cells

The epidermal transit time of keratinocytes in normal human skin is about 1 month, whereas it may be reduced to 4 days in inflammatory human skin, such as when psoriasis is present.

More than 90% of the normal human epidermal cells consists of keratinocytes, the remainder being melanocytes, *Langerhans cells*, and Merkel cells.

Functional aspects of the epidermis involve the retention of water inside the body and a barrier of defense against bacterial, viral, chemical, or physical pathogens. In inflammatory skin diseases such as *atopic dermatitis*, the function of the *epidermal barrier* is decreased.

EPINEPHRINE

A catecholamine produced by the adrenal medulla (also known as *adrenaline*).

EPISTASIS

This means that the expression of *genes* at one *locus* depends upon the *genotype* at another locus (gene interaction).

EPITHELIAL CELL

Epithelial cells in the airways can be ciliated (see *cilia*) or nonciliated (see *Clara cells* and *goblet cells*). The traditional view of the bronchial epithelium was that of a passive physical barrier to the external environment.

Epithelial cells play an important role in the regulation of airway *inflammation*.

For instance, epithelial cells are able to generate *cytokines*, lipid *mediators*, and reactive *oxygen metabolites*, and may therefore contribute to the *recruitment of inflammatory cells*, as well as *apoptosis* regulation and effector functions of these cells. Table 45 summarizes cytokines, including *chemokines*, which have been shown to be expressed by bronchial epithelial cells under inflammatory conditions.

TABLE 45
Epithelial-Derived Cytokines and Chemokines

1. Colony-stimulating factors	*GM-CSF*, *G-CSF*, M-CSF, CSF-1
2. Growth factors	TGF-α, *TGF-β, SCF*, bFGF
3. Other cytokines	*IL-1*, *IL-6*, *IL-10*, IL-11, *IL-16*, *TNF-α*
4. *CXC chemokines*	*IL-8*, GRO-α, GRO-γ
5. *CC chemokines*	*Eotaxin*, *RANTES*, *MCP-1*, MCP-4, *MIP-1α*

Bronchial epithelial cells can also express *MHC class II molecules* and may, therefore, like other epithelial cells such as *keratinocytes* or *M cells*, be able to function as *antigen-presenting cells* (APCs). However, their capacity to present *antigen* might be very limited compared to *dendritic cells*.

Besides their role in maintaining inflammation, it appears that epithelial cells have antiinflammatory properties.

Such *immunosuppressive mechanisms* are important for the limitation and resolution of inflammatory processes (see *resolution of inflammation*). For instance, neutral metalloen-dopeptidase 24.11 and aminopeptidase M reduce the effects of *peptide* mediators by actively degrading them. Substrates of these peptidases include *tachykinins* and *bradykinin*. Rapid degradation of these mediators may limit *airway obstruction* in *asthma*. In addition, epithelial cells produce a range of protease inhibitors that can prevent tissue damage (see *epithelial damage*) by enzymes such as elastase, *cathepsin G*, or *chymase*.

EPITHELIAL DAMAGE

Shedding of *epithelial cells* in *asthma* was described in the 19th century. Clusters of epithelial cells can be found in the *sputum* and are often referred to as Creola bodies.

> Epithelial damage is a feature of all grades of asthma and is seen even in patients with extremely mild disease.

The surface layers of the epithelium strip off, leaving a thin layer of basal cells attached to the basement membrane. The mechanism of epithelial damage is not entirely clear, but it is known that *eosinophil granule proteins* (such as *eosinophilic cationic protein*) cause shedding of the epithelium in animal models, at concentrations that are found in human airways. Moreover, *nitric oxide* (NO) and reactive *oxygen metabolites* may also directly damage airway tissue.

> Epithelial damage is thought to contribute to the irritability of the airway that is manifested clinically as *airway hyperresponsiveness*.

EPITOPE

An epitope is a single antigenic determinant of a segment or a portion of an *antigen* that binds to the *antibody* or *T cell antigen receptor*. The *T cell* and *B cell epitopes* were found to be distinct. In principle, *B cells* recognize *conformational epitopes* that are related to the structure of an antigen, whereas *T cells* recognize linear *amino acid* sequences (*linear epitopes*, see also *epitope mapping*) that are processed and presented by *antigen-presenting cells* (APCs).

EPITOPE MAPPING

T cell epitope mapping is the process of determining the dominant T cell binding sequences (= *epitopes*) of an *allergen* or *antigen*. In order to become activated, *T cells* have to recognize processed *antigenic peptides* (see *antigen recognition*) presented in the antigen-binding groove of *MHC class II molecules* of *antigen-presenting cells* (APCs), and at the same time receive obligatory co-stimulatory signals (see *co-stimulation*). By the nature of antigen presentation via MHC class II molecules, where short (13 to 17-mer) *peptides* are presented to the *T cell antigen receptor*, linear sequences constitute the majority of important T cell epitopes (see *linear epitopes*). Most strategies involve purifying or cloning allergenic material (see *cloning of allergens*), *amino acid* sequencing it (see *primary structure*), and manufacturing a series of short overlapping peptide sequences.

> Overlapping peptides are tested for their ability to induce *CD4+ T cell proliferation* from *peripheral blood mononuclear cells* (PBMC) or *T cell clones*, which exhibit that allergen specificity.

B cells and *immunoglobulins* recognize larger *conformational epitopes* because their antigen binding structures are considerably larger than those of the *major histocompatibility complex* (MHC), but similar methods can be adopted to define them. Major epitopes have been mapped for *house-dust mite* (Der p 1 and Der p 2), *pollen, animal dander, fungal allergens*, as well as food and bee venom allergens (see *food* and *hymenoptera allergy*).

EROSION

One of the basic dermatologic lesions, defined as a loss of the *epidermis*, which heals without scarring.

ERS

European Respiratory Society.

ERYTHEMA

One of the basic dermatologic lesions, defined as a nonpalpable redness of the skin produced by vascular congestion or perfusion.

ERYTHEMA EXSUDATIVUM MULTIFORME (EEM)

EEM is a clinically defined reaction pattern of the skin with characteristically target-shaped lesions, predominantly on the hands and lower arms. A recurrent subtype of EEM is frequently associated with a preceding herpes simplex virus infection (postherpetic EEM). In all these cases, any fresh episode of herpes should be treated with antiviral chemotherapy (e.g., acyclovir) immediately. In severe and recurrent cases, acyclovir prophylaxis should be considered.

ERYTHEMA MULTIFORME

(See *erythema exsudativum multiforme*.)

ERYTHEMA NODOSUM

Erythema nodosum is a clinically defined reaction pattern of the skin with extremely painful cutaneous–subcutaneous nonulcerating nodules and a histological correlate of septal panniculitis. Besides *sarcoidosis*, a wide spectrum of bacterial, viral, and fungal agents as well as various drugs have been described as causative for these skin lesions. A basic workup should include a drug history, laboratory parameters for *inflammation*, and a chest X-ray for exclusion of sarcoidosis.

EUROGLYPHUS

Genus of *house-dust mite*. Along with the genus *Dermatophagoides*, species of Euroglyphus, especially E. maynei, are a common component of the indoor environment (see *allergens* and *aeroallergens*).

EUROPEAN NETWORK ON ASPIRIN-INDUCED ASTHMA (AIANE)

A group of European scientists formed a network to investigate pathogenic mechanisms in *aspirin-sensitive asthma*. They have established the so-called AIANE database, in which clinical data of more than 450 aspirin-sensitive patients are registered.

EXACERBATION OF ASTHMA

(See *asthma exacerbation*.)

EXCORIATION

An excoriation is any loss of substance of skin produced by scratching, which reaches the dermal layer.

EXERCISE-INDUCED ASTHMA (EIA)

EIA is a transitory *airway obstruction* which follows exercise or participation in sports.

It occurs in patients with *asthma*, but it has also been reported in nonasthmatic individuals, in particular in athletes. EIA is more frequently associated with moderate to severe asthma, and it occurs more often in asthmatics whose *lung function tests* are below the normal predicted values. In children, EIA appears to be an early manifestation of asthma and needs a careful check-up. EIA is enhanced after exposure to *allergens* during the *pollen* season or to environmental *pollutants* (e.g., *sulfur dioxide*). The magnitude of airway obstruction is also influenced by the climate. Breathing cool and dry air increases the severity of EIA.

The *bronchoconstriction* in EIA is caused by water loss from the respiratory tract.

There are two main hypotheses to explain EIA. The first one favors vascular hyperemia and airway obstruction following mucosal cooling and rapid rewarming. The second hypothesis describes airway *smooth muscle* contraction subsequent to *mediator* release from *mast cells* (e.g., *leukotrienes*) following mucosal dehydration and increased osmolarity.

Diagnosis
The diagnosis can often be made on the patient's history. Moreover, a fall of >15% of the pre-exercise values in *peak expiratory flow rate* (PEFR) and *forced expiratory volume* (FEV_1) following exercise is regarded as diagnostic. The major drop in lung function occurs 5 to 10 minutes after stopping exercise. EIA is considered to be mild if there is a 10 to 25% drop in PEF/FEV_1, moderate up to 50%, and severe when the drop is >50%. A post-exercise drop in the *forced expiratory flow* (FEF_{25-75}) over 26% also indicates EIA. Different types of exercise (e.g., bicycling, running) under laboratory conditions can be used to assess the severity of EIA. Medications that could affect the test should be withheld (short-acting *β2-agonists* for 6 hours, long-acting β2-agonists for 24 hours, *corticosteroids* in the morning of the test day, *cromoglycates* for 6 hours, *antihistamines* for 48 hours).

Therapy
EIA can be prevented or reversed by *bronchodilator* medication, especially β2-agonists. Cromoglycate and *nedocromil* protect against EIA if given before exercise. Long-term treatment with corticosteroids may decrease the incidence of EIA. *Leukotriene antagonists* have also been reported to be effective. EIA in asthmatics results in unfitness when patients avoid exercise. Although it is uncertain whether physical training significantly decreases *airway hyperresponsiveness*, it can restore normal levels of fitness. Asthmatics should choose the right sport (e.g., swimming), prepare with a warm-up period, and use an appropriate medication just before starting exercise.

EXERCISE-INDUCED BRONCHOSPASM

(See *exercise-induced asthma*.)

EXOCYTOSIS

Mast cells, *eosinophils*, *basophils*, and *neutrophils* have the regulated ability to release preformed secretory *granule* constituents to the extracellular environment as the result of fusion of the granule membranes with the plasma membrane. This process is termed exocytosis or degranulation.

As it is highly energetically unfavorable, exocytosis takes place only at a very slow rate in unstimulated cells.

In order to overcome this energy hurdle, cells must synthesize either specialized proteins or lipids that can form non-bilayer membrane structures, which facilitate membrane fusion but do not result in loss of integrity of either the plasma membrane or granule membrane. Recent work suggests that a number of physiologically relevant lipids, called "fusogens," can act in this capacity.

> The activation of *signal transduction* pathways responsible for exocytosis is often mediated via
> *G protein-coupled receptors* and involves *phospholipase C* activation and *calcium mobilization*.

However, additional *priming* is usually required. Important ligands, which frequently stimulate exocytosis, include *complement factors* and several *lipid mediators*. In mast cells, *allergens* stimulated mediator release by *cross-linking* of the *high-affinity IgE receptor* (see also *endocytosis*).

EXOGEN-ALLERGIC ALVEOLITIS

(See *extrinsic allergic alveolitis*.)

EXON

This is a *DNA* sequence of a *gene*, which is present in mature *RNA*.

EXPERIMENTAL ALLERGIC ENCEPHALOMYELITIS (EAE)

EAE is a *CD4+ T-cell*-mediated disease of the central *nervous system* induced in rodents by the injection of myelin basic protein (MBP; please note that for the *eosinophil*-derived *major basic protein* the same abbreviation is used), and is used as a model for multiple sclerosis (MS) in humans. MS is an inflammatory autoimmune disease (see *autoimmunity*) of the central nervous system.

> T cell clones derived from MS patients specific for MBP are *Th1 cells*.

Moreover, Th1, but not *Th2*, cells are able to transfer EAE. Spontaneous recovery correlates with the appearance of Th2 *cytokines*. Treatment with *IL-4*, *IL-10*, Th2-*T cell clones* (see *cytokine therapy*), or neutralizing anti-*TNF-α* or anti-*IL-12 antibodies* (see *antibody therapy* and *anticytokine therapy*) ameliorates the disease.

EXPOSITION TEST

A test for *allergy* or *intolerance* that exposes the original target organ of the reaction (e.g., conjunctiva, nasal mucosa, bronchial or gastrointestinal system) with the supposed causative agent of allergic or pseudoallergic reactions. Exposition tests give more reliable information as compared to skin testing or in vitro *IgE* diagnostics (see *RAST, Phadiatop, CAP-system*), but are laborious to perform and have a higher risk of systemic reaction (see *anaphylaxis*) for the patient. Therefore, *skin tests* should always precede exposition tests. There are standard procedures described for exposition tests with *food additives*, preservatives, *antibiotics*, and *nonsteroidal antiinflammatory drugs* (NSAID) (see also *allergen challenge* and *bronchial provocation tests*).

EXTRACELLULAR MATRIX

The extracellular matrix (= intercellular tissue matrix) is a framework of a heterogenous group of proteins and glucoproteins that provides mechanical support to tissues. Besides that, the extracellular matrix guides the localization, *migration*, differentiation, and activation of inflammatory cells. For instance, matrix proteins (e.g., *fibronectin*) can stimulate specific *adhesion molecules*. Moreover, the matrix can accumulate inflammatory *mediators* as complexes with matrix components (e.g., *TGF-β*). At least some components of the extracellular matrix undergo specific changes in *asthma* (see *airway remodeling* and *subepithelial fibrosis*). Extracellular matrix proteins can be degraded by *metalloproteases*.

EXTRINSIC ALLERGIC ALVEOLITIS (EAA)

People who work with hay, especially moldy hay, can become sensitized to thermophilic actinomycetes (see *fungal allergens*), which cause an *immune complex* reaction (see *Coombs and Gell classification*, type III) as well as cell-mediated responses (*delayed hypersensitivity*, type IV) in the parenchyma of the lung.

> Patients may present with an acute illness or with a more chronic form of *allergic alveolitis*.

The acute form is relatively easy to recognize; the patient experiences repeated episodes of influenza-like illness accompanied by *cough* and breathlessness a few hours after exposure to the relevant dust. The systemic features tend to dominate, including malaise, fever, aches, pains, headaches, anorexia, and tiredness. If the patients exert themselves, they will notice a dry cough and difficulty in taking a deep breath. In the *bronchoalveolar lavage* (BAL) fluid, many *granulocytes* are found at this stage.

The chronic form is more difficult to identify and in some ways more serious, because the patient develops gradual loss of effort tolerance due to diffuse *pulmonary fibrosis*. Immunophenotyping of BAL *lymphocytes* (see *flow cytometry*) often helps to establish the diagnosis.

> EAA is associated with an accumulation of *CD8⁺ T cells* in the lung.

Moreover, increased *NK cell* numbers are also often observed. Once the fibrosis is established, it can be very difficult to eradicate it, and the patient could proceed to develop *hypoxia* and pulmonary hypertension, eventually leading to right heart failure. Chronic EAA is more often seen in patients who keep birds, e.g., budgerigars or pigeons (see *pigeon fancier's lung*), than in farm workers. This is thought to be due to the chronic low level of exposure as opposed to the acute high level of exposure seen in farmers. In addition to the thermophilic actinomycetes associated with farmer's lung, a huge range of microorganisms, animal proteins, chemicals, and vegetable dusts have been associated with forms of EAA. Most of these are occupational diseases and are recognized in the context of affected workers.

EXTRINSIC ASTHMA

This is another term for *allergic asthma*. Extrinsic *asthma* is the result of external causes such as *aeroallergens*. The converse is *intrinsic asthma*.

EXTRINSIC ATOPIC DERMATITIS

This is the common subtype of *atopic dermatitis*. In contrast to *intrinsic atopic dermatitis*, the patients demonstrate positive *prick tests* toward *allergens* and have high allergen-specific (see *RAST*, *Phadiatop*, and *CAP-system*) and total *IgE levels* in serum.

EXUDATION

Exudation is defined as the penetration of serum through the skin to the skin surface, a frequent event in acute *dermatitis*. The subsequent drying of the exudate leads to formation of *crusts* covering the inflammatory skin.

F

Fab

Fab is the fragment of an *antibody* that contains an *antigen*-binding site. It consists of a light chain and an enzyme-digested part of an *immunoglobulin* (Ig) heavy chain.

FAMILIAL

This term is used to describe any condition that is more common in relatives of an affected individual than in the general population.

FARMER'S LUNG

(See *extrinsic allergic alveolitis*.)

Fas LIGAND

Fas ligand is a 40-kDa cell surface glycoprotein belonging to the *TNF superfamily* of *cytokines*. It activates cells via the *Fas receptor* to induce *apoptosis*.

Fas ligand is expressed by *T cells* after several days of activation.

Fas ligand is also expressed by cells in immune "privileged" tissues (e.g., Sertoli cells in the testis, corneal epithelium in the eye, tumor cells — see *immune surveillance*). There are efforts to express Fas ligand in transplants to prevent rejection. Interestingly, Fas ligand itself transduces signals into cells (e.g., cell cycle arrest in T cells).

Fas RECEPTOR (APO-1, CD95)

The Fas *receptor* is a 45-kDa cell surface *death receptor* and belongs to the *TNF receptor superfamily*.

Fas receptors are expressed by many cells; however, not all cells are susceptible to killing.

Functional Fas receptors (see *functional receptors*) are expressed by *T cells* when they become activated during an *immune response*. Functional Fas receptors are also expressed by *neutrophils*, *eosinophils*, and *mast cells*. *Cross-linking* of Fas receptors by cells expressing *Fas ligand* results in *caspase* activation and subsequent *apoptosis* in susceptible cells. This apoptotic process appears to be important in the downregulation of an immune response (see *resolution of inflammation* and *immunosuppressive mechanisms*). Defects in Fas receptor expression or functional Fas receptor resistance by activated T cells may result in *T cell lymphoma* and *hypereosinophilia*.

Fc

Fc is the fraction of an *antibody* that functions for binding to antibody *receptors* (see *Fc receptor*) and *complement factor* C1$_q$.

Fc RECEPTOR

The Fc *receptor* is a receptor for the *Fc* piece of various *immunoglobulin* (Ig) *isotypes*. They include *IgG* and *IgE* receptors (see *Fcγ receptors, FcεRI*, and *FcεRII*).

FcεRI

(See *high-affinity IgE receptor.*)

FcεRII/*CD23*

(See *low-affinity IgE receptor.*)

Fcγ RECEPTORS

They include FcγRI, RII, and RIII, and bind the *Fc* domain of *IgG antibodies*. Most Fcγ *receptors* only bind aggregated IgG, allowing them to discriminate bound antibody from free IgG. They are expressed on *phagocytes, B cells, natural killer cells*, and follicular *dendritic cells*. Fcγ receptors play a key role in humoral immunity, linking antibody binding to effector cell functions.

FENOTEROL

Fenoterol is a *β2-agonist.*

FEV₁

FEV_1

(See *forced expiratory volume in first second.*)

FIBROBLASTS

Fibroblasts are structural cells that produce important components of the *extracellular matrix*. The recognition of the basement membrane thickening (see *subepithelial fibrosis*) in *asthma* led to the search for the origin of this material.

> Specialized fibroblasts (*myofibroblasts*) produce increased amounts of subepithelial *collagen* in asthmatic subjects.

Fibroblasts from different anatomical locations, and sometimes from the same tissue, can be heterogeneous in terms of collagen production, proliferation rate, morphology, response to specific inflammatory *mediators*, accumulation of intracellular lipids, and expression of cell *surface molecules* including *integrins*. *Mast cells* affect fibroblast properties and hence modulate the process of tissue *remodeling*. For instance, *histamine, heparin, tryptase*, and mast cell-derived *IL-4* and *TGF* stimulate fibroblast proliferation and collagen synthesis. In contrast, therapeutically applied *IFN-γ* may inactivate fibroblasts in *cryptogenic fibrosing alveolitis.*

FIBRONECTIN

In addition to *collagen* and *laminin*, fibronectin is an important component of the *extracellular matrix*, which stimulates *T cells* and *eosinophils* via β1-*integrins*. For instance, fibronectin contributes to delayed *eosinophil apoptosis* in *allergic diseases* associated with *eosinophilia.*

FIBROSIS

Fibrosis is a pathologic condition associated with deposition of increased amounts of *collagen* and other *extracellular matrix* proteins that are produced by *fibroblasts*.

> Several lines of evidence suggest that *mast cells* participate in the activation of fibroblasts.

Fibrotic processes are seen in many diseases associated with *allergic inflammation*, including *asthma* (see *airway remodeling*) and *atopic dermatitis*. However, clinical fibrotic situations are also seen in nonallergic diseases such as cirrhosis of the liver, *cryptogenic fibrosing alveolitis*, *scleroderma*, *graft-versus-host disease* (GVHD), or *wound healing*.

FILARIASIS

Infection by Onchocerca volvulus (river blindness), Wuchereria bancrofti, and Brugia malayi (lymphatic filiariasis) account for most human filarial disease (see *parasitic diseases*). The *immune response* is characterized by *IgE*-mediated *immediate hypersensitivity*, but this response appears to be polyclonal since much of the specificity of the IgE is not directed at parasite *antigens*. *Th2 cytokine* production dominates *T cell* responses, and high levels of *IL-5* induce filarial-associated *eosinophilia*. Allergic reactivity to parasite antigens is rare, and high levels of *IgG* subclasses may account for this. Inability to clear an infection is related to the ability of the parasite to induce immune hyporesponsiveness by mechanisms which may involve specific *anergy*, active suppression by *monocytes*, suppressor T cell activity, or soluble suppressive parasite products (see *immunosuppressive mechanisms*).

FINN CHAMBERS

Finn chambers are a common system used to apply *allergens* in *patch tests*. The chambers consist of small aluminum discs mounted on a nonocclusive, hypoallergenic tape.

FISH ALLERGY

Fish is one of the most common allergenic foods (see *food allergy*). The consumption of fish or inhalation of cooking vapors from fish frequently cause *IgE*-mediated *immediate hypersensitivity* reactions. Molecular characterization of the codfish *allergen* Gad c 1 revealed that the molecule is parvalbumin. The existence of structurally related parvalbumins in different fish species may explain cross-reactivity in fish-allergic individuals (see *cross-reacting allergens*).

FIXED DRUG ERUPTION (FDE)

An FDE is an adverse cutaneous reaction to an ingested drug (see *drug allergy*), characterized by the formation of solitary, sometimes multiple, skin lesions. The morphology of the lesion ranges from a dusky-red to violaceous plaque to a bulla or an erosion.

> Upon rechallenge with the drug, the FDE recurs at the identical skin site within hours and persists for a few weeks.

Lesions are usually asymptomatic but may be pruritic or burning. The diagnosis is often made following an accidental rechallenge with the drug. Patch testing (see *patch test*) with the drug at the site of the lesion may give positive results.

FK506

(See *tacrolimus*.)

FLAP

(See *5-lipoxygenase activating protein*.)

FLEXURAL ECZEMA

The most important manifestation form of *atopic dermatitis* in adult patients.

FLOUR ALLERGENS

The majority of cases of *baker's asthma* are related to wheat, rye, and barley. The water-soluble albumin and globulin fractions as well as wheat *α-amylase inhibitor protein* were identified as *major allergens* of wheat flour.

FLOW CYTOMETRY

Method for measuring the expression of surface and intracellular proteins using fluorescence-labeled *antibodies* and a flow cytometer. For instance, the numbers of *CD4+* and *CD8+ T cells*, *B cells*, or *NK cells* can be determined in blood and *bronchoalveolar lavage* (BAL) fluids for clinical diagnosis (e.g., *extrinsic allergic alveolitis, sarcoidosis, T cell lymphoma, acquired immunodeficiency syndrome*).

FLOW VOLUME LOOP

A representation of the forced expiratory and inspiratory maneuvers plotting the flow of air in liters per second against the volume expired. The expiratory part of the flow volume loop is useful for diagnosing mild forms of *airflow obstruction*, while the inspiratory part of the loop is used mainly to study central airways and obstruction due to tracheal tumors or extrathoracic obstructions such as retrosternal goiters (see *lung function tests*).

FLUNISOLIDE

A powerful topical *corticosteroid*.

FLUORESCENT IN SITU HYBRIDIZATION (FISH)

This is a special form of *in situ hybridization* that is used to determine the chromosomal localization of a *gene*.

FLUTICASONE

This is an *inhaled corticosteroid* (ICS) which is almost completely metabolized during its first pass through the liver.

FOOD ADDITIVES

Several chemicals are used as preservatives, antioxidants (bisulfites, metabisulfites, see *sulfites*), colorings (tatrazine), or flavor enhancers (glutamate) in foods or drugs. They can cause non-*IgE*-mediated *adverse food* or *drug reactions*. They may play a role in chronic *urticaria* or provoke *airway obstruction* in patients with *asthma*.

FOOD ALLERGY

Food *allergy* is defined as a pathologic immune reaction to food or food components. Food allergy can result in one or a number of interrelated signs and symptoms including *urticaria* or erythematous flares, eczematous lesions (see *eczema*), vomiting, diarrhea, abdominal colics, laryngeal *edema, rhinitis, airway obstruction*, and *wheeze. Anaphylactic reactions* have been reported after ingestion of peanuts (see *peanut allergy*), seeds, seafood (see *Crustacea* and *fish allergy*), eggs (see *egg allergy*), and *celery*.

The most common food allergy reaction is the *oral allergy syndrome*, which resembles a contact urticaria of the lips and the oropharynx.

The oral allergy syndrome can often be seen in patients with allergies against *pollen* that cross-react with fruits, nuts, vegetables, or spices (see *cross-reacting allergens*).

Mechanisms

The role of *IgE*-mediated reactions in food allergy is best established. However, there is some evidence that *IgG, immune complexes* (see *Coombs and Gell classification*, type III), or cell-mediated mechanisms (*delayed hypersensitivity*, type IV) may also provoke food allergy. Although sharing some common endpoints, it is distinct from *food intolerance* or toxic reactions. It can be difficult to identify the *allergens* due to primary food processing in the stomach and intestine before absorption. *T cell sensitization* is thought to occur across damaged or immature intestinal mucosa or via specialized *M cells* in *gut-associated lymphoid tissues* (GALT) in susceptible individuals.

Diagnosis

The diagnosis is based on the patient's history. Diet diaries (see *allergy diet*) may help to review the relationship between the symptoms and the ingested food. Skin *prick tests* using food extracts (see *allergen extracts*) or fresh food, and the measurement of specific IgE levels (see *CAP-system, Phadiatop, RAST*) should be done. To prove the relevance of positive or negative test results, food *provocation tests* are suitable (see *allergen challenge* or *exposition test*). The double-blind placebo-controlled *food challenge* test is here the gold standard. Food challenge tests are not recommended in cases of clear history and diagnostic results, as well as after severe, anaphylactic reactions following an isolated ingestion of a specific food.

Therapy

Avoiding relevant food allergens is the only therapeutic tool (see *allergen avoidance*). After severe reactions, a set of emergency medications (*corticosteroids, antihistamines, adrenaline*) should be prescribed.

FOOD CHALLENGE

Double-blind placebo-controlled food challenges (see *allergen challenge* or *exposition test*) are recommended in diagnosing *adverse food reactions*. The results take priority over *allergy diets*, open challenges, or single-blind challenges.

FOOD-INDUCED PULMONARY HEMOSIDEROSIS

This is a rare syndrome characterized by recurrent pneumonias, hemosiderosis, gastrointestinal blood loss, and iron-deficiency anemia. It is frequently associated with a *hypersensitivity* to cow's milk, egg, or pork. Both *immune complex* (see *Coombs and Gell classification*, type III) and *delayed hypersensitivity* (type IV) reactions have been suggested in the pathogenesis of this disorder. The diagnosis is based on peripheral blood *eosinophilia* and precipitating *antibodies* to the responsible *antigen*. Treatment consists of strict elimination of the responsible food (see *diet*).

FOOD INTOLERANCE

In contrast to *food allergy*, food *intolerances* are the consequence of nonimmunological mechanisms following the ingestion of food. They may be due to toxic contaminants (e.g., *histamine* in scombroid fish, bacterial toxins), pharmacological properties (nonspecific histamine release, see *food additives*), or metabolic disorders (e.g., lactase deficiency; see also *adverse food reactions*).

FORCED EXPIRATORY FLOW (FEF$_{25-75}$)

This parameter is derived from the *forced vital capacity* (FVC) maneuver and indicates the forced expiratory flow between 25 and 75% of the vital capacity. The FEF$_{25-75}$ is not more sensitive and much more variable than the *forced expiratory volume in first second* (FEV$_1$).

FORCED EXPIRATORY MANEUVER

A *lung function test* originally described by Tiffeneau in which the subject takes a maximal breath in, then blows out as fast as possible for as long as possible. The amount of air expired in the first second is the *forced expiratory volume in first second* (FEV$_1$), and the total amount of air expired is *forced vital capacity* (FVC). Characteristic changes are observed in obstructive and restrictive lung diseases. The forced expiratory maneuver forms part of the *flow volume loop*.

FORCED EXPIRATORY VOLUME IN FIRST SECOND (FEV$_1$)

The amount of air that can be blown out in the first second, starting from full lung capacity in a *forced expiratory maneuver*.

FORCED VITAL CAPACITY (FVC)

The maximum amount of air that can be forced out in a single *forced expiratory maneuver* starting from full lung capacity. The ratio of *forced expiratory volume in first second* (FEV$_1$) to FVC gives some indication of the degree of *airway obstruction*. However, many patients find it difficult to complete the forced expiratory maneuver, and therefore FVC is often underestimated.

FORMALDEHYDE

Formaldehyde is used in hospitals, furniture manufacture, and as insulation in buildings. It has been reported to cause *occupational asthma*. Formaldehyde is also known as a potent contact *allergen* (see *contact dermatitis*).

FORMOTEROL

This is a long-acting *β2-agonist*.

FRAGRANCE

Fragrances are found in perfumes, cosmetics, household cleaners, air fresheners, detergents, and in foods and beverages. Contact *allergy* to fragrances is very common (see *contact dermatitis*).

FRAMESHIFT MUTATION

This is a *mutation* involving a *deletion* or *insertion* within a coding sequence which is not a multiple of 3 bp and thus destroys the *reading frame* of a *gene*.

FRC

(See *functional residual capacity.*)

FUNCTIONAL RECEPTORS

This term is used to indicate that activation of a *receptor* is associated with a specific cellular response. Some receptors are expressed at the *mRNA* and the protein level, but they do not transduce signals or their initiated *signal transduction* pathway is somehow disrupted (nonfunctional receptors).

FUNCTIONAL RESIDUAL CAPACITY (FRC)

The amount of gas left in the lungs at the end of normal tidal breathing. FRC is increased in *emphysema* and in acute *asthma*, but is usually normal in patients with stable asthma.

FUNGAL ALLERGENS

Fungi mainly cause respiratory *allergies*, but eczematous skin lesions (see *eczema*) due to fungal *allergens* have also been described. *Molds* play an especially important role as *aeroallergens*. Penicillium and Cladosporium are the most common indoor molds. Warmth, dampness, and low air ventilation facilitate the growth of molds, particularly in bathrooms, basements, and on wooden panels and painted walls. Moreover, fruits and vegetable stored in the kitchen can be a source of molds. Air-conditioning systems colonized by molds disperse them throughout buildings. The occurrence of fungal spores in the outdoor air depends on the season and weather. The spores of Alternaria and Cladosporium represent important outdoor allergens. Molds may play an important role in developing *occupational asthma* (agriculture, dairy, tobacco industry). *Aspergillus* fumigatus is an example of a mold growing in the human body with allergenic potency causing *allergic bronchopulmonary aspergillosis* (ABPA). Thermophilic actinomycetes can cause *extrinsic allergic alveolitis* (EAA). Dermato-phytes are also known to induce *allergies*. Dermatophyte-induced *asthma* has been observed in podiatrists and in individuals with athlete's foot or onychomycosis. In patients with *atopic dermatitis*, a worsening of the skin lesions in the head and neck area is often associated with the growth of Pityrosporum ovale.

FUNGUS

Fungi are eukaryotic organisms that live as saprotrophs or parasites, because they lack chlorophyll. There are more than 100,000 different species in our environment, but only 10 to 20 of them are known to cause *allergies* (see *fungal allergens*). Fungi provoke *IgE*-mediated (see *Coombs and Gell classification*, type I) responses, *immune complex*-mediated allergies (type III), or *delayed hypersensitivity* reactions (type IV).

FUROSEMIDE

Furosemide, a loop diuretic, has been shown to be beneficial in *asthma*. Inhaled furosemide effectively prevents *airway obstruction* caused by *allergens* and a number of nonallergic stimuli. The mechanism involves an inhibitory effect on the release of *histamine* and the biosynthesis of *leukotrienes*.

FVC

(See *forced vital capacity*.)

G

GALACTOSIDASE

β-D-Galactosidase belongs to the group of *acid hydrolases* and catalyzes the hydrolysis of terminal nonreducing residues in β-D-galactosides with release of D-galactose. *Leukocytes* and *mast cells*, as well as skin and lung *fibroblasts*, are sources of β-D-galactosidase. In mast cells, it is released in parallel with *histamine* upon *IgE*-dependent activation.

GALT

(See *gut-associated lymphoid tissue*.)

GAMMA/DELTA (γ/δ) T CELLS

γ/δ T cells are a minor subset of *CD3+* T cells (from 1 to 10% of T cells emerging from the *thymus*) and express γ and δ chains to form the *antigen*-binding portion of the *T cell antigen receptor* (TCR). γ/δ T cells often have low intrinsic antigen specificity and generally do not express either *CD4* or *CD8* on their surface. This is in contrast to the α/β variable chain arrangement in the antigen binding region of CD4+ and CD8+ T cells.

> γ/δ T cells are stimulated by *antigen-presenting cells* (APCs), which present antigen via *CD1*, but not via *MHC class II molecules* (see Figure 27).

An implicated co-stimulatory pathway (see *co-stimulation*) involves *CD28* on the T cell and *CD86* on APCs. γ/δ T cells are most commonly associated with *epithelial cells* of intestinal and nasal mucosal surfaces (see *mucosa-associated lymphoid tissues*) and have been described as overrepresented in the bronchial mucosa of patients with *asthma*.

> γ/δ T cells may be involved in allergic *sensitization* because of their possible role in recognizing *allergen* presented by activated *macrophages* in the absence of the normally circulating α/β T cells and their ability to release intracellular stores of *IL-4* on activation.

This may initiate or maintain *Th2 cytokine* production of infiltrating CD4+ (or CD8+) α/β T cells. Mice lacking γ/δ T cells were unable to induce a Th2-mediated airway *inflammation* in response to antigen stimulation.

GANGLIOSIDES

Gangliosides are members of a group of galactose-containing cerebrosides. They are known to modulate *receptor*-dependent processes in various cell types. For instance, gangliosides augment anti-*IgE*-induced *mediator* release in *mast cells*, perhaps by optimizing *high-affinity IgE receptor*–ligand interactions.

GAS EXCHANGE

The primary function of the lung is gas exchange. It allows oxygen to move from the air into the venous blood. For carbon dioxide the process is reversed. The movement of gas across the blood–gas interface is by passive diffusion. The gas exchange area of the lung is 50 to 100 m^2. The blood–gas barrier is extremely thin (less than 0.5 μm). Gas exchange in patients with *asthma* cannot be predicted from *spirometry*. Despite asthma severity, most patients are likely to have abnormal gas exchange. When *forced expiratory volume in first second* (FEV$_1$)

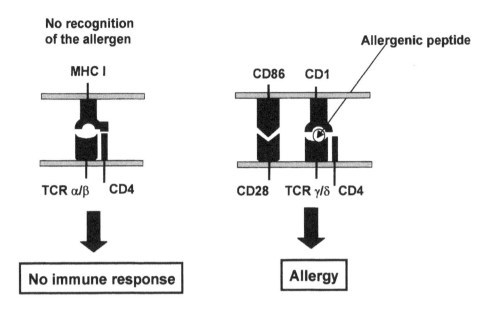

FIGURE 27   Recognition of allergenic peptides by γ/δ T cells via CD1.

decreases below 40%, the *ventilation–perfusion mismatch* becomes clinically alarming. The ventilation/blood flow mismatching appears to be due to both peripheral *airway obstruction* and pulmonary vascular involvement.

GASTROENTERITIS

Gastroenteritis is an *inflammation* of the gastrointestinal tract. This is commonly due to infection but can also be caused by *allergy.* Symptoms may include vomiting, diarrhea, and abdominal colics. Common *food allergens* are peanuts (see *peanut allergy*), seeds, seafood, eggs, and celery. Gastroenteritis can also be the consequence of *food intolerance. Eosinophilic gastroenteritis* is characterized by *eosinophil* infiltration of the wall of the digestive tract.

GASTRO-ESOPHAGEAL REFLUX

This is a free-flow of stomach contents back into the esophagus. It may be due to a weak cardiac sphincter or to a hiatus hernia, which allows the gastro-esophageal junction to sit above the diaphragm. Anti-asthmatic medications such as *β2-agonists* and *corticosteroids* tend to further decrease the tone of the gastro-esophageal sphincter. Gastro-esophageal reflux causes vagal stimulation, which has been associated with nocturnal *airway obstruction*, especially in children. Aspiration of gastric contents is another possible mechanism.

GATA

(See *guanine–adenine and thymine–adenine repeats.*)

GATA-1

This is a *transcription factor* found to be required for *eosinophil* differentiation and the activation of *eosinophil granule protein* (MPO, EPO) *genes.*

GATA-3

This is a *transcription factor* found to be required for *transcription* of the *T cell antigen receptor β* and *δ genes.* GATA-3 is expressed in naive *T cells*, and its expression seems to be involved in the development and maintenance of the *Th2* specific *cytokine* expression pattern. GATA-3 is selectively suppressed during *Th1* development. Inhibition of GATA-3 by transfection of an *antisense* GATA-3 construct prevented *IL-4* expression. Conversely, transgenic expression (see *transgenic mice*) of GATA-3 induced IL-4 expression in developing Th1 cells. The IL-4 *promoter* carries two GATA-3 binding elements, and it was postulated that GATA-3 is sufficient for IL-4 gene expression in T cells, at least in the mouse system studied. In humans, *mRNA* levels of the GATA-3 transcription factor were found to be higher in the airways of *asthma* patients compared to healthy individuals.

> Elevated GATA-3 mRNA levels correlate with *airway obstruction*, *airway hyperresponsiveness*, and the numbers of *IL-5*-expressing cells of the *bronchoalveolar lavage* (BAL) fluid.

Coexpression of both IL-5 and GATA-3 was found in *CD3⁺* cells by double *in situ hybridization*. Moreover, the IL-5 promoter also provides a bona fide GATA-3 binding element, and transcription of IL-5 is increased by GATA-3. Thus, the GATA-3 gene encodes a strong candidate for the *genetic predisposition* of atopic diseases.

G-CSF

(See *granulocyte colony-stimulating factor.*)

GELL AND COOMBS CLASSIFICATION

(See *Coombs and Gell classification.*)

GENE

A gene is a sequence of bases in *DNA* that codes for a polypeptide chain. The human *genome* harbors an estimated 100,000 genes. Most eukaryotic genes have an *exon–intron* organization, where only the exon sequences are present in the mature *mRNA* and are translated into a polypeptide (see *translation*). In addition, the genome also codes for structural *RNA* molecules (class I and class III genes). The correct initiation and enhancement of transcripts of genes are controlled by the *promoter* and *enhancer* regions. In humans, three different types of DNA-dependent *RNA polymerases* exist, according to which three classes of genes are designated. Class I genes are transcribed by RNA polymerase I (pol I) and encode multicopies of the 5.8 S, 18 S and 28 S ribosomal RNAs (rRNA). Class III genes are the genomic regions coding for transfer RNA (tRNA) and additional small structural RNA molecules. Protein encoding genes are transcribed by RNA polymerase (pol II) and thus named class II genes (see *transcription*).

GENE ENVIRONMENTAL INTERACTIONS

It is clear that *allergic diseases* have a genetic background (see *genetic predisposition*). However, the clinical expression of *allergy* is not only genetically determined. For instance, people from Papua New Guinea were nonallergic until modern civilization brought them in contact with blankets, and hence one of the most important *allergens*, the *house-dust mite*. Since *genes* cannot simply change within one generation, environmental exposures may determine the clinical expression of allergy to a large extent. Gene environmental interactions may occur during a whole lifetime, including the intrauterine development of the fetus. Many different exposures may occur, such as allergens, viruses, bacteria, and *pollutants*. Moreover, certain *diets* may constitute environmental triggers (see *risk factors*).

GENERAL TRANSCRIPTION FACTORS

These *transcription factors* are found active in all mammalian cells and are necessary for any *gene transcription*. Examples are the *RNA polymerase* complex, which consists of a large number of different proteins: TATA motif binding protein (TBP), the multisubunit complex TFIID, TFIIA, -B, and additional cofactors which include TFIIE, -F, -H, -J, which can collaborate with the *RNA* polymerase II complex to initiate transcription. From the initiation site, the *DNA*-dependent polymerase II starts to slide along the DNA molecule, exerting RNA polymerase activity.

GENE REARRANGEMENT

Gene rearrangement is a process of somatic recombination of gene segments to form a unique *exon*. Such recombinations physiologically occur during the development of *T cells* and *B cells* to create large numbers of different *antigen receptors*. Increased identical antigen receptor rearrangements can be detected by several molecular biology techniques and are used to diagnose lymphoproliferative diseases (see *T cell lymphoma* and *hypereosinophilia*). A so-called "second gene rearrangement" occurs during *immunoglobulin class switching*.

GENE THERAPY

Gene therapy is a set of approaches to the treatment of human diseases based on transfer of genetic material into an individual.

In contrast to *DNA vaccination*, the goal of gene therapy in *allergic diseases* is to prevent an *immune response*.

However, acute inflammatory reactions usually occur and are one of the many problems associated with gene therapy. Another problem is that repeated injections are frequently needed. Therefore, suitable *vectors* for gene therapy are not available at the moment. For *IgE*-mediated allergic diseases, *IL-10, IL-12, IL-18, IFN-α, IFN-γ, TNF-α* antagonists, *IL-1 receptor antagonist, IL-4* antagonist, or *IL-5* antagonist might be suitable candidates for gene therapy (see *cytokine therapy* and *anticytokine therapy*).

GENETIC CODE

The triplets in *DNA* and *mRNA* that specify the 20 different *amino acids*.

GENETIC HETEROGENEITY

Different *genotypes* result in the same or similar *phenotype*.

GENETIC LOCUS

This is a specific position on a *chromosome*.

GENETIC MARKER

A genetic marker represents a *genetic locus* whose *alleles* can be easily detected. It may be localized either inside or outside a *gene*.

GENETIC POLYMORPHISM

In a population, the occurrence of two or more *alleles* (genetically determined alternative *phenotypes*) at such a frequency that the rarest could not be maintained by recurrent *mutation* alone. Commonly, a genetic locus is considered polymorphic when the rare allele has a frequency of at least 0.01, such that *heterozygotes* carrying this allele occur at a frequency greater than 2%. The *major histocompatibility complex* (MHC) is the most polymorphic *gene* cluster known.

GENETIC PREDISPOSITION

The existence of an important genetic component in *allergic diseases* was first suggested by the presence of familial aggregation for total serum *IgE levels* and by *twin studies*. Segregation analysis has shown that there are at least two major loci (see *locus*) involved in determining an individual's total serum *IgE* levels (see *linkage studies* and *genome-wide screening studies*). The second strategy is to investigate *candidate genes* based on the available knowledge regarding the pathogenesis (see *allergic inflammation*). Efforts have focused on *genes* involved in the regulation of IgE production. Some of our current knowledge regarding the genetic predisposition of allergic diseases is summarized below.

HLA associations

The association of certain *human leukocyte antigen* (HLA) alleles with disease susceptibility has been appreciated for more than 20 years. In this approach, the question is whether the presentation of the majority of *allergens* to *T cells* is mediated by only a few HLA *phenotypes* (see *MHC restriction*). Such associations have been found for inflammatory diseases such as ankylosing spondylitis, psoriasis, and *celiac disease*. This has led geneticists to search for particular HLA alleles associated with allergic diseases. For instance, rye *grass pollen allergen* responses are associated with DR3 and DR5 HLA alleles, and responses to *house-dust mite* are restricted to DR2, DR5, DR52b, and DR51. Moreover, HLA-DP restriction has been shown to be an important component of T cell responses to *cat* (Fel d 1), *mold* (Alt a 1), house-dust mite (Der p 1, Der p 2), and certain *pollen* allergens. These data suggest that allergenic recognition (see *antigen recognition*) by T cells is associated with HLA restriction.

High-affinity IgE receptor

Almost one decade ago, a genetic linkage between *chromosome* 11q and elevated serum IgE levels in *allergic rhinitis* and *asthma* patients was reported. The gene encoding for the β-subunit of the *high-affinity IgE receptor* (FcεRIβ) was suggested as a candidate. A variant differing in *amino acid* position 181 (Ile to Leu) was found to be transmitted from the mother in atopic families, thus leading to the hypothesis that the Leu 181 variant could be a susceptibility *allele* for atopy. Further studies on variant amino acids in positions 181, 183, 237, and other markers of chromosome 11q13 partly obtained conflicting results in Australian, Dutch, Italian, and Japanese populations. Thus, association of chromosome 11q, and particularly of FcεRIβ, to atopic diseases has to be evaluated in new sample groups of atopic patients and should not be regarded as pivotal for elevated serum IgE levels and atopic disease today.

Promoter of the IL-4 gene

Investigators have focused on *genetic polymorphisms* in the *promoter* region of *Th2 cytokine* genes. One single base exchange (T → C) of the *IL-4* promoter/*enhancer* region at position −590 bp relative to the *transcription* initiation site was reported to be associated with higher serum total IgE levels, asthma, and positive skin *prick tests* in American individuals carrying the T-mutation. It is speculated that this substitution influences the transcriptional activity. The *mutation* in the allele associated with higher serum IgE levels was suspected to generate an additional *DNA*-binding element for the *nuclear factor of activated T cells* (NF-AT) which can transactivate IL-4 transcription. Studies performed in Japan confirmed the association of the T-allele with asthma and *atopic dermatitis*, but not with increased serum total IgE levels. One group of investigators reported nine point mutations, different from the −590 bp alleles, within the proximal IL-4 promoter. One base pair exchange involves part of a functional DNA-binding element at position −81 bp. Examination of the functional impact revealed that the A to G mutation increased binding of the *transcription factor activator protein 1* (AP-1). These results may point to an enhanced IL-4 synthesis due to stronger collaborative binding of the transcription factors AP-1 and NF-AT. So far no family (linkage) or population (*association*) study has addressed this hypothesis. Most recently, another polymorphism (C → T) in the 5′ flanking region of the human IL-4 gene was described in position +33 bp, a position in which binding of proteins of the initiation complex might be involved. Again, no data related to atopic diseases are provided for this *genetic polymorphism* so far.

IL-4 receptor mutation

A variant of the IL-4 receptor β-chain (Q576R) has been reported to be associated with *atopy* and the *hyper-IgE syndrome*. However, another study involving 82 families neither observed increased frequencies of the Q576R allele in patients with allergic asthma or atopy, nor confirmed the association of increased serum IgE levels with two genetic markers located near the β-chain.

Th2 cytokine gene cluster

An association between total serum IgE levels and genetic markers in the chromosomal segment 5q31–q33 containing many cytokine genes has been described (see *Th2 cytokine gene cluster*). For the *IL-3* gene, a diallelic polymorphism in position –68 bp (T → C) with a frequency of 0.25 for the C-mutation was described. For the IL-9 gene, a diallelic polymorphism within the promoter region in position –351 bp (A → C) with a frequency of 0.83 for the A-mutation was described. So far, no association to the transcriptional regulation or atopic status is known.

β-adrenergic receptor gene

The *intron*-less gene encoding the β2-adrenoreceptor was cloned and located on the long arm q of human chromosome 5 (5q31–33), a region of highest interest, encoding candidate genes for atopic diseases. To date, nine polymorphisms have been found, four of which lead to amino acid exchanges in the *G protein-coupled receptor*. Mutations of the nucleic acid sequence in positions 46 (A → G), 79 (C → G), 100 (G → A), and 491 (C → T) result in the amino acid exchanges Arg16Gly, Gln27Glu, Val34Met, and Thr164Ile. The 164 Ile mutation was found to lead to a significant decrease in binding *affinity* for *catecholamine* ligands. The Gln 27 allele was associated with elevated IgE levels in a family study, while in another study, the Gly 16 allele has been shown to be associated with severity of asthma. Furthermore, an *RFLP* at nucleic acid residue 523 (C → A) creates a new *endonuclease* recognition site and was found to be associated with increased incidence of allergic asthma in a Japanese population. Further studies of clinically and genetically well-characterized patients will be needed to perform an extended *haplotype* analysis at this candidate gene *locus* within the so-called cytokine gene cluster on chromosome 5q31–33.

Transcription factors

(See *c-Maf*, *GATA-3*, *AP-1*, and *STAT*.)

GENOME

The genome is the complete *DNA* sequence of an organism, containing the entire genetic information.

GENOME-WIDE SCREENING STUDIES

The whole *genome* is scanned with a dense collection of *genetic markers* (typically about 360 polymorphic markers). Upon statistical *linkage* analysis, regions are identified that may carry *genes* that contribute to the pathophysiology of a certain disease. A genome-wide study revealed a number of regions that are linked to *asthma* and *atopy* (Table 46) (see *genetic predisposition*).

GENOMIC DNA

Chromosomal *DNA* contained within the nucleus, in contrast to the DNA in organelles (e.g., mitochondria).

GENOTYPE

The genotype is the genetic constitution of the organism. For a given *allele*, it can be *heterozygous* or *homozygous*.

TABLE 46
Regions Linked to Asthma and Atopy

Chromosome	Region	Candidate Genes
2	2q33	?
5	5p15	?
	5q23-p31	*IL-3, IL-4, IL-5, IL-9, IL-13, GM-CSF,*
		β2-adrenergic receptor
6	6p21.3-p23	*MHC, TNF*
11	11p15	?
12	12q14-q24.2	*IFN-γ, NO synthase, STAT6*
13	13q21.3	Esterase D
14	14q11.2-13	*NF-κB, TCR*
17	17p11.1-q11.2	?
19	19q13	?
21	21q21	?

GIANT PAPILLARY CONJUNCTIVITIS

This *conjunctivitis* is due to a combination of chronic low-grade trauma and a *hypersensitivity* reaction to foreign material (or to surface biodeposits on top of such material). It is commonly caused by wearing contact lenses, particularly soft lenses. The conjunctiva is infiltrated by *mast cells, eosinophils, basophils, neutrophils,* and *lymphocytes,* including *plasma cells.* Patients complain of itching, watering, blurring of vision, and reduced lens tolerance. Giant papillary conjunctivitis is completely reversible after avoiding the provoking factor.

GLEICH SYNDROME

This term is used for a subgroup of patients with *hypereosinophilic syndrome* (HES) associated with *angioedema.* The association was first reported by Gleich.

GLIADIN

Gliadin is the alcohol-soluble portion of *gluten* found in wheat, rye, barley, and oat. In patients with *gluten-sensitive enteropathy,* gliadin is the gluten component responsible for the development of the disease.

GLUCOCORTICOSTEROIDS

(See *corticosteroids.*)

GLUCOCORTICOSTEROID RECEPTOR

(See *corticosteroid receptor.*)

GLUCOCORTICOSTEROID RESPONSIVE ELEMENT (GRE)

(See *corticosteroid responsive element.*)

β-GLUCURONIDASE

β-Glucuronidase belongs to the group of *acid hydrolases* and catalyzes the reaction occurring between β-D-glucuronide and water, producing alcohol and glucuronate. The enzyme exists in microsomal and lysosomal isomeric forms, which differ predominantly in their carbohydrate content. In *mast cells*, the majority of the enzyme is found in the primary lysosomes. In *eosinophils*, it is stored in the secondary *granules*. The enzyme is also expressed in *neutrophils* and skin as well as lung *fibroblasts*. In mast cells, it is released parallel with *histamine* upon *IgE*-dependent activation.

GLUTATHIONE

Glutathione is an important *antioxidant*. Reduced glutathione levels increase tissue damage caused by reactive *oxygen metabolites*. This pathomechanism appears to be relevant in *cryptogenic fibrosing alveolitis*, and perhaps other chronic *inflammations*.

GLUTATHIONE TRANSFERASE

(See *leukotriene C4 synthase*.)

GLUTEN

Gluten is a mixture of *gliadin*, the major prolamin protein of wheat, and glutenin, the major glutelin protein of wheat.

GLUTEN-SENSITIVE ENTEROPATHY

This disease is also called "celiac disease." It is characterized by malabsorption with diarrhea, and consequent weight loss and malnutrition. Patients develop a *gluten*-specific *T cell sensitization*. Gluten-activated *T cells* cause a *delayed hypersensitivity* reaction (see *Coombs and Gell classification*, type IV).

Celiac disease should be considered a *food allergy*, but in practice it is not.

The T cell response leads to tissue damage, especially atrophy of the jejunal mucosa. Therefore, the disease can be diagnosed by intestinal biopsy, showing villous atrophy as a characteristic feature. Glutens are proteins found in wheat, barley, oats, and rye. A gluten-free *diet* is the only therapeutic tool (see *allergen avoidance*).

GLYCOLIPIDS

Glycolipids are lipids containing carbohydrate groups, usually galactose, but also glucose, inositol, and others. They may modulate functional responses initiated via the *high-affinity IgE receptor* in *mast cells*.

GM-CSF

(See *granulocyte/macrophage colony-stimulating factor*.)

GOBLET CELLS

Goblet cells are *mucus*-producing bronchial *epithelial cells*.

GOLD

Gold salts are used as *immunosuppressive drugs*.

G PROTEIN

This is a signaling molecule which binds GTP and converts it into GDP in the process of *signal transduction* via many cell surface *receptors*. Trimeric (α,β,γ) G proteins transduce signals initiated via *G protein-coupled receptors*. G proteins activate *phospholipase C* (PLC) and *adenylate cyclase*. Small G proteins, such as *Ras*, act distal to many transmembrane signaling events.

G PROTEIN-COUPLED RECEPTOR

G protein-coupled *receptors* represent a family of receptors with seven transmembrane domains that are linked to *G proteins*. The activation of G proteins can be blocked by pretreatment of the cells with Bordatella *pertussis toxin* before ligand stimulation.

> G proteins activate *phospholipase Cβ*, which generates *inositol-1,4,5-trisphosphate* (IP$_3$). As a consequence, an intracellular *calcium mobilization* occurs.

In addition, G proteins activate *adenylate cyclase* and, therefore, increase intracellular *cAMP* levels. G protein-coupled receptors are also linked to the *mitogen-activated protein kinase* (MAPK) pathway via *arrestin*.

GRAFT-VERSUS-HOST DISEASE (GVHD)

Chronic GVHD is a complication occurring in up to 30% of long-term survivors of *bone marrow* transplantation. It is an autoimmune-like disorder (see *autoimmunity*), resulting in skin manifestations resembling idiopathic scleroderma, and is associated with *mast cell* activation. Mast cell activation due to GVHD has a slow onset with morphologic characteristics of a *piecemeal degranulation* (PMD) rather than an anaphylactic *degranulation* (see *anaphylactic reaction* and *exocytosis*). Treatment with *cromones* may improve the clinical situation of GVHD patients.

GRANULES

Granules are intracellular structures within inflammatory effector cells, such as *neutrophils*, *eosinophils*, *basophils*, or *mast cells*. They contain *mediators* for host defense mechanisms. The release of granular products occurs via *exocytosis*. In *allergic inflammations*, this process is associated with *hypersensitivity* reactions and subsequent tissue damage (see *epithelial damage*) and *remodeling*. Paul Ehrlich observed that granule proteins take up certain dyes due to their physicochemical properties. Such fixation and staining techniques allow identification of *granulocytes* as eosinophils, basophils, and neutrophils.

GRANULOCYTES

Important inflammatory effector cells involved in host defense. This group of *leukocytes* includes *neutrophils*, *eosinophils*, and *basophils*.

GRANULOCYTE COLONY-STIMULATING FACTOR (G-CSF)

G-CSF is a *cytokine* involved in the differentiation, activation, and survival (see *survival factors*) of *neutrophils* but not *eosinophils*. During inflammatory processes, it is expressed by *epithelial cells*, *macrophages*, *fibroblasts*, and neutrophils.

GRANULOCYTE/MACROPHAGE COLONY-STIMULATING FACTOR (GM-CSF)

GM-CSF is a *cytokine* involved in the differentiation, activation, and survival (see *survival factors*) of myeloid cells, including *dendritic cells*, *monocytes*, *macrophages*, and *granulocytes*. GM-CSF is produced by a variety of cells such as *T cells*, monocytes, macrophages, *fibroblasts*, *endothelial cells*, and granulocytes. It has a potential role in enhancing *eosinophil* survival in *asthma* (see *eosinophil apoptosis*).

GRANULOCYTE/MACROPHAGE COLONY-STIMULATING FACTOR RECEPTOR

The *receptor* of *GM-CSF* is a heterodimer of α- and β-subunits. The α-chain is specific for this *cytokine receptor*, whereas the β-chain is shared by *IL-3*, *IL-5*, and GM-CSF receptors.

GM-CSF receptors are expressed by pluripotent stem cells in the *bone marrow*, but also by mature *granulocytes*, *monocytes*, *macrophages*, and *dendritic cells*. For *signal transduction*, see *interleukin-5 receptor*.

GRANULOCYTE PRIMING

Preexposure of *eosinophils*, *neutrophils*, and *basophils* to subactivating doses of certain agonists results in an enhanced functional response to a second activator. *Cytokines* such as *IL-3*, *IL-5* (for eosinophils and basophils only), and *GM-CSF* are especially able to initiate such a priming process. In addition to soluble agonists, molecular interactions between *granulocyte adhesion molecules* and *endothelial cells*, *matrix* proteins, or airway *epithelial cells* may also result in functional upregulation of the inflammatory cells. Priming for increased *leukotriene* synthesis may involve cytokine-mediated *mitogen-activated protein kinases* (MAPK) activation (ERK-1/ERK-2) and/or serine 505 *phosphorylation* of *phospholipase A_2* (PLA$_2$).

GRANULOMATOUS VASCULITIS

A synonym of *Churg–Strauss syndrome.*

GRASS POLLEN

Allergenically (see *allergen*) important grass *pollens* include bermuda grass (Cynodon dactylon), rye grass (Lolium perenne), timothy grass (Phleum pratense), and orchard grass (Cactylis glomerata; see also *aeroallergens*).

GUANINE

A purine base that is an essential component of *DNA*.

GUANINE–ADENINE AND THYMINE–ADENINE REPEATS (GATA)

Family of *transcription factors*. In contrast to many other transcription factors, *GATA-3* specifically promotes *Th2 cytokine* expression. Moreover, GATA-3 directly represses *Th1 cytokine* development and *IFN-γ gene* expression by a mechanism that is independent of *IL-4* and that may disrupt *IL-12 signaling*.

GUIDELINES OF ASTHMA THERAPY

(See *management guidelines* and *asthma treatment strategies*.)

GUT-ASSOCIATED LYMPHOID TISSUE (GALT)

The GALT plays an important role in the induction of oral *tolerance* and in the immune suppression of adverse reactions (e.g., *adverse food reactions*). The intestinal tract is exposed to a variety of foreign materials, mainly foods, but also viruses and bacteria. The mucosal barrier is formed by the mucosal lining (*epithelial cells*, intraepithelial *lymphocytes*) and nonspecific factors such as peristalsis, digestion, degradation, and *mucus*. The underlying lamina propria contains large numbers of immune cells including *mast cells*, *eosinophils*, *T cells*, *antigen-presenting cells* (APC), and *NK cells*. In the small intestine, the microfold (M) cells (see *M cells*) in the epithelium play an important role in *allergen* presentation to the organized lymphoid tissue, called Peyer's patches (see *lymph node*). *Sensitization* to *allergens* is thought to occur in damaged or immature intestinal mucosa (see *food allergy* and *gluten-sensitive enteropathy*).

H

HAIR ANALYSIS

Method to diagnose *allergic diseases* that belongs to *complementary procedures.*

HANIFIN AND RAJKA CRITERIA

In 1980, John Hanifin and George Rajka published a list of diagnostic criteria for *atopic dermatitis.* These criteria have become the standard for identification of atopic dermatitis patients in clinical trials. To be diagnosed, patients must fulfill three out of the four major criteria (Table 47) and at least three of the many minor criteria (Table 48).

TABLE 47
Hanifin and Rajka Major
Criteria of Atopic Dermatitis

Pruritus
Lichenification
Chronic course
Personal and/or family history of *atopy*

HAPLOID

This is the number of *chromosomes* of gametes: in man 22 *autosomes* and one sex chromosome either the X or Y chromosome.

HAPLOTYPE

This is the set of *chromosomes* inherited from one parent (see *haploid*).

HAPTEN

A hapten is a small molecule, which alone is unable to initiate an *immune response.* However, following binding to a carrier molecule, the hapten-carrier complex is able to initiate immune responses. For instance, phthalic anhydride may induce *IgE*-mediated reactions by acting as a hapten, with complete immunologic recognition being dependent on binding to albumin.

Most of the contact *allergens* leading to allergic *contact dermatitis* are haptens (e.g., *nickel*).

HARDY–WEINBERG EQUILIBRIUM

This is an equation that relates *gene (allele)* frequencies to *genotype* frequencies. It allows us to determine whether homozygotic and heterozygotic *carriers* are at equilibrium in a population or whether a specific allele is more frequent in a group of individuals sharing a *trait.*

HAY FEVER

A form of seasonal *allergic rhinoconjunctivitis* due to *grass* and *tree pollens.* Strictly speaking, hay fever is grass pollen *allergy*, but the term is in vernacular use for all forms of seasonal *allergic rhinitis.* The use of hay fever to describe year-round symptoms is not standard, but

---

TABLE 48
Hanifin and Rajka Minor Criteria
of Atopic Dermatitis

Xerosis
Ichthyosis
Positive *immediate hypersensitivity skin test* reactions
Elevated serum *IgE*
Early age of onset
Tendency toward cutaneous infections
Nonspecific hand or foot *dermatitis*
Nipple *eczema*
Cheilitis
Recurrent *conjunctivitis*
Dennie–Morgan infraorbital fold
Keratoconus
Anterior subcapsular cataracts
Orbital darkening
Facial pallor/facial *erythema*
Pityriasis alba
Anterior neck folds
Itch when sweating
Adverse food reactions
Influenced by environmental or emotional factors
Wool intolerance
Perifollicular accentuation
White *dermographism*

---

sometimes people with *perennial rhinitis* describe themselves as having hay fever all year. More often, they will describe themselves as having a cold all year round.

HELMINTHIC INFECTIONS

(See *parasitic diseases*.)

HEMATOGENOUS ALLERGIC ECZEMA

In addition to the allergic *contact dermatitis* at the site of *allergen* exposure, the eruption of multiple small satellite lesions is characteristic of this disease. Mostly follicular *eczema* lesions tend to develop in distant locations, leading to hematogenous allergic eczema. Chronic *dermatitis* in multisensitized patients with chronic leg ulcers is a frequent basis for the development of such eczema.

HEMIZYGOTE

This term describes a loss of one *allele* or *chromosome* in a *diploid* individual.

HEP

(See *histamine-equivalent prick*.)

HEPARIN

Heparin is an important *proteoglycan* produced by *mast cells*, which store it in secretory *granules*.

Heparin is essential for the storage of *neutral proteases* in these granules.

Released heparin is a potent anticoagulant, but it may also express anticomplement and antikallikrein autoactivation activities. Moreover, it inhibits the production of *IL-1*, *TNF-α*, *GM-CSF*, and IL-11 by *fibroblasts* and *monocytes*. In mast cells, heparin inhibits preferentially TNF-α and *IL-4* production after both immunologic and nonimmunologic *mast cell activation*, without having any significant effect on *degranulation*.

> These data suggest that heparin may act, at least under certain circumstances, as an antiinflammatory *mediator*.

HEREDITARY ANGIOEDEMA

(See *angioedema*.)

HERITABILITY

The heritability is the proportion of the total variation of a *trait* attributable to genetic, as opposed to environmental, factors.

HERTOGHE'S SIGN

This is a more or less complete loss of the lateral part of the eyebrows, which is one of the most important *atopy stigmata* (see *Hanifin and Rajka criteria*).

5-HETE

5S-hydroxyeicosatetraenoic acid is derived from *5-HPETE*. This intermediate in *eicosanoid* metabolism (see *leukotrienes*) can act as an inflammatory *mediator*. It shares some biological activities with LTB_4, although it is less potent.

HETEROZYGOTE

This is a *diploid* individual having two different *alleles* at a given *genetic locus* on a pair of homologous *chromosomes* (*autosomes*).

HETEROZYGOUS

(See *heterozygote*.)

HEVEA BRASILIENSIS (H.b.)

The rubber tree H.b. provides most of the latex milk used as a source of natural rubber (see *latex allergy*).

β-HEXOSAMINIDASE

Human *mast cells* are one of the richest sources of *granule*-associated β-hexosaminidase. This enzyme, a hexoglycosidase, cleaves *N*-acetyl-hexosamine residues (glucosamine or galactosamine) from glycosphingolipids. β-Hexosaminidase exists as two isomers, each composed of four subunits, α4 (type A) and α2 β2 (type B). This enzyme is also found in skin *fibroblasts* and *eosinophils*.

HFA PROPELLANTS

Hydrofluoroalkane (HFA) propellants have been developed as alternatives to the *CFC propellants* formerly used in *metered dose inhalers*. They are thought to be less damaging to the *ozone* layer.

HIGH-AFFINITY IgE RECEPTOR (FcεRI)

Mast cells express about 2 to 3×10^5 FcεRI per cell, which bind monovalent *IgE* with a K_a of 2.8×10^9 mol/l. In addition to mast cells, *basophils* and *Langerhans cells* also demonstrate clear evidence for FcεRI surface expression.

> FcεRI *cross-linking* by *allergen* in mast cells and basophils with consequent *mediator* release (e.g., *histamine*) is an important mechanism in *immediate hypersensitivity* reactions.

The FcεRI *receptor* is composed of one α-chain, one β-chain, and two γ-chains (αβγ2). Some cells (e.g., *eosinophils* and Langerhans cells) have been described to express a functional FcεRI without a β-chain (αγ2) (see *eosinophil surface molecules*). Moreover, *knockout mice* lacking the β-chain were able to develop *anaphylaxis*. These data stimulated intense research on the function of the β-chain.

> It appears that the β-chain increases the total FcεRI receptor expression per cell and might function as an amplifier of *signal transduction*.

The α-chain is readily accessible on the cell surface and contains the IgE-binding domain. In addition to this extracellular part, it contains transmembrane and cytoplasmic domains. *Antibodies* against the α-chain are of pathogenic importance in a subset of patients with *urticaria*. These autoantibodies (see *autoimmunity*) do not cross-link the IgE receptor but cause complement activation (see *complement system*). The β- as well as the two γ-chains are not accessible on the surface and are involved in signal transduction through the receptor. Signal transduction pathways involve *tyrosine kinases* (e.g., *Lyn* and Syk), *phospholipase C*, and *calcium mobilization*.

HIGH-ALTITUDE CLIMATE THERAPY

(See *climate therapy*.)

HISTAMINE

Histamine [2-(4-imidazolyl)-ethylamine, MW 111] is the sole major biogenic amine in *mast cells* and *basophils* from normal subjects. It is synthesized in the Golgi apparatus of mast cells by decarboxylation of the precursor *amino acid*, histidine, and stored in *granules*. As an extracellular *mediator*, histamine is rapidly metabolized by methylation (70%) or oxidation (30%). Human mast cells contain 3 to 8 pg of histamine per cell. Secretion is initiated by *mast cell activation*. *Histamine release* is a trigger for histamine resynthesis. Histamine has wide-ranging biologic activities mediated through activation of specific cell surface *receptors* (see *histamine receptors*). The use of selective antagonists (see *antihistamines*) of the pharmacological action of histamine has led to the classification of histamine receptor subtypes H_1, H_2, and H_3.

HISTAMINE CHALLENGE

Histamine is used as a positive control in many *skin tests* and *exposition tests*.

HISTAMINE-EQUIVALENT PRICK (HEP)

The classical approach to labeling *allergen extracts* is to standardize the amount of protein used for extraction, resulting in a labeling in "Noon units." Alternatively, the protein content of the resulting solution can be determined by biochemical methods, resulting in a labeling with "protein nitrogen units" (PNU). However, the response of patients with *IgE*-mediated *allergic diseases* to allergen extracts does not exactly correspond to the protein content. In order to standardize allergen extracts on a biological basis, the HEP was proposed in 1972 by Aas and Belin. This approach requires the performance of skin *prick tests* in a population of allergic subjects. The standardization is made in the comparison of the *allergen*-induced wheal to the response with a standardized positive control solution (e.g., *histamine* at 1 mg/ml). This technique is regarded as highly useful and reliable. There are many modifications of this approach in use, involving the concentration, test reading method, and control substance. For practical reasons, HEPs are often transformed to "biological units" (BU), with a concentration of 1 HEP/ml corresponding to 1000 BU/ml.

HISTAMINE RECEPTORS

Histamine is involved in many physiological and pathological processes and is a neurotransmitter of the central *nervous system*. Its actions are mediated by three *receptor* types — H_1, H_2, and H_3 — and can be opposed by *antihistamines*. The most important effects in *allergic diseases* are mediated through the H_1 receptor. In general, histamine induces *edema, smooth muscle* contraction, and reflex vasodilatation. Table 49 gives a more detailed overview about the known histamine-mediated effects initiated via the different histamine receptors.

TABLE 49
Biological Effects of Histamine

Receptor	Effects
H_1	Pruritus
	Bronchial smooth-muscle contraction (see *bronchial provocation tests*)
	Increased vascular permeability
	Tachycardia
	Activation of vagal reflexes (glandular *mucus* secretion in the nose is indirectly mediated, explaining why unilateral nasal *histamine challenge* results in controlateral glandular secretion that is inhibited by *atropine*)
	Dilation of the precapillary lung arterioles
	Increased leakage of the postcapillary lung venules (responsible for histamine-induced skin wheal)
H_2	Esophageal contraction
	Gastric acid secretion
	Increased lower airway secretion
	Inhibition of H_1-mediated effects
	Inhibition of effector functions of *basophils* and *T cells*
H_3	Inhibition of histamine synthesis and release in the central nervous system

---

Histamine has also been claimed to be a *chemotactic factor* for *eosinophils*. However, this has not been confirmed under in vivo experimental conditions.

HISTAMINE RELEASE

The amount of *histamine* found in urine from control individuals ranges from 5 to 15 µg per 24 hours, and normal plasma levels are between 0.05 and 0.2 ng/ml, suggesting continuous secretion of histamine. Indeed, histamine is secreted spontaneously at low levels by *mast cells* and *basophils*. The precise mechanism by which this occurs is not known, but it may include *piecemeal degranulation* (PMD). *Exocytosis* of mast cells and consequent release of high histamine amounts in *allergic diseases* occurs via specific surface *receptors*, such as *high-affinity IgE receptor* and many *G-protein-coupled receptors* (e.g., *complement factor* receptors). Histamine release is rapid and depends on intracellular *calcium mobilization*, but does not depend on extracellular calcium.

HISTAMINE-RELEASING ASSAY

The *histamine release* from peripheral blood *basophils* in vitro, as induced by *allergen*-mediated *cross-linking* of *IgE* bound to *high-affinity IgE-receptors* on the cell surface, may be used as an additional diagnostic tool in *allergic diseases* (see *skin test* and *immunoassay*). The advantage of this assay is that the *histamine*-releasing capacity of various *pseudoallergens* that induce an IgE-independent release of histamine may be assessed as well.

HISTAMINE-RELEASING FACTORS (HRF)

Besides activation via the *high-affinity IgE receptor*, other mediators that activate *G-protein-coupled receptors*, such as *complement factors*, *platelet-activating factor* (PAF), and *leukotrienes*, can also act as HRF in *mast cells* and *basophils*. For instance, most *CC chemokines* may also have *histamine*-releasing activity in basophils. However, *cytokines* such as *IL-3*, *IL-5*, and *GM-CSF* are required to prime basophils for *chemokine*-induced *degranulation* (see *granulocyte priming*). In contrast to basophils, only *MIP-1α* appears to be an HRF in mast cells. Interestingly, the *CXC chemokine IL-8* blocks *histamine release* under certain experimental in vitro conditions (see also *mast cell activation*).

HISTONE

Histones are small proteins rich in basic *amino acids* (lysine and arginine) which form the core structure of a *nucleosome* that constitutes the *chromatin* organization in the nucleus.

HISTORY OF ALLERGY RESEARCH

The modern history of *allergy* research (Table 50) dates back to 1873 when Charles Blackley showed that windborne *pollen* grains caused the symptoms of June *hay fever*. He also demonstrated that aqueous pollen extracts (see allergen extracts) caused immediate wheal and flare reactions when scratched into the skin (see *skin test*) of a hay fever sufferer (himself). At the turn of the century, the causative agents of this *immediate hypersensitivity* reaction were defined as *allergens* (von Pirquet), and this form of immunity was shown to be mediated by homocytotropic (or "reaginic") *antibody* (Prausnitz and Küstner, see *Prausnitz–Küstner reaction*).

> By the 1920s, it was known that inhalation of allergens derived from pollens, *house-dust mites*, and *animal dander,* or the ingestion of foods was associated with the clinical symptoms of hay fever, *asthma*, *atopic dermatitis*, or *food allergy,* and that these conditions affected 10 to 20% of the population.

This was a "golden era" of research on *allergic disease* and, indeed, the first edition of the *Journal of Immunology* contained an article of about 100 pages by Robert Cooke on the genetics of asthma, showing that the disease had strong hereditary links (see *genetic predisposition*). The second golden era was in the 1960s, when the first allergens were purified from ragweed and rye *grass pollen*, and *histamine-releasing assays* were developed. Also at this time, the landmark studies by the Ishizakas established that immediate hypersensitivity reactions are mediated by *immunoglobulin E* (IgE). In 1988, the first *major allergen*, Der p 1, was cloned from a house-dust mite *cDNA* library, and since then over 200 allergen sequences have been elucidated (see *cloning of allergens*). Most recently, the three-dimensional structures (see *X-ray crystallography*) of two important allergens have been determined: birch pollen allergen, Bet v 1, and mite allergen, Der p 2. For both Bet v 1 and Der p 2, *amino acids* that are important in binding antibodies (see *epitopes*) have been identified. In addition to these studies, there have been numerous studies on *T cell epitopes* on allergens.

> Important issues in current research are, in particular, the immunological mechanisms responsible for *delayed hypersensitivity* reactions and chronic *allergic inflammation*.

TABLE 50
A Brief Synopsis of the History of Our Understanding of Allergic Diseases

1873	Blackley	Showed that windborne pollen grains caused hay fever and that pollen extracts caused wheal and flare reactions when "scratched" into the skin.
1906	Von Pirquet	Defined "allergy" as supersensitivity to foreign antigens or "allergens."
1911	Noon and Freeman	Used desensitizing injections of pollen extracts ("pollen toxin") to treat hay fever.
1916	Cooke	Demonstrated familial inheritance of hay fever/asthma, i.e., a genetic trait.
1921	Prausnitz and Kustner	Passive transfer of immediate skin test reactivity using serum from an allergic patient (the P-K test).
1940	Loveless	Production of "blocking antibodies" during *immunotherapy.*
1963	Osler and Lichtenstein	Development of histamine-releasing assay.
1963	Coombs and Gell	Classification of allergic diseases.
1964	Voorhorst and Spieksma	Discovery of house-dust mites.
1965	King, Marsh, and Norman	First allergens purified from ragweed (Antigen E) and rye grass.
1967	Ishizaka and Ishizaka; Johansson	Discovery of IgE.
1970	Norman and Lichtenstein	Controlled trials of ragweed immunotherapy.
1980	Chapman and Platts-Mills	Purification of dust mite allergen, Der p 1.
1988	Chua and Thomas	First allergen to be cloned, Der p 1.
1992	Robinson and Kay	Delayed hypersensitivity reactions and chronic airway *inflammation* in asthma are associated with activated *Th2 cells.*
1997	Simon	Tissue *eosinophilia* associated with allergic diseases is mostly the consequence of delayed *eosinophil apoptosis.*

HIV

(See *acquired immunodeficiency syndrome.*)

HLA

(See *human leukocyte antigen.*)

HMC-1

HMC-1 is a leukemic human *mast cell* line established from the peripheral blood of a patient with mast cell leukemia. It grows independently of *stem cell factor* (SCF).

HMC-1 cells are important tools for current research on mast cells.

Although these cells lack *high-affinity IgE receptors*, they share *cytokine receptors* and other important *surface molecules* of human lung mast cells. They contain *tryptase* and small amounts of *chymase*. HMC-1 cells generate and release a variety of different *mediators* including *cytokines* (see Table 51).

HOMEOPATHY

Homeopathy is a treatment method of *allergic diseases* that belongs to *complementary procedures.*

HOMING

Tissue-specific *migration* of activated immune cells has long been believed, following the discovery of *lymphocyte* recirculation in the early 1960s. This dogma suggests that lymphocytes,

---

TABLE 51
HMC-1 Mediators

mRNA Expression	Protein Expression
TNF-α[a], *TGF-β*[a], M-CSF[a]	TNF-α[c], *heparin*[c], *chondroitin sulfate*[c], *histamine*[c], *IL-16*[c]
IL-1[b], *IL-3*[b], *IL-4*[b], *IL-6*[b], *IL-8*[b], *GM-CSF*[b], *TNF-β*[b], PDGF-A[b]	IL-3[d], IL-4[d], IL-8[d], GM-CSF[d]
Tryptase	I-309[e], *MCP*-1[e], *MIP-1α*, MIP-1β,
Chymase	*RANTES*

[a] *mRNA* constitutively expressed
[b] induced mRNA
[c] prestored
[d] protein after activation
[e] constitutively expressed protein

---

for example, home to tissues either from which they originated or in which they were activated. There appears to be a functional advantage in such a system, as lymphocytes would be recruited back to sites where they may be more likely to encounter the specific *antigen* that activated them. Pursuing this hypothesis has led to the suggestion that organ- or tissue-specific homing molecules (e.g., *cutaneous lymphocyte antigen*) may be activated and expressed as a result of the microenvironmental developmental conditions encountered during *T cell activation* or *B cell activation* and differentiation. Evidence to support such a scenario has come from the discovery of molecules expressed on the surface of lymphocytes and their respective ligands on *endothelial cells*, the so-called addressins, which form part of the *adhesion molecule* system. Early results on which these assumptions were based now appear to be somewhat flawed, and the tissue-specific migration of lymphocytes may have been severely biased by the use of animal models in which bacterial or parasitic infections (see *parasitic diseases*) were present.

There remains the question of cause and effect. For instance, *immunoglobulin* (Ig) A-secreting *B cells* appear to home specifically to mucosal surfaces. The addressin hypothesis would suggest that this is due to specific homing *receptors* imprinted on those cells when undergoing Ig *isotype* selection. However, it is just as likely that the preferential migration to specific sites is more closely linked to the functional characteristics of such B cells, which accumulate slowly over time, but are not often found in sites where Ig secretion across mucosal surfaces cannot occur. The same situation occurs with *T cells* and appears to be orchestrated by the *Th1* and *Th2* functional phenotypes (and related phenotypes for *CD8*+ and *gamma/delta (γ/δ)-T cells*). Moreover, in models where naive animals (newborns or fetuses) were challenged with antigen, no tissue-specific homing could be detected, and it has been demonstrated that the distribution of antigen-specific *memory T cells* is independent of the site of antigen immunization.

> In conclusion, the expression of adhesion molecules and *chemokines* induced by inflammatory cytokines appears to be a more functionally likely mechanism of memory or activated lymphocyte recruitment than of homing by tissue-specific receptors.

HOMOLOGOUS RECOMBINATION

This term describes the *recombination* (*crossing-over*) between identical or very similar (homologous) *DNA* sequences.

HOMOLOGY

(See *sequence homology.*)

HOMOZYGOTE

This is a *diploid* individual with two identical *alleles* at a given autosomal locus.

HOMOZYGOUS

(See *homozygote.*)

HORSE ALLERGENS

Allergen extracts of horse hair and dander (see *animal dander*) contain three *allergens* (Equ c 1, Equ c 2, and Equ c 3). Horse serum albumin exhibits only weak allergenicity.

HOTSPOT

A mutational hotspot is any *DNA* sequence that is associated with an abnormally high frequency of *mutation* or *recombination* (see *recombination hotspot*).

HOUSE-DUST MITES (HDM)

HDM are the most important source of *allergens* associated with the indoor environment (see *indoor air pollutants* and *aeroallergens*). Mites of the genus *Dermatophagoides* are most common in Europe and North America, whereas mites of the genus Europhlyphus and Blomia are more common in Central and South America and Southeast Asia.

> HDM are found in association with human habitation and are a major cause of *IgE*-mediated *allergic diseases* including *asthma*, particularly in developed countries where human social behavior and the creation of suitable environments provide conditions for HDM population explosions.

HDM require a warm and humid environment (22° to 26°C, >7 g water/g dry air), and they feed on human skin scales. Microscopic examination of dust samples has shown that mites infest carpet, upholstered furniture, and bedding. In regions of the U.S. that experience warm, humid summers, there appears to be a seasonal rise in mite infestation during this period and a decrease in the drier winter months. In tropical and subtropical areas of the world, the levels of mites remain constant year round. In high-altitude areas (in Europe, 1500 m above sea level), the mite concentrations are dramatically reduced (see *climate therapy*). Barrier avoidance, washing, *vacuuming*, and the use of *acaricides* are all useful methods of HDM avoidance (see *allergen avoidance*).

> *Major allergens* have been identified from both D. pteronyssinus (Der p 1 [24 kDa], Der p 2 [14 kDa]) and D. farinae (Der f 1, Der f 2) and have been sequenced and cloned.

The allergens are digestive enzymes to which human *T cells* mount predominantly *Th2* responses (see *allergen-induced immune responses*). The production of *recombinant allergens* has enabled investigators to produce *monoclonal antibodies* (mAbs) and develop sensitive *immunoassays* for the assessment of allergens in the indoor environment. *Epitope* and restriction mapping have shown that *allergy* to HDM is *major histocompatibility complex* (MHC) restricted, principally by HLA-DR but also HLA-DP and possibly others. Specific allergen *immunotherapy* has been shown to be efficacious in HDM *allergy*.

HOUSEKEEPING GENES

These are *genes* whose expression is essential for the function of all or most cells of the body. Constitutively expressed genes encode enzymes and proteins of basic functions, e.g., metabolism, cytoskeleton proteins) necessary for the survival of cells. Their *promoters* are constitutively active, but not inducible.

5-HPETE

5-hydroperoxyeicosatetraenoic acid is an unstable intermediate in *eicosanoid* metabolism. It is the first product of *5-lipoxygenase* (5-LO) made from *arachidonic acid*. It is either reduced to the alcohol *5-HETE* or further metabolized by 5-LO to generate *leukotriene* A_4 (LTA_4).

12-HPETE

12-hydroperoxyeicosatetraenoic acid is produced by activated *platelets* and can stimulate *5-lipoxygenase* (5-LO) in *leukocytes*.

H_1 RECEPTOR ANTAGONISTS

(See *antihistamines*.)

HUMAN IMMUNODEFICIENCY VIRUS (HIV)

HIV is the virus that causes *acquired immunodeficiency syndrome*.

HUMAN LEUKOCYTE ANTIGEN (HLA)

HLA is the genetic designation for the human *major histocompatibility complex* (MHC).

HUMIDIFIERS

Patients with *asthma* who are sensitive to *house-dust mites* should not use humidifiers or evaporative (swamp) coolers. The increased humidity from these devices can encourage growth of dust mites and *molds* (see *fungal allergens*), and improperly maintained humidifiers may foster growth of mold spores and aerosolize them (see *air conditioning system*).

HYALURONIDASE

This is an important *allergen* of bee and wasp venoms (see *hymenoptera allergy*).

HYBRIDIZATION

This is a general method of pairing *complementary* nucleic acid strands, either *DNA*–DNA or *RNA*–DNA (hybrid) in molecular genetics. Techniques to detect specific DNA or RNA sequences are based on hybridization of a labeled probe to the target nucleic acid (see *in situ hybridization* and *Southern blot*).

HYDROCHLOROCHINE

This is an *immunosuppressive drug*.

HYDROCORTISONE

(See *cortisol*.)

HYDROGEN PEROXIDE (H_2O_2)

H_2O_2 is an *oxygen metabolite*. It is generated from *superoxide anion* (O_2^-) by *superoxide dismutase*. H_2O_2 is scavenged by *catalase* or *peroxidases*.

HYDROXYZINE

This is a first-generation H_1 antagonist (see *antihistamines*).

HYMENOPTERA ALLERGY

Allergic responses to venoms of the hymenoptera range from limited cutaneous to systemic *anaphylactic reactions* with fatal end (see *anaphylaxis*).

> These allergic reactions are *IgE*-mediated but are not related to *atopy*.

As a general rule, there are cross-reactions between honeybee (Apis mellifera) and bumblebee (Bombus) on one hand, as well as between wasp (Vespula vulgaris) and hornet (Vespa crabro) on the other hand (see *cross-reacting allergens*). The *major allergen* in bee venom is *bee venom phospholipase A$_2$* (PLA$_2$), whereas *phospholipase A$_1$* represents the major *allergen* in wasp venom.

> *Immunotherapy* in hymenoptera-allergic patients has the highest success rate of all immunotherapy regimens performed at present.

Therefore, immunotherapy with commercially available lyophilized venom proteins from bee and wasp should be offered to all patients with systemic reactions. In addition, an "emergency kit," consisting of at least liquid formulations of *antihistamines* and *corticosteroids*, eventually supplemented with an *adrenaline* inhaler, should be carried by each patient diagnosed with hymenoptera *allergy*.

HYPERCAPNIA

Elevated arterial CO$_2$ gas tension (p_aCO_2). Hypercapnia always represents alveolar hypoventilation. This may be due to respiratory center depression, mechanical problems at the chest wall, exhaustion, or may be a compensatory mechanism for metabolic alkalosis. In acute *asthma*, hypercapnia is a very poor prognostic sign and an indication for elective *ventilation*.

HYPEREOSINOPHILIA

> Any blood *eosinophilia* of greater than 1500/µl is called hypereosinophilia.

Allergic or *parasitic diseases* may be associated with hypereosinophilia. The apparent etiology involves an *allergen/antigen*-induced *immune response* that involves high *Th2 cytokine* expression, especially *IL-5*. Drugs may also induce hypereosinophilia (see *drug-induced eosinophilia*). In other cases, the reason for the hypereosinophilia might be unclear (see *hypereosinophilic syndrome*).

HYPEREOSINOPHILIC SYNDROME (HES)

> HES is defined as a persistent *hypereosinophilia* of unclear pathogenesis.

Therefore, HES is also called "idiopathic hypereosinophilic syndrome." Table 52 shows the defining features of HES.

TABLE 52
Criteria of HES

Blood *eosinophilia* of greater than 1500/µl present for longer than 6 months.
Unclear pathogenesis (e.g., *allergic diseases* and parasitic infections must be excluded).
Organ involvement.

HES is more common in men than women (9:1). Only a few cases have been reported in children. Although the etiology is unknown, HES is likely to include a range of different diseases. Subgroups may include patients with a clonal expansion of *IL-5*-expressing *T cells* (see *T cell lymphoma*) and patients with an *intrinsic defect of apoptosis* in *eosinophils*, which is at least partially due to an upregulation of the *Bcl-2 gene* in these cells. Hypereosinophilic patients may develop *angioedema* as a consequence of *complement system* and subsequent *eosinophil activation* (*Gleich syndrome*).

HYPER-IgE SYNDROME (HIES)

> HIES is a complex disorder characterized by high levels of serum *IgE*, chronic *dermatitis*, and recurrent serious infections.

HIES patients have large numbers of circulating IgE-secreting *B cells* (1/100,000 compared to 0.4/100,000 in normal subjects). This suggests that clonal expansion of IgE-producing B cells might be a major mechanism underlying elevated IgE production in HIES. However, there is also evidence to suggest that the syndrome might be *T cell*-mediated. For instance, most circulating B cells from HIES patients bear *CD23* on their membrane, which suggests high *IL-4* and/or *IL-13* activity in vivo. Thus, *Th2* activation but deficient *Th1 cytokine* production, which explains the immune deficiency in these patients, might be an important feature in the pathogenesis of the disease. A monoclonal T cell expansion (see *T cell lymphoma*) of *gamma/delta (γ/δ) T cells* that helped B cells to produce very large amounts of IgE has also been described. On the other hand, IL-4 responsiveness might be enhanced in HIES patients. Indeed, a novel IL-4 *receptor α allele* was identified in which *guanine* was substituted for *adenine* at *nucleotide* 1902, causing a change from glutamine to arginine at position 576 in the cytoplasmic domain. The R576 allele was associated with higher levels of expression of CD23 by IL-4 than the wild-type allele. It enhanced *signal transduction* due to a change in the binding specificity of the adjacent tyrosine residue at position 575. The R576 allele also appears to be more frequent in atopic individuals (see *genetic predisposition*).

> Taken together, similar to the *hypereosinophilic syndrome*, HIES appears to be a heterogeneous group of diseases.

HYPER-IgM SYNDROME (HIMS)

> HIMS is an immunodeficiency characterized by recurrent infections in patients with very low levels of serum *IgG*, IgA, and *IgE*, but with normal or elevated IgM, and a normal number of circulating *B cells*.

It was originally thought that B cells from HIMS patients had an intrinsic inability to undergo *immunoglobulin class switching*. However, the observation that patients with HIMS, and particularly those with the X-linked form of the disease (X-HIMS), are prone to opportunistic infections was suggestive of a *T cell* defect, in spite of laboratory evidence for a humoral immune deficiency.

> Indeed, *mutations* of the CD40 ligand (CD40L, see *CD154*), which is expressed on activated T cells, account for X-HIMS.

A total of 68 mutations of the CD40L *gene* have been identified in different X-HIMS families. Although mutations may affect the entire CD40L gene, they are, however, unequally distributed, and the majority fall in *exon* 5, which contains most of the *TNF*-homology domain (see

TNF superfamily). The phenotype of *knockout mice* with targeted disruption of the *CD40* and CD40L genes paralleled that of X-HIMS patients.

HYPERLINEAR PALMS

Hyperlinearity of the palms is a major diagnostic feature of the autosomal dominant genodermatosis *ichthyosis vulgaris*, but is also one of the most important *atopy stigmata*.

HYPERRESPONSIVENESS

(See *airway hyperresponsiveness*.)

HYPERSENSITIVITY

Hypersensitivity is a general term used to describe an adverse clinical reaction to an *antigen* (*allergen*) or *pseudoallergen*.

Some authors differentiate hypersensitivity from the term *allergy* (always pathologic, see *allergic diseases*), since some protective immune responses (e.g., tuberculin) are also associated with hypersensitivity reactions. However, most hypersensitivity reactions are caused by allergens (see *immediate* and *delayed hypersensitivity*). The *Coombs and Gell classification* of hypersensitivity reactions is still in use.

HYPERSENSITIVITY PNEUMONITIS

(See *extrinsic allergic alveolitis*.)

HYPERVENTILATION

Patients who over-breathe (deliberately or subconsciously) will reduce their p_aCO_2 and alkalinize the blood. This leads to symptoms of tingling, weakness, and sickness. Hyperventilation is usually obvious when it occurs at rest, but less obvious when it occurs on exercise. Measurement of end-tidal CO_2 can be useful if assessing whether the respiratory response to exercise is appropriate or excessive. Breathlessness and discomfort associated with hyperventilation are usually excluded from the definition of *dyspnea*.

HYPNOSIS

Hypnosis is a treatment method of *allergic diseases* that belongs to the *complementary procedures*.

HYPOSENSITIZATION

(See *immunotherapy*.)

HYPOXIA

Reduced arterial oxygen tension (p_aO_2). Hypoxia may be due to reduced partial pressure of oxygen in the inspired air, e.g., at high altitude, *ventilation–perfusion mismatch*, or hypoventilation. Tissue hypoxia occurs when insufficient oxygen reaches the tissues, and this may be due to all the above plus failure to deliver oxygen from the lungs to the tissues caused by poor circulation, anemia, hemoglobinopathies, or *carbon monoxide* (CO) poisoning.

I

IAACI

International Association of Allergology and Clinical Immunology.

ICAM-1

(See *intercellular adhesion molecule-1*.)

ICHTHYOSIS HAND

(See *hyperlinear palms*.)

ICHTHYOSIS VULGARIS

Being the most common of all inherited skin disorders, ichthyosis vulgaris is characterized by dry scales at the trunk and extremities, sparing the flexures. Many patients are unaware of their disease, since the symptoms are generally mild and tend to improve under a proper skin-care regimen. *Hyperlinear palms* are the diagnostic hallmark of this frequently undiagnosed skin disease. About 50% of the affected patients suffer from *atopic dermatitis*.

IDEC

(See *inflammatory dendritic epidermal cells*.)

IDIOPATHIC RHINITIS

(See *vasomotoric rhinitis*.)

IDIOPATHIC HYPEREOSINOPHILIC SYNDROME

(See *hypereosinophilic syndrome*.)

IDIOPATHIC THROMBOCYTOPENIC PURPURA

(See *thrombocytopenic purpura*.)

IDIOSYNCRASY

Idiosyncrasy is a *hypersensitivity* reaction with no immunological basis.

The symptoms are also not related to the pharmacological effects of a given substance. *Pseudoallergy* is a common synonym for idiosyncrasy. If there is an immunological background for the reaction, an *allergic disease* is diagnosed. If there are symptoms resembling the pharmacological (toxic) effects of the substance at higher doses, an *intolerance* reaction is diagnosed (see *adverse drug* and *food reactions*)

IDIOTYPE

When an *immunoglobulin* is used as an *antigen*, it will be treated like any foreign protein. The hypervariable regions of *antibodies* act as single antigenic determinants (see *epitope*) and elicit an antibody response.

IDIOTYPIC NETWORK

When it was shown that *antibodies* can be raised against hypervariable regions of other antibodies, it was assumed that anti-*idiotype* antibodies can mimic *epitopes* of the original *antigen*. Anti-idiotype antibodies were shown to suppress the *B cells* producing the original antibody. Therefore, Jerne proposed a network to control the antibody responses by anti-idiotype antibodies.

> Today, there is only little evidence that anti-idiotype antibodies play an important role in downregulation of *immune responses*.

IFN

Standard abbreviation for *interferon*.

Ig

Standard abbreviation for *immunoglobulin*. Different immunoglobulin *isotypes* are called IgM, IgD, *IgG*, IgA, and *IgE* (see *immunoglobulin class switching* and *antibody*). Ig is also used to describe the following molecules:

Igα and Igβ: co-receptors of the *B cell antigen receptor*
Igμ: heavy chain of IgM
Igδ: heavy chain of IgD
Igγ: heavy chain of IgG
Igα: heavy chain of IgA
Igε: heavy chain of IgE

IgE

IgE is an *immunoglobulin* (Ig) molecule independently discovered by the Ishizakas and Johansson (see *history of allergy research*). The heavy chain of the molecule has four constant domains. This is in contrast to other Igs, which have only three constant domains. IgE is found primarily bound to *high-affinity IgE receptors*, and therefore it was called homocytotropic *antibody*. Moreover, due to its capacity to sensitize skin (see *Prausnitz–Küstner reaction*), it was called reaginic antibody.

> The primary role of IgE seems to be related to the *immune response* to parasites.

Once IgE is cross-linked (see *cross-linking*) on the surface of *mast cells* or *basophils* by an *antigen*, it induces *degranulation* and *mediator* release, leading to an *immediate hypersensitivity* reaction. Mast cells in the gut are sensitized with IgE and migrate to the gut mucosa, where they are triggered to degranulate following contact with worm antigen. Since approximately 30% of the world's population has *parasitic diseases*, the evolutionary pressure might have initiated the development of a specific Ig class for host defense against parasites.

> *Allergic diseases* appear to be an unfortunate by-product of this evolutionary step.

IgE is a direct target of new therapeutic strategies in such diseases (see *anti-IgE therapy*).

IgE LEVELS

Normal total serum concentration of *IgE* is in the range of 10 to 100 IU/ml (25 to 250 ng/ml), which is 10^5 times less than *IgG*, and comprises less than 0.001% of the total *immunoglobulin*. IgE levels are often raised in IgE-mediated *allergic diseases*, but also in *parasitic diseases*.

Highest levels are found in patients with *hyper-IgE syndrome* (HIES). *Atopy* is often associated with high IgE levels, but normal levels do not exclude atopy. High IgE levels (up to 100 times normal levels) are usually found in *atopic dermatitis* patients. In *hay fever* and *asthma*, elevation of IgE in serum is observed in about half of the patients (up to 2 to 10 times normal levels).

> Normal total IgE levels do not exclude the possibility of elevated *allergen*-specific IgE *antibodies* (see *RAST, Phadiatop, CAP-system*).

The presence of specific IgE antibodies can also be investigated using *skin tests*.

IgE RECEPTORS

(See *high-affinity IgE receptor* and *low-affinity IgE receptor*.)

IgE REGULATION

> Selection of *IgE* is mediated by the *Th2 cytokines IL-4* and/or *IL-13*.

The role of *T cell sensitization* and *allergen* recognition is central to the regulatory effects of these cells on IgE production. The effect of IL-4 interaction with its *receptor* on *B cells* (see *IL-4 receptor signaling*) is the preferential appearance of epsilon (ε) germ-line transcripts during the process of *antibody affinity maturation* and *gene rearrangement* associated with *immunoglobulin class switching*. IL-4 is also important in sustaining the population of Th2 cells necessary for this process, by positive feedback. In contrast to Th2 cytokines, *Th1* cytokines such as *IFN-γ* and *IL-12* are inhibitory.

> In addition to cytokine release, Th2 cells also provide cognate help (see *cognate/noncognate interactions*) to B cells.

For instance, direct interactions between T and B cells occur via the *T cell antigen receptor* and *MHC class II molecules* on B cells (B cells can act as *antigen-presenting cells*). Moreover, *co-stimulations* involving *CD28/B7* or *CD40/CD40 ligand* also contribute to the signals necessary to induce IgE selection and production (see Figure 28).

Moreover, the *low-affinity IgE receptor* (CD23) can influence the regulation of IgE by two distinct mechanisms. First, it can act as an *adhesion molecule* between T and B cells during cognate interactions, and this interaction may contribute to IgE selection in much the same way as the co-stimulatory interactions mentioned above. Second, membrane-bound CD23 can undergo spontaneous proteolysis (by constitutive membrane serine proteases) to release several soluble fragments. There is evidence that certain of the human soluble CD23 fragments have a modulatory (usually reported as enhancing) effect on IgE production. However, as the expression of CD23 is initially regulated by Th2 cytokines (particularly IL-4), it is not clear what the relevance of CD23 is in IgE production.

IgG

IgG is the principal *immunoglobulin* (Ig) *isotype* in the blood and extracellular fluid. It efficiently opsonizes pathogens for engulfment by *phagocytes* and activates the *complement system*. There are four IgG subclasses. Lack of IgG causes humoral immunodeficiency. Some patients with *asthma* are primary or secondary *(corticosteroids!)* IgG-deficient. *Intravenous immunoglobulin (IVIG) preparations* might be especially beneficial in these patients.

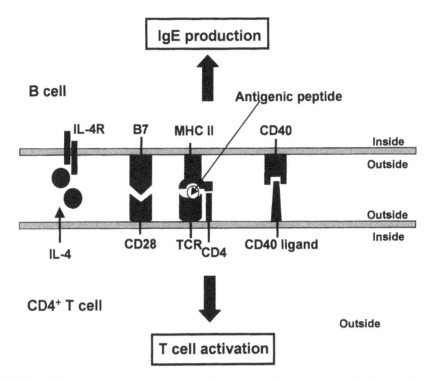

FIGURE 28 Molecular interactions between Th2 cells and B cells to induce IgE production. IL-13 can replace IL-4 in the induction of immunoglobulin class switching.

IgG$_4$

IgG$_4$ is the least abundant among the four human *IgG* subclasses, with serum levels that average 0.2 to 1 g/l in adults. Lack of IgG$_4$ is perhaps the most common *immunoglobulin* (Ig) *isotype* deficiency. IgG$_4$ has been reported to be involved in mucosal immunity, and particularly in the response to protein *antigens* and prolonged antigenic challenge. Among children with recurrent severe respiratory infections, up to 26% of the patients had selective IgG$_4$ deficiency. On the other hand, IgG$_4$-deficient adults are often asymptomatic. *Immunotherapy* is associated with an increase in *allergen*-specific IgG$_4$ (see *immunotherapy: effects on IgE and IgG isotypes*).

IL

IL is the standard abbreviation for *interleukin*.

IMMEDIATE HYPERSENSITIVITY

Immediate *hypersensitivity* reactions have a rapid onset. They occur within a few minutes following *allergen* contact. The reaction reaches its peak about 15 or 20 minutes after the initial trigger and clears by 1 hour, unless it is followed by a *late-phase response* (LPR).

Role of mast cells

The *mast cell* is a central player involved in orchestrating the immediate hypersensitivity reaction. In allergic reactions, mast cells are activated by an *IgE*-dependent mechanism (classical allergic reaction, see *Coombs and Gell classification*, type I). However, mast cells can also be activated directly by non-IgE mediated mechanisms (e.g., *complement factor receptors*).

Clinical symptoms are the consequence of either IgE or non-IgE-mediated *mast cell activation*, leading to the release of preformed *mediators* from their cytoplasmic *granules* (see *exocytosis*).

These mediators include *histamine, leukotrienes, platelet-activating factor* (PAF), *eotaxin*, and various *neutral proteases* and reactive proteins.

IgE-mediated mechanisms

Mast cells or *basophils* bind IgE via *high-affinity IgE-receptors*. *Cross-linking* of IgE receptor molecules due to allergen binding initiates a signal at the cell membrane that is transduced into the cell (see *signal transduction*), leading to mediator release.

T cell sensitization of individuals to allergens and specific IgE antibody production by *B cells* is a prerequisite for IgE-mediated immediate hypersensitivity reactions.

The most *common allergens* include *house-dust mite, animal dander*, and *grass pollens*. Some drugs (e.g., penicillin) can also induce an allergic response (see *drug allergy*). Some lectins, which are found in fruits such as strawberries, are also able to cross-link high-affinity IgE receptors.

Non-IgE-mediated mechanisms

Mast cells can be triggered in the absence of IgE (see Figure 29). For instance, the *anaphylatoxins C3a* and *C5a* can bind to specific *G protein-coupled receptors* and consequently activate mast cells. Other receptor-mediated degranulation mechanisms are the consequence of *platelet-activating factor* (PAF), *leukotriene*, or *chemokine* stimulation (see *histamine-releasing factors*). In addition, opiates, such as *morphine,* cause cellular activation and mediator release in a non-receptor-mediated manner (see *anesthetic allergy*). Mast cells can

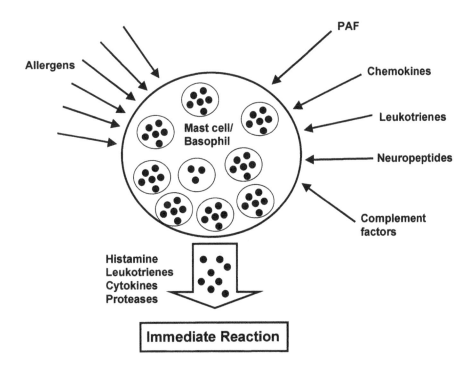

FIGURE 29 IgE and non-IgE-mediated mechanisms of immediate hypersensitivity reactions.

also be activated by mediators from the granules of *neutrophils* or by *neuropeptides*, such as norepinephrine and *substance P*.

> Unlike IgE-dependent hypersensitivity, non-IgE-mediated reactions can occur during the first exposure to such agents.

Symptoms and localization

The release of mast cell mediators can have several effects such as vasodilation, *smooth muscle* contraction, acute *inflammation*, sensory nerve stimulation, *mucus* hypersecretion, and tissue damage. These biological effects cause symptoms such as itching eyes, runny nose, and sneezing, as well as *airway obstruction* and *wheeze* as is frequently observed in *allergic rhinoconjunctivitis* and *asthma*.

> Immediate allergic reactions can be localized to a particular organ, such as the lung or skin, or they can be systemic, in which case they are called *anaphylaxis*.

Route of allergen exposure, number of mast cells at the location, phenotype of the mast cells resident at that location (see *mast cell heterogeneity*), and the sensitivity of the local tissue to mast cell mediators determine the location and the intensity of the immediate hypersensitivity reaction. The onset of either a localized or systemic allergic reaction can prove fatal as a result of asphyxiation or cardiac failure (see *death from asthma*).

Skin reaction

If the allergen is injected into the skin, a classical wheal and flare response is seen (see *immediate hypersensitivity skin test*). The raised wheal is pale and soft with a spreading flare that is maximal in 15 to 20 minutes and fading within a few hours. The effects of histamine in the immediate allergic response have been understood using *antihistamines*. The *edema* (wheal) is caused by contraction of *endothelial cells* of the postcapillary venules, mediated by activation of histamine H_1 receptors, with consequent exudation of plasma fluid. The local *erythema* (flare), which does not contain a cellular infiltrate immediately after triggering, is caused by arteriolar vasodilation due to the interaction of histamine with H_2 receptors, resulting in an increased blood flow.

Lung reaction

If an allergen is inhaled, an immediate allergic reaction occurs in the lung. In this event, mast cell mediators act on both blood vessel and bronchial smooth muscle cells. The smooth muscle cells in the airways of asthmatics are frequently "hyperreactive" to mast cell mediators such as histamine (see *airway hyperresponsiveness* and *bronchial provocation tests*).

Anaphylaxis

Inoculation by a stinging insect, for example bee venom (see *hymenoptera allergy*), or parenteral administration of an *antibiotic* such as *penicillin* can result in anaphylaxis. *Tryptase* and histamine levels in the serum of subjects with systemic anaphylaxis are elevated in the majority of cases, indicating that mast cells or basophils are involved. In fact, the serum concentrations of these two mediators have been shown to correlate with the decline in mean arterial pressure.

Pharmacological inhibition

At therapeutic doses, H_1 receptor antagonists (e.g., terfenadine and astemizole) can inhibit up to 75% of the wheal and flare response to an intradermal allergen and approximately 50% of the immediate allergen-induced *airway obstruction* in the lung. *Cromoglycate* sodium and *nedocromil* sodium can inhibit immediate allergic reactions in the airways and gastrointestinal tract, but have little effect on such reactions in the skin. *β2-Agonists* are also potent inhibitors of immediate hypersensitivity reactions. They inhibit the release of mediators from mast cells and also antagonize the contractile effects of mast cell mediators. β2-Agonists have also been shown to inhibit the wheal and flare reaction in the skin, as well as the allergic symptoms following nasal *allergen challenge*. In contrast, *corticosteroids* have only little direct effect on immediate hypersensitivity reactions.

IMMEDIATE HYPERSENSITIVITY SKIN TEST

There are two types of *immediate hypersensitivity* skin test: (1) *prick tests* and (2) *intradermal tests*. Wheal and flare reactions develop 15 to 20 minutes after injection in allergic individuals. This reaction is caused by *degranulation* of skin *mast cells* following *cross-linking* of *high-affinity IgE receptors* by *allergen* via bound *IgE* molecules. Mast cell *granules* contain *histamine*, which is responsible for the *edema* and *erythema*. The reaction usually resolves within 1 hour.

Immediate hypersensitivity skin tests form the basis of *allergy* diagnosis.

Patients can be tested with a battery of *allergen extracts*, depending on the clinical history. The diameter of the wheal and flare is an indication of the degree of hypersensitivity to a given allergen.

IMMUNE COMPLEX

Immune complexes are *antigen–antibody* aggregates. They are usually formed to eliminate antigens and are taken up by *phagocytes*. In the case of antigen excess, small immune complexes are created that tend to deposit in blood vessel walls, where they can activate the *complement system* or activate *leukocytes* via *Fc receptors*, causing inflammatory *mediator* release (see *allergic vasculitis*). The *hypersensitivity* reactions caused by immune complexes are called *type III reactions* (see *Coombs and Gell classification*).

IMMUNE RESPONSE

(See *allergen-induced immune responses*, *primary immune response*, and *secondary immune response*.)

IMMUNE SURVEILLANCE

With the exception of some immune "privileged" organs such as the testes, all compartments of the human body are controlled by the *immune system*. The capacity of the immune system to detect tumor cells is called immune surveillance. However, many tumors use escape mechanisms to prevent anti-tumor *immune responses*. Interestingly, these mechanisms are at least partially similar to those seen in immune "privileged" tissues (e.g., *Fas ligand* expression).

IMMUNE SYSTEM

The immune system is a collection of cells and proteins that protects the body from potentially harmful, infectious microorganisms, such as bacteria, viruses, and *fungi*. A *hypersensitivity* reaction occurs when an *antigen*-induced *secondary immune response* results in tissue damage and *inflammation*.

IMMUNOASSAY

A test for measuring *antigen* (*allergen*) or *antibody*. The *radio allergo sorbent test* (RAST) utilizes ^{125}I-conjugated anti-*IgE* antibody and provides a measure of *allergen*-specific IgE in

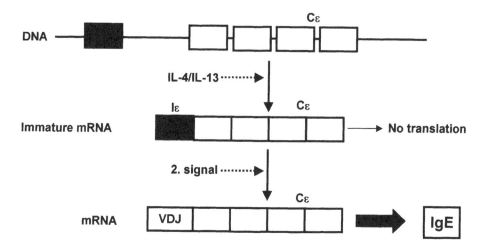

FIGURE 30 Mechanisms of immunoglobulin class switching in the generation of IgE antibodies. Under the influence of IL-4 or IL-13, an immature IgE mRNA is induced. A mature mRNA is generated only if the B cell receives a second activation signal (e.g., via CD40).

serum. The *enzyme-linked immunosorbent assay* (ELISA) uses an enzyme-base reaction (usually hydrogen *peroxidase* or alkaline *phosphatase*) to generate a colorimetric test for quantifying antigen or antibody (see also *Phadiatop and CAP-system*).

IMMUNOGLOBULIN (Ig)

(See *Ig* and *antibody.*)

IMMUNOGLOBULIN CLASS SWITCHING

During a *T cell*-mediated *immune response*, a *B cell* can undergo *immunoglobulin* (Ig) *isotype* switching (Figure 30), which results in the expression of a different heavy chain in association with the same rearranged variable region.

The newly generated Ig has the same *antigen*-binding specificity but acquires new effector functions.

Therefore, isotype class switching is one of the mechanisms that permit modulation of humoral immune responses. Igs are encoded by heavy chain (C_H) *genes*, which are associated with rearranged VDJ genes, which encode for antigen specificity. Switching to a particular isotype is an irreversible *recombination* event, directed by *cytokines* and *B cell* activation signals. Several molecular changes in the 5′ flanking regions of the switch regions correlate with targeting of switch recombination. These include the induction of *DNase hypersensitivity*, and consequent germline *transcription* of the implicated *genes*. Germline transcripts share a similar structure: they initiate from a *TATA box*-less *promoter* a few kB upstream of the switch region and proceed through one or more short *exons* (I exons) that are spliced to the first exon of the C_H gene that will be expressed. They do not contain a VDJ region and have stop codons in all three reading frames, so they are not able to code for any *peptide* of significant length. For this reason germline transcripts are also called "sterile." The I exons are shorter than VDJ so that germline transcripts are shorter than mature transcripts.

IMMUNOGLOBULIN GENE REARRANGEMENT

(See *gene rearrangement.*)

IMMUNOGLOBULIN SUPERFAMILY

Immunoglobulin (*Ig*) domains are the characteristic feature of proteins of the immunoglobulin superfamily that include *antibodies*, *adhesion molecules*, *T cell antigen receptor*, *MHC molecules*, *cytokine receptors*, etc. The immunoglobulin domain comprises two β-pleated sheets held together by a disulfide bond, called the immunoglobulin fold. All members of the family have at least one immunoglobulin domain.

IMMUNOHISTOCHEMISTRY

Technique to detect *antigens* in tissues using specific *antibodies*. It allows the analysis of *gene* expression at the protein level under in vivo conditions.

IMMUNOMODULATORS

Based on the pathomechanisms in *asthma* and other *allergic diseases*, target sites for immunomodulation include the inhibition of *T cell activation* or production of *cytokines*, *eosinophil* accumulation (see *eosinophilia*), *IgE* production, and effector functions of inflammatory cells (see *mast cell activation* and *eosinophil activation*). Modulation of the *immune system* can be done by nonselective (see *corticosteroids, cyclosporin A, theophylline, intravenous immunoglobulin* (*IVIG*) *preparations*) or more selective (see *immunotherapy, anti-IgE-therapy, cytokine* or *anticytokine therapy*) approaches (see also *anti-allergic/asthmatic drugs*).

IMMUNORECEPTOR TYROSINE-BASED ACTIVATION MOTIF (ITAM)

Many components of the *T cell antigen receptor*, *B cell antigen receptor*, and *high-affinity IgE receptor* contain a common sequence motif in their cytoplasmic tails. This motif consists basically of two YxxL *amino acid* sequences, which are precisely spaced over an approximately 26-amino-acid sequence. The sequence is as follows:

$$D/Exxxxxxx D/Exx\textbf{Y}xx\textbf{L}xxxxxxx\textbf{Y}xx\textbf{L}$$

This sequence is important for *signal transduction* via the above-mentioned *antigen receptors*. It is essential for *calcium mobilization* induced by *cross-linking* of these *receptors*. In general, it appears that *Src tyrosine kinases* phosphorylate the ITAM, which allows the recruitment of other tyrosine *kinases*, such as ZAP-70 (in *T cells*) or Syk (in *B cells* and *mast cells*). These kinases then activate, directly or indirectly, *phospholipase C* by *tyrosine phosphorylation*.

IMMUNORECEPTOR TYROSINE-BASED INHIBITION MOTIF (ITIM)

Most studies in the last few decades focused on the mechanisms that induce *inflammation*. This means that we understand quite well how an *immune response* is initiated.

> However, it is clear that the activation of the *immune system* has to be limited, otherwise *hypersensitivity* reactions and subsequent *allergic diseases* develop.

Such *immunosuppressive mechanisms* are, compared to the above-mentioned activation events, less well understood. In addition, they may also play a role in the *resolution of inflammation*. The discovery of ITIMs present in several surface *receptors* has generated a broader interest in this area. The ITIM motif consists basically of one YxxL *amino-acid* sequence, whereby the tyrosine residue is critical for the initiation of distal *signal transduction* events. The sequence is as follows:

$$T/Sxx\textbf{Y}xx\textbf{L}$$

In general, it appears that *tyrosine kinases* phosphorylate the ITIM, which allows the recruitment of inhibitory *tyrosine phosphatases*. The inhibitory *phosphatases* prevent or terminate an induced *signaling* cascade initiated via activation receptors by rapid *dephosphorylation* of tyrosine-phosphorylated proteins. ITIMs are present in *CTLA-4*, CD32 (FcγRIIb), CD22, CD122, *CD131*, and CD158 (see *CD antigens*). Therefore, ITIMs appear to play a role in the termination of signaling events initiated via *antigen receptors* and *cytokine receptors*, as well as in the limitation of *NK cell* activity.

IMMUNOSUPPRESSIVE DRUGS

Immunosuppressive drugs are widely used in transplantation and autoimmune diseases (see *autoimmunity*). *Allergic diseases* are associated with chronic *T cell activation* that maintains the inflammatory process in allergic tissues, e.g., in the airways of patients with *asthma*.

Immunosuppressive drugs are used to downregulate *T cell* responses.

For instance, *corticosteroids* are used to decrease *cytokine* expression in T cells (see *asthma treatment strategies*). However, some patients are steroid-resistant (see *corticosteroid-resistant asthma*), and therefore other immunosuppressive drugs have been used to control *inflammation* in asthma. These drugs include anti-*CD3* and anti-*CD4 monoclonal antibodies* (see *antibody therapy*), *methotrexate*, as well as *cyclosporin A* (CsA). Moreover, a few studies using gold, azathioprine, and hydrochlorochine have shown a steroid-sparing effect in *corticosteroid-dependent asthma*. Some *anticytokine* (e.g., anti-*TNF-α*) and *cytokine therapies* (e.g., *IFN-α*) may also be immunosuppressive. Anti-*CD25* antibodies may also be used to target activated T cells.

IMMUNOSUPPRESSIVE MECHANISMS

The *immune system* has the capacity to upregulate certain cell numbers and functions during host defense mechanisms.

When the pathogen has been eliminated, the normal condition has to be reestablished, indicating that immunosuppressive mechanisms must exist.

Moreover, when the immune system is activated (e.g., during *antigen* exposure in *inflammation*), mechanisms have to exist that limit the *immune response*. Table 53 summarizes some of the inhibitory molecules that may also play a role in *allergic diseases*.

IMMUNOTHERAPY

Definition
Allergen-specific immunotherapy is the practice of administering gradually increasing quantities of an *allergen extract* to an allergic subject to ameliorate the symptoms associated with subsequent exposure to the causative allergen.

In contrast to *allergen avoidance* and pharmacological intervention (see *anti-allergic/asthmatic drugs*), immunotherapy is a causal therapy of *allergic diseases*.

Immunotherapy was introduced by Noon and Freeman in 1911 to treat *hay fever* (see *history of allergy research*).

Indications
Immunotherapy should be offered to a patient if there are severe symptoms caused by an *IgE*-mediated reaction (see *immediate hypersensitivity*) to an allergen that cannot be avoided (see Table 54). It has proven efficacy in *hymenoptera allergy*, in certain respiratory *allergies*,

---

TABLE 53
Extracellular and Intracellular Molecules with Inhibitory Effects on Immune Functions

Extracellular

1. *Fas ligand* and other factors that activate *death receptors*
2. *Cortisol*
3. *TGF-β*
4. *IL-10*
5. *Antigens* in the absence of co-stimulatory signals (*see anergy*)
6. Ligand-induced *receptor* internalization
7. *IL-4*
8. Soluble receptors (e.g., soluble *TNF receptor*)
9. *IL-1 antagonist*
10. Ligands that stimulate receptors with an intracellular *immunoreceptor tyrosine-based inhibition motif* (ITIM) (e.g., *CTLA-4*)
11. Peptidases on the surface of *epithelial cells*
12. Protease inhibitors produced by epithelial cells that prevent tissue damage and invasion of inflammatory cells
13. *Lipoxins*

Intracellular

1. Src-homology 2 (SH2)-domain-containing *tyrosine phosphatases* (e.g., SHP-1)
2. *C-terminal tyrosine kinase* (CSK)
3. Suppressor of *cytokines* signaling (SOCS) family
4. Signal-regulatory protein (SIRP) family
5. *Corticosteroid receptor*
6. SMAD protein family (*TGF-β* signal transducers)
7. *Caspases* (execute cells that are no longer needed for host defense, see *apoptosis*)
8. Degradation of signaling molecules
9. Naturally occurring dominant negative variants of signaling molecules (e.g., *STAT5*)
10. *cAMP*
11. *Heparin*

---

such as those to *pollens* and *house-dust mites*, and has been tried in a wide range of other allergies including those to *animal dander* and *fungal allergens*. However, there are several interrelated factors that make this a potentially dangerous form of therapy (see *anaphylactic reaction*). Therefore, it is now usually only conducted in controlled clinical environments where resuscitation equipment is immediately at hand.

Contraindications

Immunotherapy is contraindicated in cases of moderate to severe *allergic asthma*, where pathological mechanisms can be exacerbated by exposure to even minute amounts of specific allergen (see *asthma exacerbation*). Contraindications also include chronic infections, autoimmune diseases (see *autoimmunity*), or a therapy with β-blockers. Immunotherapy should not be started in pregnancy, but may be continued when it has been started before pregnancy.

Guidelines

The treatment consists of establishing an exposure dose of allergen to which a subject does not react (usually by titration using *skin test* methods) to use as a starting dose for subcutaneous injection. Gradually increasing the dose of allergen administered over a number of injections renders the subject desensitized, that is, nonresponsive to successively higher doses of allergen. The time course and incremental doses are determined by the immunotherapy regimen being

---

TABLE 54
Indications and Contraindications for Immunotherapy

Indications

1. Hymenoptera allergy
2. *Allergic rhinitis, rhinoconjunctivitis, asthma*
   - Pollen allergy
   - House-dust mite allergy
   - Allergy to animal dander
   - *Mold* allergy

Contraindications

1. Treatment with β-blockers
2. Other immunologic diseases or malignancies
3. Poor *compliance*
4. Severe asthma (uncontrolled by pharmacotherapy, irreversible *airway obstruction*)
5. Cardiovascular diseases
6. Children under the age of 5 years

---

followed and range in time from an injection course over several months and maintenance injections lasting for years, to an induction phase of 24 hours to reach high but tolerated allergen doses, followed by maintenance. The effects of immunotherapy can last for years (or even indefinitely), but more data are required to accurately assess the long-term effectiveness of this treatment.

The most severe side effect of immunotherapy is the induction of anaphylaxis.

These symptoms are usually effectively treated by the administration of *adrenaline* and *corticosteroids*. There are many contributory factors that affect the efficacy of immunotherapy, and among the most important is the nature of the allergenic material used for treatment. Where purified, recombinant, or synthetic *peptide* allergens (see *recombinant allergen* and *peptide immunotherapy*) have been used, results are generally more favorable than with poorly standardized or crude allergenic fractions. Thus, allergen standardization is a major issue in this field of treatment. *DNA immunotherapy* is a new development in this direction.

Mechanisms

The immunological mechanisms of effective hyposensitization are complex and involve an initial phase, where IgE-mediated reactions are circumvented, as well as a later phase, where *T cell* mechanisms become altered. Gradual and subclinical depletion of preformed *mediators* from *mast cells* and *basophils* in response to increasing concentrations of allergen during immunotherapy has been postulated, but anecdotal evidence showing that systemic reactions can occur at any point during immunotherapy suggest that this is not a major mechanism of desensitization. The potential for *histamine* release and *prostaglandin* production from basophils falls during successful immunotherapy, but not rapidly enough to account for the onset of desensitization. This leaves the question open as to how rapid desensitization of inflammatory effector cells occurs. There is the intriguing possibility that the effects of increasing concentrations of allergen interacting with IgE initially serve to directly inhibit the signals transduced via the *high-affinity IgE receptor*. However, the exact mechanism by which *degranulation* of mast cells and basophils is prevented remains to be elucidated.

Several other mechanisms have been proposed to explain the long-term clinical improvement of immunotherapy. For instance, the induction of blocking *antibodies* directed against the causal allergen and/or of anti-*idiotype* antibodies directed against the IgE antibody was one of the earlier explanations (see *immunotherapy: effects on IgE and IgG isotypes*). Moreover, a shift from *Th2* to a *Th1 cytokine*-pattern as well as the induction of *T suppressor/cytotoxic cells* are still under discussion.

> However, recent data suggest that induction of a state of specific *anergy* (only T cells expressing the allergen-specific *T cell antigen receptor* are affected) represents the key mechanism of immunotherapy.

Specific anergy is characterized by suppressed allergen-induced proliferative responses (see *lymphocyte transformation test*) and reduced both Th1 and Th2 cytokine production. Reduced Th2 cytokine expression then leads to decreased IgE levels and lower *eosinophil* numbers. Anergy is associated with increased basal *tyrosine kinase* and/or decreased *tyrosine phosphatase* activity. Moreover, the induction of anergy in allergen-specific Th2 cells represents an active process that is associated with the induction of *IL-10* and *IL-2 receptor* (CD25) *genes*. Increased IL-10 expression has been demonstrated during immunotherapy in T cells, *B cells*, and *monocytes*.

> IL-10 appears to be important for the induction and maintenance of anergy.

Interestingly, *allergen-specific immune responses* can be reestablished in anergic T cells by cytokines from the microenvironment. For example, *IL-2* and/or *IL-15* can restore proliferative responses as well as *IFN-γ* secretions. On the other hand, *IL-4* and/or *IL-13* reestablish Th2 cytokine expression in anergic cells (see Figure 31). These data explain why and when an immunotherapy might not be successful: an allergen-induced anergy may not last long in a polyallergic individual (see *polysensitization*) where the anergic cells are in a Th2 environment. In contrast, immunotherapy appears to be a promising therapeutic option in mono- or oligoallergic patients. These new insights may also explain why immunotherapy is especially successful in children and in patients with hymenoptera allergy.

IMMUNOTHERAPY: EFFECTS ON IgE AND IgG ISOTYPES

While peripheral *anergy* has been demonstrated in allergen-specific *T cells*, the capacity of *B cells* to produce *allergen*-specific *IgE* and *IgG₄ antibodies* does not appear to be abolished during conventional *immunotherapy*. Serum-specific IgE levels initially rise and gradually fall to normal over a period of months. Moreover, increases in IgG_1 and large increases in IgG_4 specific for the allergen have been detected. In ultrarush bee venom immunotherapy (see *hymenoptera allergy*), specific serum levels of both IgE and IgG_4 increase during the early phase of treatment.

> However, the increase in specific IgG_4 is more pronounced, and the ratio of specific IgE to IgG_4 decreases by 10- to 100-fold.

Also, the in vitro production of *bee venom phospholipase A_2* (PLA_2)-specific IgE and IgG_4 antibodies by *peripheral blood mononuclear cells* (PBMC) changes in parallel with the serum levels of specific *isotypes*. Reciprocal production of allergen-specific IgG_4 vs. IgE by B cells appears to be favored at high and low *IFN-γ* to *IL-4* ratios, respectively. Furthermore, *IL-10*, which is induced and increasingly secreted during allergen-specific immunotherapy, appears to counterregulate antigen-specific IgE and IgG_4 antibody synthesis.

IMPRINTING

Differential expression of an *allele* depending on whether it was inherited from the mother or father.

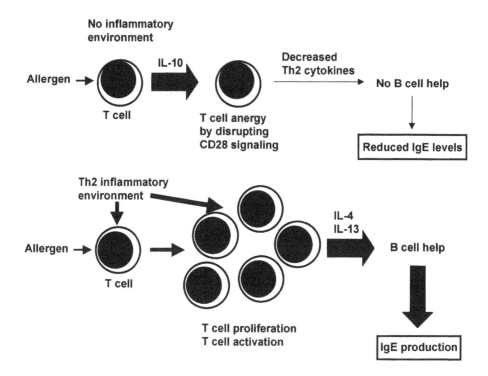

FIGURE 31 Immunological mechanisms of specific immunotherapy (upper panel). In the presence of inflammation, T cells receive cognate (CD80, CD86) and noncognate (IL-2, IL-4, IL-15) co-stimulatory signals, which lead to T cell activation in the presence of allergen (lower panel). The figure may also explain why individuals with an IgE-mediated allergy develop more and more allergies in life.

INDETERMINATE CELLS

Indeterminate cells describe a rare epidermal cell population of non-*keratinocytes* in normal skin. The name was suggested by G. Rowden in 1979, describing an inhomogenous mixture of probably immature, *Langerhans cell*-related cells and immature melanocytes. However, since *Birbeck granules* could be detected in serial sections of many of the indeterminate cells, and because it is questionable to describe cells that do not represent a biological entity, most researchers decided to discontinue its use. If encountered in a more recent paper, the term is most likely to refer to a cell somehow related to a Langerhans cell.

INDOOR AIR POLLUTANTS

In addition to *outdoor air pollutants*, people are also exposed to a wide variety of agents indoors. These agents range from *allergens* to combustion *pollutants* to *irritants* in consumer products. A number of substances found in indoor air may cause *asthma*, and several indoor pollutants are known to precipitate and increase asthma symptoms upon exposure. The following classes of indoor pollutants are relevant to respiratory diseases: (1) *aeroallergens*, (2) agents used in occupational environments (see *occupational asthma*), and (3) irritants. Indoor *aeroallergens* include *animal dander, house-dust mite, cockroach,* and *fungal allergens*. Occupational exposures range from irritants to organic dusts. Irritants include tobacco smoke (see *smoking*), ambient pollution such as *ozone* and *sulfur dioxide*, formaldehyde, and other compounds found in fabrics, carpets, and furniture, as well as fumes, sprays, and strong odors (see also *air conditioning, air-duct cleaning, allergen avoidance, dehumidifiers, humidifiers, indoor air cleaning devices, vacuuming*).

INDUCED CYTOKINE PRODUCTION

The *transcription* of *cytokine genes* can be induced by activation of cell surface *receptors* in many different cells. *Cross-linking* of receptors activates *signal transduction* pathways that stimulate *transcription factors*. The induction of *Th2* cytokine genes is a characteristic feature of *allergic inflammation* (see *cytokine gene activation*).

INDUCIBLE NITRIC OXIDE (NO) SYNTHASE

(See *nitric oxide synthase*.)

INFLAMMATION

> Inflammation is traditionally defined by heat, pain, redness, and swelling (in Latin: calor, dolor, rubor, and tumor) as a consequence of bacterial infection.

These symptoms are the result of *cytokines* on the blood vessel that mediate dilation and increased permeability. Cytokines also increase the expression of *adhesion molecules* on *endothelial cells* of the blood vessel wall, allowing *migration* of inflammatory cells into the tissue. The classical view is that inflammation is a process responsible for host defense against bacteria. The main cell types seen in such an inflammatory response in its initial phase are *neutrophils* and *macrophages* (innate immunity). Inflammatory responses later in a bacterial infection involve *lymphocytes* (adaptive immunity).

> Today, the term "inflammation" is used in a broader way, since an *immune response* can also be initiated by *antigens* that are not bacteria.

When the antigen represents an *allergen*, the immunological response, which occurs in patients with *allergic diseases*, is called *hypersensitivity* reaction resulting in *allergic inflammation*.

INFLAMMATORY DENDRITIC EPIDERMAL CELLS (IDEC)

IDEC are epidermal *dendritic cells* that accumulate within inflamed *epidermis*. Unlike *Langerhans cells*, they have no *Birbeck granules* and no *LAG antigen*, but they do express *CD1*b and CD11b. IDEC have been observed for many years, but ultrastructural and immunophenotypic delineation of the two cell types has only recently been achieved. The ontogeny of this cell type is unclear, but there is some evidence for a *monocyte*-derived origin of these cells. In *atopic dermatitis*, these cells express very high levels of the *high-affinity IgE-receptor*.

INFLAMMATORY LUNG DISEASES

This term could be used to describe a heterogeneous group of diseases associated with *inflammation* in the lungs. The many diseases differ as to their etiology and pathogenesis. Therefore, each disease could be characterized using the classification presented in Table 55.

In clinics, the term "inflammatory lung disease" is usually less broadly used.

> Instead, it is used as a synonym for "idiopathic pneumopathy," which means that the differential diagnosis of the lung disease is unclear.

TABLE 55
Possible Classification of Inflammatory
Lung Diseases

1. Based on the pathogen
   - Infectious (bacteria, virus, fungi, parasites)
   - Noninfectious (e.g., *allergen*, autoantigen)
2. Based on the course of the disease
   - Acute
   - Chronic
3. Based on the inflammatory cell infiltrate
   - Neutrophilic (see *neutrophils*)
   - Eosinophilic (see *eosinophils*)
   - Lymphocytic (see *lymphocytes*)
   - Mixed
4. Based on the localization of inflammation
   - *Alveolitis*
   - Bronchiolitis
   - *Bronchitis*
   - Tracheitis
   - Interstitial
5. Based on the response of the *immune system*
   - Immunodeficient
   - Allergic (see *hypersensitivity*)
   - Autoimmune (see *autoimmunity*)

Bronchoalveolar lavage (BAL) fluid investigations are often useful to differentiate between *sarcoidosis, extrinsic allergic alveolitis, cryptogenic fibrosing alveolitis*, and other chronic inflammatory diseases.

INFRAORBITAL EYELID FOLD

(See *Dennie–Morgan infraorbital fold*.)

INHALATION SYSTEMS

Today, inhalation is the preferable route of delivery for *anti-allergic/asthmatic drugs*. It reduces systemic effects and may have additional effects on superficial inflammatory cells. *β2-Agonists, corticosteroids*, sodium *cromoglycate, nedocromil*, and *ipratropium* are available as inhaled preparations.

> Four different inhalation systems can be used: *metered dose inhalers* (MDI), MDI with spacers (see *spacer devices*), *dry powder inhalers* (DPI), and *nebulizers*.

There are marked differences between these systems in output characteristics, deposition pattern of the inhaled particles, optimal inhalation technique, and ease of use.

INHALED CORTICOSTEROIDS (ICS)

The recognition of the chronic inflammatory nature of *asthma* (see *allergic inflammation*) has led to a fundamental change in our thinking about how best to manage asthma. When asthma was thought of as a disorder of excessive, intermittent contraction of *smooth muscle*, the logical way to treat it was with short-acting *bronchodilators*. Inhaled corticosteroids were generally considered as second-line agents to be used when bronchodilators were insufficient.

> Now we believe that the optimum strategy is to relieve the *inflammation* first, and thereby reduce the triggers of *airway obstruction*.

The early 1990s saw an increasing emphasis on the use of ICS, which in turn raised concerns about possible long-term side effects of ICS, especially when started in childhood. It is clear that inhaled corticosteroids are very effective agents in most patients with asthma, but it is becoming clear that up to 30% of asthmatic patients show little or no response to ICS, even though they have reversible airflow obstruction and appear to be asthmatic by all other criteria. At the same time, we now realize that the dose–response curve for ICS is relatively flat. In other words, ICS can achieve a certain amount of improvement, but increasing the dose beyond 800 mg beclomethasone per day (or equivalent) confers only limited additional benefit in most asthmatic patients.

> Concerns about possible adverse effects of ICS on children's growth have attracted publicity, but all the evidence indicates that asthmatic children grow better if their asthma is properly treated.

Even if they fail to grow as rapidly as normal children, they seem to continue growing for longer and eventually reach the same height. These limitations on the beneficial role of ICS have been highlighted by the introduction of long-acting *β2-agonists* (salmeterol, formoterol), which provide relief over and above that achievable with high-dose ICS (see *asthma treatment strategies*).

INHIBITORY FACTOR OF κB (IκB)

IκB is an intracellular physiologic inhibitor of *nuclear factor-κB* (NF-κB).

INITIATION SITE OF TRANSCRIPTION

Synonymous with *transcription* start site or cap site, representing the first transcribed *nucleotide* of the *gene* sequence.

INNER-CITY ASTHMA

Asthma in the inner city has been identified as an important public health problem.

> While a number of factors may contribute to the increased frequency and severity of asthma in the inner city, socioeconomic status (SES) and *cockroach allergens* are of particular interest.

Low SES has been correlated with increased prevalence of asthma and increased asthma severity. Race seems not to be a factor per se, as studies show no ethnic differences in asthma severity when SES factors are taken into consideration. Studies in the U.S. have also indicated that cockroach allergen may be a principal *risk factor* in *childhood asthma* in the inner city. *Allergy* to cockroach, but not *house-dust mite* or cat (see *cat allergen*), correlates with increased risk of hospitalization for asthma.

INOSITOL-1,4,5-TRISPHOSPHATE (IP$_3$)

IP$_3$ is an intermediary metabolite of the *inositol polyphosphate cascade* that is directly responsible for intracellular *calcium mobilization*.

INOSITOL POLYPHOSPHATE CASCADE

Activation of the inositol polyphosphate cascade starts with the generation of *inositol-1,4,5-trisphosphate* (IP$_3$) by *phospholipase C* (PLC), which is activated either by *G proteins* or *tyrosine kinases*. PLC activation results in activation of *protein kinase C* (PKC) and *calcium mobilization*. The control of intracellular calcium ion concentration [Ca^{2+}]$_i$ is very tightly regulated, and an integral and important component of intracellular *signaling* pathways leading to cell activation.

INSERTION

An insertion is the integration of a *DNA* sequence into a defined DNA sequence.

IN SITU HYBRIDIZATION

This is a laboratory technique to analyze *mRNA* expression of specific *genes* in tissue sections. A labeled nucleic acid (probe) hybridizes (see *hybridization*) to target nucleic acids in tissue sections. It allows a qualitative and quantitative detection of *DNA* or *RNA* molecules in cells or tissues in a physiological context. It can be combined with *immunohistochemistry* to identify the cell type which expresses the particular mRNA. This technique has been used to demonstrate the predominant expression of *Th2 cytokines* in bronchial tissues from patients with *asthma* (see also *fluorescent in situ hybridization*).

INTEGRINS

Integrins are molecules found on the surface of *leukocytes* involved in cell–cell and cell–*extracellular matrix* interactions. They are dimers composed of α and β subunits.

Integrins can be grouped into subfamilies based on their β subunit.

β1 integrins, also known as very late antigens (see *VLA-4*) proteins, have a common β-chain (*CD29*) paired with α-units of the α1 group (see below). β2 integrins, also known as leukocyte cell-*adhesion molecules*, share the β-chain (*CD18*) paired with α-units of the α2 group (see below).

The α-subunits include three subfamilies.

The α1 group is expressed with six variants of the α-chain (CD49a-f). The ligands for these molecules include *laminin, fibronectin, collagen*, and *VCAM-1*. CD49d/CD29 is VLA-4 found on *eosinophils* and is thought to be important in mediating *allergic inflammation*. The α2 group is expressed on *leukocytes, macrophages, monocytes*, and *granulocytes* and is co-expressed with one of three variants of CD11: CD11a (LFA-1, see *lymphocyte function-associated antigen-1*), CD11b (Mac-1), or CD11c (p150,95).

Failure of *neutrophils* to express CD11b/CD18 is the basis for *leukocyte adhesion deficiency*, in which neutrophils cannot adhere to *endothelial cells* and therefore are unable to respond to tissue infection.

The α3 integrins are involved with adhesive events between platelets and molecules such as fibronectin and fibrinogen. α-Subunits associated with this group are *CD1* and CD51.

INTERCELLULAR ADHESION MOLECULE-1 (ICAM-1)

ICAM-1 or CD54 mediates adhesion and *migration* between cells by molecular interactions with its specific ligand *lymphocyte function-associated antigen-1* (LFA-1), a member of the β2 *integrin* family of *adhesion molecules*.

ICAM-1 is a member of the *immunoglobulin superfamily* of molecules. It is constitutively expressed on bronchial *epithelial cells* and *endothelial cells*, and can be upregulated by *IFN-γ*,

TNF-α, IL-1β, IL-4, and other inflammatory *mediators* released upon cell activation. It can be considered as an early marker of *inflammation.* Raised levels of soluble ICAM-1 are associated with bronchial *asthma, allergic rhinoconjunctivitis,* and viral infection. ICAM-1 expression is downregulated by *corticosteroids* and *antihistamines.*

INTERDIGITATING RETICULAR CELLS

These are *dendritic cells* that have matured and successfully migrated to the *lymph node,* where they accumulate in *T cell*-rich regions. Interdigitating reticular cells are *antigen-presenting cells* (APCs) that present their *antigens* to naive T cells (see *naive lymphocytes*).

INTERFERONS (IFNs)

IFNs can be classed into either type I IFNs, such as *IFN-α* and IFN-β, or type II IFNs, such as *IFN-γ.* IFNs are particularly important in the first line of defense against viruses, as well as exerting immunoregulatory effects on other cells. For instance, IFNs induce the expression of *major histocompatibility complex* (MHC) antigens, as well as *macrophage, T cell, B cell,* and *NK cell* activity. IFN-γ is the *cytokine* that was identified first, and it typifies a *Th1 cell* response.

INTERFERON-α (IFN-α)

IFN-α is a family of several closely related proteins. It is synthesized by many cell types after viral infection, and induces a state of resistance to viral replication in all cells. IFN-α and IFN-β bind to a common cell surface *receptor* (see *cytokine receptors*).

> IFN-α is an interesting therapeutic option in severe *asthma* and in the *hypereosinophilic syndrome* (see Table 56).

TABLE 56
Effects of IFN-α Related to Allergic and Eosinophilic Diseases

- Inhibitory effect on *IL-4* expression in *Th2 cells* and consequent reduced *IgE* synthesis in *B cells.*
- Inhibitory effect on *IL-5* expression in *Th2 cells* and consequent reduction of *eosinophil* numbers.
- Inhibitory effects on eosinophil effector functions.
- Activation of *NK cells* with possible *IFN-γ* release.
- Upregulation of the *Fas receptor* in several cells — this may help to resolve *inflammation* by induction of *apoptosis.*
- May increase the effect of *corticosteroids* in steroid-resistant patients (see *steroid-resistant asthma*).

INTERFERON-γ (IFN-γ)

> IFN-γ is a classical *Th1 cytokine.*

However, IFN-γ production is not restricted to *CD4+* Th1 cells. *NK cells, CD8+ Tc1 cells,* and *γ/δ T cells* are also able to generate large amounts of IFN-γ. Recently, *mast cells* and *eosinophils* (see *eosinophil cytokines*) have also been reported to be able to generate IFN-γ, although the biological significance of these findings is not clear at the moment.

> NK cell-derived IFN-γ is crucial in controlling viral infections before *T cells* have been activated to produce this cytokine.

IFN-γ *receptors* (see *cytokine receptors*) are present on virtually all cell types, with the exception of erythrocytes, and are abundantly expressed by neural cells. The IFN-γ receptor is comprised of a ligand-binding transmembrane glycoprotein, and a less characterized accessory protein necessary for *signal transduction*. The antiviral activity of IFN-γ is mediated by induction of reactive *oxygen metabolites* and *nitric oxide* (NO) in *macrophages* and *neutrophils*. Besides antiviral activity, IFN-γ activates macrophages to kill tumor cells and intracellular parasites (*see parasitic diseases*).

> IFN-γ or IFN-γ receptor *knockout mice* succumb to infection with a range of intracellular pathogens.

On the other hand, autoimmune diabetes has been observed in IFN-γ *transgenic mice*. IFN-γ upregulates *major histocompatibility complex* (MHC) expression (both class I and II molecules) on *antigen-presenting cells* (APCs) and other *leukocytes*. Furthermore, IFN-γ can influence proliferation, differentiation, and effector functions of T cells. For instance, IFN-γ inhibits *Th2* cytokine expression and *IgE* synthesis.

> Peripheral blood mononuclear cells (PBMC) from patients with IgE-mediated *allergic diseases* often have a reduced capacity to generate IFN-γ upon pan-*T cell activation*.

IFN-γ *gene* expression is modulated by various cytokines and drugs (see Table 57).

TABLE 57
Factors that Modulate IFN-γ Gene Expression

Factors that induce IFN-γ gene expression
IL-1
IL-2
IL-12
IL-18
TNF-α
Antigens
Mitogens (PHA, ConA)

Factors that inhibit IFN-γ gene expression
Corticosteroids
IL-4
IL-10
Cyclosporin A (CsA)
2,5-Dihydroxyvitamin D3
Genetic predisposition of patients with allergic diseases

The antiviral, antitumor, and antiparasitic activities displayed by IFN-γ suggest that this cytokine may have therapeutic value in a broad spectrum of diseases. Indeed, IFN-γ is being used as an antineoplastic agent for a variety of cancers, although initial results have not been encouraging. IFN-γ also has demonstrable efficacy in treating viral diseases such as hepatitis B. Moreover, IFN-γ is a treatment for *cryptogenic fibrosing alveolitis* and *rheumatoid arthritis*.

> In contrast, the clinical efficacy of IFN-γ appears to be marginal in *asthma* and *atopic dermatitis* (see *cytokine therapy*).

INTERLEUKINS (ILs)

The term IL was created during a time when researchers believed that *cytokines* were molecules produced by *leukocytes* that act on leukocytes. However, this is now known not to be the case, since cytokines act upon many different cell types (see *pleiotropism*). However, the terminology persists. There are 18 described ILs that have been cloned (see *DNA cloning*). Many of the ILs are produced by *T cells*, and play an important role in *allergic inflammation*.

INTERLEUKIN-1 (IL-1)

The IL-1 family is a group of three related polypeptide hormones that includes IL-1α, IL-1β, and *IL-1-receptor antagonist* (IL-1ra). *IL-18* is a related *cytokine* that may also belong to the IL-1 family.

> IL-1 is an endogenous pyrogen and induces fever.

IL-1 is also involved in muscle proteolysis, bone resorption, wound healing, and hematopoiesis.

> Moreover, IL-1 induces *adhesion molecules* on *endothelial cells*.

Therefore, IL-1 is involved not only in inflammatory diseases such as diabetes, periodontitis, and *rheumatoid arthritis*, but also in *IgE*-mediated and non-IgE-mediated *allergic diseases*. For instance, production of IL-1 by *Langerhans cells* and *lymph node dendritic cells* is an early and characteristic response during *contact sensitization*. Numerous other cell types also produce IL-1, including astrocytes, *B cells*, endothelial cells, *keratinocytes*, *epithelial cells*, and *monocytes*. IL-1 *gene* expression is modulated by various *cytokines*, inflammatory *mediators*, and drugs (see Table 58).

TABLE 58
Factors that Modulate IL-1 Gene Expression

Factors that induce IL-1 gene expression
LPS
IL-1
TNF-α
Leukotrienes
C5a
GM-CSF
Zymosan
Phorbol ester

Factors that inhibit IL-1 gene expression
Corticosteroids
cAMP
IL-4
IL-10
TGF-β
PGE_2
Retinoic acid

IL-1 is synthesized as a biologically inactive precursor molecule lacking a signal *peptide*.

> IL-1 precursor requires cleavage into an active, mature molecule by the intracellular *IL-1-converting enzyme* (ICE), which is also known as *caspase* 1.

Therefore, inhibitors of ICE may be useful as *immunosuppressive drugs*. On the other hand, overexpression of IL-1 may block *Fas receptor*-mediated *apoptosis*.

INTERLEUKIN-1-CONVERTING ENZYME (ICE)

ICE is a protease with at least two functions: (1) activation of *IL-1*, and (2) activation of distal *caspases* in the process of *apoptosis*. An alternative name is caspase 1.

INTERLEUKIN-1 RECEPTORS

Two distinct *IL-1 receptors* (IL-1R) have been identified, termed type I (80 kDa) and type II (68 kDa) (see *cytokine receptors*). Both receptors bind IL-1α and IL-1β with high affinity (10^{-10} M). Receptor density ranges from 0 to 30,000 per cell, with *fibroblasts* and *keratinocytes* displaying the highest levels. Both IL-1RI and IL-1RII are members of the *immunoglobulin superfamily*.

INTERLEUKIN-1-RECEPTOR ANTAGONIST (IL-1ra)

IL-1ra is a naturally occurring *IL-1 receptor* antagonist. Clinical trials have shown that recombinant IL-1ra is effective in treating several inflammatory diseases including *asthma* (see *anticytokine therapy*).

INTERLEUKIN-2 (IL-2)

IL-2 and the IL-2 *receptors* are primarily expressed by *Th cells* which have been activated via the *T cell antigen receptor*, resulting in clonal expansion of *antigen*-specific T cells.

> IL-2 is an autocrine factor driving the expansion of antigen-specific cells, a mechanism which is also important in *allergic inflammation*.

In addition, IL-2 may act as a paracrine factor, influencing the activity of other cells, both within the *immune system* and outside of it. *B cells* and *NK cells* respond to IL-2 when suitably activated. The so-called lymphocyte-activated killer (LAK) cells appear to be derived from NK or NK-like cells under the influence of IL-2. Moreover, *eosinophils* express high-affinity IL-2 receptors following stimulation with *IL-5* (for IL-2 receptor, see *cytokine receptors*).

INTERLEUKIN-2 GENE ACTIVATION

(See *cytokine gene activation*.)

INTERLEUKIN-3 (IL-3)

> IL-3 is produced primarily by activated *T cells*.

This is in contrast to *GM-CSF*. The largely exclusive production of IL-3 by activated T cells has led to the concept that IL-3 may only be involved during *immune responses*, and does not play a role in normal hematopoiesis. However, in *inflammation*, its main effects are on the development of pluripotent stem cells in the *bone marrow*, where it can stimulate the generation and differentiation of *monocytes*, *neutrophils*, *eosinophils*, *basophils*, *mast cells*, and erythroid cells.

INTERLEUKIN-3 RECEPTOR

The *receptor* of *IL-3* is a heterodimer of α- and β-subunits. The α-chain is specific for this *cytokine receptor*, whereas the β-chain is shared by IL-3, *IL-5*, and *GM-CSF* receptors. IL-3 receptors are expressed by pluripotent stem cells in the *bone marrow*, but also by mature *granulocytes* and *monocytes*. For *signal transduction*, see *interleukin-5 receptor*.

INTERLEUKIN-4 (IL-4)

IL-4 is a potent multifunctional *cytokine* that can stimulate growth and differentiation and maintains the viability of subsets of *B cells* and *T cells*.

IL-4 is characteristically produced by *Th2 cells*.

Mast cells, *basophils*, and *eosinophils* can also generate significant amounts of IL-4.

IL-4 is one important factor for *immunoglobulin class switching* and subsequent *IgE isotype* selection and synthesis in B cells.

It has approximately 30% homology with *IL-13* and shares some functions with it, such as IgE selection.

IL-4 induces naive T cells to develop into a Th2 functional phenotype, which is reciprocally antagonized by *IFN-γ*.

In addition, it induces expression of *vascular adhesion molecule-1* (VCAM-1) on *endothelial cells* and *low-affinity IgE receptor* (CD23) on B cells, and may be involved in the development of *fibrosis* during tissue repair processes in chronic *allergic inflammation* (see *airway remodeling*).

Moreover, IL-4 directly induces *IL-10 gene* expression in Th2 cells.

This mechanism may explain some of the antiinflammatory effects of IL-4 that may also limit *allergic inflammation* (see *immunosuppressive mechanisms*).

INTERLEUKIN-4 CYTOKINE GENE CLUSTER

(See *T helper 2 cytokine gene cluster*.)

INTERLEUKIN-4 RECEPTOR

Immunoglobulin class switching to *IgE* and subsequent synthesis of IgE *antibodies* by *B cells* form the basis of IgE-mediated *allergic diseases*. Given the critical role of *IL-4* and *CD40* in inducing IgE synthesis, an understanding of the IL-4 *receptor* (IL-4R) and CD40 *signaling* complexes is essential for the design of anti-allergic strategies that interfere with *isotype* switching to IgE.

The α-chain of the IL-4 receptor (IL-4Rα) is also part of IL-13 receptors.

To determine the *signal transduction* events mediated via this shared receptor component, chimeric receptors, consisting of the extracellular and transmembrane domains of the erythropoietin (Epo) receptor, were fused to the intracellular domain of IL-4Rα. Treatment of these cells with Epo induced the activation of Jak1 (see *Janus kinases*) and STAT6 (see *signal transducer and activator of transcription*), and Cε germline *transcription* in the absence of the IL-4R γ-chain and of Jak3. Moreover, deletion of the so-called box 1-motif in IL-4Rα abolished its signaling capacity, indicating that Jak1 is critical for the induction of Cε germline transcripts following homodimerization of the IL-4Rα chains.

Taken together, Jak1 and STAT6 activation appear to be critical signaling events following stimulation of B cells via IL-4Rα with IL-4 or IL-13.

INTERLEUKIN-5 (IL-5)

IL-5 is a classical *Th2 cytokine*.

Besides *T cells*, *mast cells* and *eosinophils* can also generate significant amounts of IL-5. IL-5 structure is closely homologous across species, and there is cross-reactivity of the protein between various mammalian species. The biologically active form is comprised of two monomeric units arranged into an anti-parallel dimer. The main target of IL-5 is the eosinophil and as such it controls eosinophil numbers and functions.

Overexpression of IL-5 leads to *eosinophilia* due to both increased generation of eosinophils in the *bone marrow* and delayed *eosinophil apoptosis*.

IL-5 also activates eosinophils for effector functions (see *eosinophil activation*). Since the eosinophil appears to be an important inflammatory effector cell in *allergic inflammation*, IL-5 represents a target for new anti-allergic drug developments (see *anticytokine therapy*).

INTERLEUKIN-5 RECEPTOR

The *receptor* of *IL-5* is a heterodimer of α- and β-subunits. The α-chain is specific for this *cytokine receptor* and, in humans, is expressed only on *eosinophils* and *basophils*.

In contrast, the β-chain is shared by *IL-3*, IL-5, and *GM-CSF* receptors.

Mutant β-subunits that lack respective cytoplasmic regions are incapable of transducing signals, suggesting that the β-chain is essential for *signal transduction* via these receptors. The cytoplasmic part of the β-chain does not contain a *kinase* domain. Therefore, it utilizes cytoplasmic *tyrosine kinases* of the *Janus kinase* and the *Src* family to phosphorylate distal molecules. In eosinophils, it has been shown that Jak2 and *Lyn* are essential for delayed *eosinophil apoptosis*. These kinases are also activated in other cells upon IL-3 or GM-CSF stimulation. In addition, the activation of *phosphatidylinositol 3-kinase* (PI3-kinase) has been reported in IL-3-stimulated *bone marrow-derived mast cells* (BMMC).

INTERLEUKIN-6 (IL-6)

IL-6 is both produced by and has effects on a broad spectrum of cell types. IL-6-mediated functions include growth promotion and inhibition, regulation of *immunoglobulin* and acute phase protein *gene* expression as well as induction of differentiation. IL-6 appears to be involved in *autoimmunity* related to polyclonal *B cell* activation and lymphoproliferative disorders. The role in *allergic inflammation* is unclear. However, it may synergize with *IL-4* and *IL-13* in upregulating *IgE* (and *IgG*) production. IL-6 can be induced by a variety of agents including LPS, *IL-1*, *TNF*, and *IFNs* (for IL-6 receptor, see *cytokine receptors*).

INTERLEUKIN-8 (IL-8)

IL-8 is a member of the *CXC chemokine* family and is a *chemotactic factor* for *neutrophils*; this appears to be the major function of this *chemokine*, although functional IL-8 receptors were also observed on a subset of *T cells* (see *chemokine receptors*). IL-8-mediated *chemotaxis* for *eosinophils* has been described, but findings are controversial. Biological activity in human cultures is restricted to a narrow concentration range between 5 and 50 ng/ml. Many cells are capable of producing IL-8 in response to appropriate stimuli, including *monocytes*, *lymphocytes*, neutrophils, and eosinophils as well as other cell types such as *epithelial cells*, *fibroblasts*, and *keratinocytes*.

IL-8 expression is increased at allergic inflammatory sites (see *allergic inflammation*), however, the role of IL-8 in *allergic diseases* remains unclear.

INTERLEUKIN-9 (IL-9)

Lung selective expression of IL-9 in *transgenic mice* has been shown to induce *airway hyperresponsiveness*, in addition to morphologic changes similar to those in *asthma*.

INTERLEUKIN-10 (IL-10)

IL-10 was described as a *Th2 cytokine*. However, this view has been corrected, because of functional aspects of IL-10, and also due to the fact that it can also be produced by *Th0* and *Th1 cells*. Other potential cellular sources of IL-10 are *B cells*, *monocytes*, and *keratinocytes*. IL-10 has been shown to exhibit profound inhibitory effects on some functional aspects of monocytes, including downregulation of *MHC class II molecules*. This might be due to a suppression of the *IFN-γ* gene by IL-10. Moreover, IL-10 suppresses many other cytokine genes, including *IL-4* and *IL-5* (see *immunosuppressive mechanisms*). In addition, IL-10 is a potent suppressor of both total and *allergen*-specific *IgE*, while IgG_4 formation increases simultaneously.

> IL-10 is currently in preclinical studies to evaluate its potential in *allergic diseases*.

Interestingly, IL-10 concentrations in *bronchoalveolar lavage* (BAL) fluids are decreased in patients with *asthma*. Moreover, IL-10 expression is induced in allergen-specific *T cells* (see *anergy*), *B cells*, and *monocytes* during *immunotherapy*. Under these conditions, it appears that IL-10 induces *anergy* by disrupting *CD28*-mediated co-stimulatory signals (see *co-stimulation*). Furthermore, under stress conditions, it has been shown that *adrenalin* and noradrenalin can stimulate IL-10 release, which is blocked by β-blockers (for IL-10 receptor, see *cytokine receptors*).

INTERLEUKIN-12 (IL-12)

> IL-12 promotes the development and expansion of *Th1 CD4+* cells and cytotoxic *CD8+* cells by the induction of *IFN-γ gene* in *T cells* and *NK cells*.

Therefore, IL-12 may have a role in modulating Th1/*Th2 cytokine* production in *allergic diseases*. The effects of IL-12 are antagonized by *IL-10* and *IL-4* (see *immunosuppressive mechanisms*). It is mainly produced by *monocytes/macrophages*, and *B cells*, and to a lesser extent by *dendritic cells*, *neutrophils*, and, perhaps, *eosinophils* (for IL-12 receptor, see *cytokine receptors*).

INTERLEUKIN-13 (IL-13)

> IL-13 can replace *IL-4* in *immunoglobulin class switching*. However, unlike IL-4, it is unable to differentiate naive *T cells* into *Th2 cells*.

Other biological activities include upregulation of *MHC class II molecules* on *monocytes* and *B cells*, and inhibition of proinflammatory *cytokines* produced by monocytes (*TNF-α*, *IL-1*, and *IL-6*). IL-13 is highly expressed in *allergic inflammation*, e.g., at the inflammatory sites in patients with *asthma* and *atopic dermatitis*. It is principally produced by activated Th2 cells, but can also be expressed by *mast cells* and *eosinophils*. IL-13 neutralization experiments demonstrated a key role for this cytokine in the pathogenesis of *asthma* in an experimental in vivo mouse model.

INTERLEUKIN-13 RECEPTOR

The α-chain of *IL-4* and *IL-13 receptors* (see *cytokine receptors*) is shared, suggesting that similar *signal transduction* pathways (see *IL-4 receptor*) are initiated by these two *cytokines* in cells which express both receptors (such as *B cells*). *T cells* do not appear to express functional IL-13 receptors.

INTERLEUKIN-15 (IL-15)

IL-15 is a more recently identified *cytokine* that shares all its activities with *IL-2*. Therefore, it can be considered as a *Th1* cytokine. In contrast to IL-2, IL-15 is produced by many different cells.

INTERLEUKIN-16 (IL-16)

IL-16 is also called *lymphocyte* chemoattractant factor (LCF).

IL-16 is a *chemotactic factor* for *CD4+ T cells, monocytes,* and *eosinophils,* but not *neutrophils.*

It also increases the expression of high-affinity *IL-2 receptors* on responding T cells. IL-16 is stored in human lung *mast cells.* Moreover, IL-16 is released from *CD8+* T cells and airway *epithelial cells* after *histamine* stimulation in vitro. Elevated IL-16 concentrations were found after *allergen challenge* in *bronchoalveolar lavage* (BAL) fluids from patients with *asthma.* These data suggest that IL-16 is one possible link between *immediate* and *delayed hypersensitivity* reactions in asthma (for IL-16 receptor, see *cytokine receptors*).

INTERLEUKIN-18 (IL-18)

IL-18 promotes the development and expansion of *Th1 CD4+* cells and cytotoxic *CD8+* cells by the induction of *IFN-γ gene* in *T cells* and *NK cells.*

IL-12 and IL-18 act synergistically to increase IFN-γ production.

Therefore, IL-18 may have a role in modulating Th1/*Th2 cytokine* production in *allergic diseases.* IL-18 is related to the *IL-1* family in terms of both structure and function. Also similar to IL-1, IL-18 is produced as a precursor molecule, which has to be activated by *interleukin-1-converting enzyme* (ICE). It is mainly produced by *monocytes/macrophages,* but also by *keratinocytes,* the adrenal cortex, and pituitary gland cells.

INTERNATIONAL STUDY OF ASTHMA AND ALLERGIES IN CHILDHOOD (ISAAC)

The rise in the prevalence of *allergic diseases* (see also *asthma epidemiology*) suggests an increase in the susceptibility to, or development of, *atopy.* Environmental factors are likely the cause for the increase in the prevalence of *asthma.* At the moment, the environmental determinants of atopy are largely unknown. Therefore, ISAAC was initiated to use the spatial distribution of disease worldwide as a tool to identify important risk factors. ISAAC provides a standardized framework for these investigations.

INTERSTITIAL LUNG DISEASES

(See *inflammatory lung diseases.*)

INTOLERANCE

A form of *hypersensitivity* reaction to a substance, intolerance has no immunological basis and resembles the pharmacological (toxic) effects of the substance at higher doses (see *Stevens–Johnson syndrome* and *food intolerance*). If the symptoms are not related to the pharmacological effects of the substance, and if there is no immunological background (see *allergic diseases*) detectable, an *idiosyncrasy* (pseudoallergy) is diagnosed.

INTRADERMAL TEST

This *skin test* is useful in diagnosing *IgE*-mediated *allergies* (see *Coombs and Gell classification*, type I). It can be used as a more sensitive alternative to the skin *prick test*. Approximately 0.03 ml of the *allergen extract* is injected into the skin. Wheal reactions above 5 mm are regarded as positive (see also *immediate hypersensitivity skin tests*).

INTRAVENOUS IMMUNOGLOBULIN (IVIG) PREPARATIONS

The passive transfer of *immunoglobulins* (Igs) provides an alternative therapy in patients with severe *corticosteroid-dependent asthma*. IVIG preparations exhibit antiinflammatory activity and may mimic some of the effects of active *immunotherapy*. It has been suggested that IVIG preparations control airway *inflammation* by affecting *cytokine* production. Moreover, IVIG preparations may contain blocking anti-*Fas receptor antibodies* (see *toxic epidermal necrosis*). In clinical trials, a reduction in *corticosteroid* dosage and an improvement in *asthma* symptom scores was demonstrated (see *antibody therapy*).

INTRINSIC ASTHMA

As early as 1918, Rackemann classified *asthma* as intrinsic or extrinsic. Intrinsic asthma occurs in individuals without evidence of *atopy*. *Skin tests* are negative and *allergen*-specific, and total *IgE levels* are low in serum. This type of asthma often begins in adult life. In intrinsic asthma, *T cells* generate *IL-5*, but compared to *allergic asthma*, decreased amounts of *IL-4*.

> Intrinsic asthma is associated with abnormal *Th2* activation and can be considered a *delayed hypersensitivity* reaction.

Moreover, and in contrast to *extrinsic asthma*, the patients often need systemic *corticosteroid* treatment (see *corticosteroid-dependent asthma*). Furthermore, patients frequently develop a *corticosteroid-resistant asthma* (CRA). Some physicians doubt that an intrinsic type of asthma exists, and suggest that all asthma is in fact extrinsic.

INTRINSIC ATOPIC DERMATITIS

A subgroup of patients with *atopic dermatitis* is known to have normal serum total *IgE levels*, undetectable *allergen*-specific IgE levels (see *RAST, Phadiatop, CAP-system*), and negative skin *prick tests* toward allergens. This form of atopic dermatitis has been termed intrinsic atopic dermatitis.

> As observed in atopic dermatitis, skin lesions of intrinsic atopic dermatitis patients are largely infiltrated by *T cells*.

Most of the skin T cells express *cutaneous lymphocyte-associated antigen* (CLA). However, and in contrast to atopic dermatitis, these skin T cells are unable to provide sufficient help for *immunoglobulin class switching*, perhaps due to decreased *IL-13* expression. Interestingly, blood T cells from both subgroups of atopic dermatitis patients have an increased capacity to produce IL-13 compared to normal control individuals (see also *intrinsic asthma*).

INTRINSIC DEFECT OF APOPTOSIS

An intrinsic defect of *apoptosis* is often observed in cancer cells. For instance, the antiapoptotic protein *Bcl-2* is upregulated in certain *B cell* lymphomas due to a chromosomal translocation, which brings the Bcl-2 gene under the control of an *immunoglobulin promoter*. A similar observation has been made in a subgroup of patients with the *hypereosinophilic syndrome*, in which delayed *eosinophil apoptosis* occurs in the absence of *eosinophil survival factors*. Therefore, this phenomenon was termed "intrinsic defect of apoptosis." In contrast, in *allergic diseases*, *delayed apoptosis* depends on the overexpression of *cytokines* such as *IL-5*. The reason for dysregulated apoptosis in these diseases is therefore "extrinsic."

INTRON

This is a noncoding *DNA* sequence in *genes*, which is initially transcribed (see *transcription*) into precursor *mRNA*, but later removed during mRNA processing by the splicing machinery; thus, mature mRNA molecules lack intronic sequences (see also *exon*).

INVARIANT CHAIN

The invariant chain is a multifunction protein with a central role in the endocytotic pathway (see *endocytosis*) of *antigen-presenting cells* (APCs). The functions include (1) *MHC class II molecule* translocation from the endoplasmic reticulum to the acidic class II-rich compartments, and (2) prevention of newly synthesized *major histocompatibility complex* (MHC) molecules from *peptide* loading inside the endoplasmic reticulum.

IN VITRO MUTAGENESIS

In vitro mutagenesis is a method to modify genetic sequences and is used to study *gene* and protein functions.

Plasmid DNA harboring the gene of interest is treated either chemically or enzymatically to alter the *nucleotide* sequence. Mutagenesis experiments may be designed to be random or targeted to specific sequences or codons. Random mutagenesis is often used when little is known about the function of a particular gene or protein. For example, chemical treatment of DNA with sodium bisulfite causes the deamination of *cytosine*, and results in a C to T base change. Such randomly substituted genes are then screened for a change in function, and sequence analysis (see *DNA sequencing*) identifies the areas that were mutated. A more detailed analysis may follow using site-specific mutagenesis, targeted to a specific region of a gene, for example *promoter* elements, or to a specific codon. The mutation of choice is generated by annealing a synthetic oligonucleotide encoding the desired mutation to the plasmid DNA. *DNA polymerase* initiates synthesis of a *complementary DNA* strand from this oligonucleotide *primer*, resulting in a copy of the gene of interest that now contains the mutation. Upon transformation of bacteria and without further selection, about 50% of the resulting colonies will harbor the wild-type gene, and 50% will contain the mutated gene. DNA sequence analysis is used to confirm the mutation. Variations of this approach have been developed that favor the recovery of the mutated sequence.

IONOPHORE

(See *calcium ionophore*.)

IPRATROPIUM

Ipratropium belongs to the group of *anticholinergic agents*. Anticholinergic drugs provide effective protection against spasmogens and are potent *bronchodilators* in *asthma* and *chronic obstructive pulmonary disease* (COPD).

IRRITANT

Besides *allergens*, low-molecular-weight reagents (= irritants) can also cause *asthm*a. The mechanisms, by which these molecules exert their effects, are not entirely understood. Many of these compounds are the cause of *occupational asthma*.

In contrast to *IgE*-mediated responses, irritants act through nonimmunological mechanisms, such as damaging the bronchial *epithelial cells* or by direct pharmacologically induced *airway obstruction*.

Damage to the epithelium (see *epithelial damage*) leads to the nerve endings being exposed to *mediators*, causing *neurogenic inflammation*. *Isocyanates* represent small molecules that clearly cause *occupational asthma* (see *isocyanate-induced asthma*); however, in most cases, they are not associated with the development of an IgE-mediated response. Other irritants associated with occupational asthma include hard metals, platinum, Western red cedar, and synthetic metals. Moreover, *ozone*, *sulfur dioxide*, and *nitrogen dioxide* are irritant gases and can elicit *airway hyperresponsiveness*.

Besides asthma, irritants are also often involved in the pathogenesis of *occupational dermatitis*.

IRRITANT CONTACT DERMATITIS

(See *occupational dermatitis*.)

IRRITANT-INDUCED ASTHMA

(See *reactive airways dysfunction syndrome* and *isocyanate-induced asthma*.)

ISAAC

(See *International Study of Asthma and Allergies in Childhood*.)

ISOALLERGEN

Isoallergens are multiple molecular forms of the same *allergen*.

They share extensive antigenic (*IgE*) cross-reactivity (see *cross-reacting allergens*). The revised *allergen nomenclature* defines an isoallergen as an allergen from a single species, sharing similar molecular size, identical biologic function, and ≥67% amino-acid sequence identity. The term "*isoform*" or "*variant*" is used to indicate allergen sequences which are polymorphic variants of the same allergen. Isoforms have been reported for Der p 1, Der p 2, Amb a 1, and Bet v 1 (for which 37 isoform sequences have been deposited in the GenBank database). Isoallergens and isoforms are denoted by the addition of four numeral suffixes to the allergen name. The first two numerals distinguish between isoallergens and the last two between isoforms. For ragweed Amb a 1, which occurs as four isoallergens, showing 12 to 24% differences in *amino-acid* sequence, the nomenclature is shown in Table 59.

TABLE 59
Nomenclature for Isoallergens and Isoforms of Ragweed Allergen

Allergen:	Amb a 1
Isoallergens:	Amb a 1.01; Amb a 1.02; Amb a 1.03; Amb a 1.04
	Three isoforms of each isoallergen occur, showing >97% sequence homology.
Isoforms:	Amb a 1.0101; Amb a 1.0102; Amb a 1.0103
	Amb a 1.0201; Amb a 1.0202; Amb a 1.0203; etc.

ISOCYANATES

This is a group of *irritants* (see *isocyanate-induced asthma*).

ISOCYANATE-INDUCED ASTHMA

Isocyanates are a group of low-molecular-weight components (methylene diphenyl diisocyanate [MDI], hexamethylene diisocyanate [HDI], toluene diisocyanate [TDI]), which commonly cause *occupational asthma*. They are used in the production of rigid and flexible foam and varnishes, as coating for electric wiring, as binder in mold and core processing in iron and steel foundries, and as *aerosols* in spray painting. The mechanism of isocyanate-induced *asthma* is not clear. Specific *IgE* and *IgG antibodies* against isocyanates can be detected in exposed workers, but are not strongly associated with the disease. A cell-mediated immune response has also been suggested (*see Coombs and Gell classification*, type IV). Both atopic (see *allergic asthma*) and nonatopic (see *reactive airways dysfunction syndrome*) individuals can be affected.

> Inhalation *exposition tests* with isocyanates induce either dual or isolated *late-phase responses.*

ISOFORM

> Isoforms are alternative forms of the same protein.

If the protein is an enzyme, the different forms are also called isozymes. Isoforms can coexist in the same individual. However, they can also be specific for tissues or cell lineages or even subcellular compartments. Isoforms can be generated by different (but highly related) *genes*, by differential use of alternative *promoters*, *alternative splicing*, or different usage of poly-adenylation sites (see *transcription*). Several isoforms may also be observed due to *polymorphism* (see *isoallergen*).

ISOTYPE

Genetic variation between a family of proteins. *IgG*, IgM, IgA, IgD, and *IgE* isotypes exist for *immunoglobulins*. The process of *immunoglobulin class switching* is controlled by *T cells*.

ISOVOLUME FLOW

Following *bronchodilator* therapy, a significant improvement in *dyspnea* may occur without improvement in the *forced expiratory flow* (FEF_{25-75}). However, when the flow volumes are plotted at the lung volumes at which they actually occurred, there is a leftward shift in the *flow volume loop* due to the reduction in the degree of hyperinflation. Such a response indicates an improved airflow at any given volume (isovolume).

ISOZYME

Isozymes are alternative forms of the same enzyme (see *isoform*).

ITAM

(See *immunoreceptor tyrosine-based activation motif.*)

ITIM

(See *immunoreceptor tyrosine-based inhibition motif.*)

ITP

(See *idiopathic thrombocytopenic purpura.*)

IUIS

International Union of Immunologic Societies (see *allergen nomenclature*).

IVIG

(See *intravenous immunoglobulin preparations.*)

J

JAK

(See *Janus kinases*).

JANUS KINASES (JAKs)

Receptors of the *cytokine receptor* superfamily do not have *kinase* domains. Therefore, cytoplasmic kinases are required for *signal transduction* through *cytokine* receptors. Many of the cytokine receptors associate with and activate members of the Jak family of *tyrosine kinases*. The family consists of four members, Jak1, Jak2, Jak3, and Tyk2. Ligand binding of cytokine receptors induces receptor dimerization and oligomerization (see *cross-linking*). This increases the affinity of the cytoplasmic domain of the receptor to bind Jaks. The importance of Jaks in vivo has been revealed by studies of genetic diseases and *knockout mice* experimental models. For instance, Jak3 deficiency results in severe immunodeficiency, because of the inability to transduce *IL-2* and *IL-4* signals. Moreover, Jak2 knockout mice are unable to transduce *IL-3, IL-5,* and *GM-CSF* signals. Table 60 lists cytokine receptors known to bind certain members of the family. *Signal transducers and activators of transcription* (STAT) molecules are direct substrates of Jaks.

TABLE 60
Jak Family Members and Their Role in Cytokine Receptor Signaling

Receptor	Jak Family Member
*G-CSF*R	Jak2
GM-CSFR	Jak2
IL-2R	Jak1, Jak3
IL-3R	Jak2
IL-4R	Jak1, Jak3
IL-5R	Jak2
*IL-6*R	Jak1, Jak2, Tyk2
IL-7R	Jak1, Jak3
*IL-9*R	Jak1, Jak3
*IL-10*R	Jak1, Tyk2
*IL-12*R	Jak2, Tyk2
*IL-13*R	Jak1, Jak2, Tyk2
*IL-15*R	Jak1, Jak3
*IFN-α/β*R	Jak1, Tyk2
*IFN-γ*R	Jak1, Jak2

JOB SYNDROME

(See *hyper-IgE-syndrome*.)

JUN-N-TERMINAL KINASES (JNKs)

The pro-inflammatory JNKs are members of the *mitogen-activated protein kinase* (MAPK) family. They are involved in the activation of the *transcription factor activator protein 1* (AP-1). Activation of JNKs is inhibited by *cyclosporin A* (see *cytokine receptor signal transduction*).

K

KALLIKREIN

There are two forms of kallikrein: plasma and tissue. Kallikrein is a kininogenase, which cleaves high- and low-molecular-weight kininogens to generate *kinins*, such as *bradykinin*.

KAPOSI'S VARICELLIFORM ERUPTION

This is a disseminated infection of inflammatory skin with viruses of the herpes group.

Atopic dermatitis is by far the most common underlying skin disease (>95%).

In these cases, the disease is also called *eczema* herpeticum or herpetic eczema. Other possible underlying skin diseases include dyskeratosis follicularis Darier, pemphigus chronicus familiaris benignus Hailey–Hailey, pityriasis rubra pilaris, mycosis fungoides, and allergic *contact dermatitis*.

kb

(See *kilobases*.)

KERATINOCYTE

Epidermal cells of the skin, keratinocytes are able to express *MHC class II molecules* and may therefore act as *antigen-presenting cells* (APCs) in *inflammation*. Moreover, keratinocytes represent an important source of various *mediators*, such as *leukotrienes*, *prostaglandins*, *cytokines*, and *chemokines*. However, the cellular interactions between keratinocytes as resident cells of the skin and *leukocytes* in *atopic dermatitis* and other inflammatory skin diseases remain to be elucidated. *T cell*-mediated *apoptosis* of keratinocytes may represent an important pathogenic event in the development of *eczema*.

KERATOCONJUNCTIVITIS

(See *allergic keratoconjunctivitis*.)

KERATOCONUS

Atopic dermatitis is sometimes associated with an expanded cornea, the so-called "keratoconus." It has been suggested that the development of keratoconus might be due to excessive eye rubbing in combination with a thinned and weakened cornea.

KERATOSIS PILARIS

Keratosis pilaris is a follicular horny thickening of the skin frequently seen in *atopic dermatitis* patients. The upper arms and upper legs are the most common location.

KETOTIFEN

An anti-asthma drug with antihistaminic properties (see *antihistamines*) and with some effect on *mast cell* stability. Ketotifen has been widely used in the Far East but has been less successful in Europe and North America.

KILOBASES

Kilobase pairs (kb), 1000 bases of *DNA* or *RNA* (see *base pairs*).

KINASE

Kinases are enzymes that phosphorylate target proteins within cells. They play important roles in *signal transduction*. Target proteins are phosphorylated on tyrosine (see *tyrosine kinases*), threonine, and serine residues. In contrast, *dephosphorylation* is performed by *phosphatases*.

KINESIOLOGY

(See *complementary procedures*.)

KININS

Kinins represent a family of vasoactive *peptides* formed during *inflammation* from kininogen by kininogenasen (see *kallikrein*). The concentrations of kallikrein and kinins are increased in *bronchoalveolar lavage* (BAL) fluids derived from patients with *asthma*, especially following *allergen challenge*. *Tryptase* and *granulocyte*-derived proteases may also act as kininogenases. *Bradykinin* is an important kinin.

KNOCKOUT MICE

Important advances in our understanding of the role of *cytokines* in *allergic inflammation* were made using knockout mice (mice deficient in a particular cytokine) and *transgenic mice* (mice overexpressing a particular cytokine). For instance, the *IL-4* and *IL-5* knockout mice clearly demonstrated the important role of these cytokines for the control of *IgE* and *eosinophil* levels. Some of the important results obtained with several cytokine-deficient mice are summarized in Table 61.

TABLE 61
Abnormalities Found in Cytokine Knockout Mice

Cytokine	Abnormalities
IL-4	Low baseline IgE levels
	Low nematode-induced IgE response
	Reduced production of *Th2* cytokines
	No *eosinophilia* following *allergen challenge* (at least in some mouse strains)
IFN-γ	Reduced expression of *MHC class II molecules*
	Increased mortality in response to sublethal infection
	Reduced *NO* and superoxide (see *oxygen metabolites*) generation
IL-5	Markedly reduced baseline eosinophil numbers
	No eosinophilia following allergen challenge
	No *airway hyperresponsiveness* to *methacholine*
IL-10	Increased eosinophilia following allergen challenge
	Airway hyperresponsiveness following allergen challenge
TGF-β	Early death due to overwhelming *inflammation*
GM-CSF	Impaired *macrophage* function
	Alveolar proteinosis1

L

LACTOGLOBULIN

An *allergen* present in cow's milk (see *cow's milk allergy*).

LACTOSE INTOLERANCE

Lactose *intolerance* is a constitutional deficiency of the enzyme lactase. Patients with lactase insufficiency cannot digest lactose. Therefore, undigested sugar is fermented in the lower bowel, causing diarrhea and flatulence (see *adverse food reactions*).

LAG ANTIGEN

The LAG (Langerhans cell *granule*) *antigen* is a protein of unknown function which is exclusively present inside the *Birbeck granules* of *Langerhans cells* (LC), but not in interstitial type *dendritic cells*. Cytoplasmic immunostaining (see *immunohistochemistry*) of LAG is frequently used to quantify or simply demonstrate the presence of Birbeck granules without the need for electron microscopy. Immunostaining for LAG delineates LAG-positive LC from LAG-negative *inflammatory dendritic epidermal cells* (IDEC).

LAMININ

Besides *collagen* and *fibronectin*, laminin is an important component of the *extracellular matrix*. It stimulates *mast cells*, which both degranulate (see *exocytosis*) and migrate (see *migration*) through laminin-rich basement membrane. Laminin may also be a *chemotactic factor* for mast cells.

LANGERHANS CELL (LC)

> The Langerhans cell is a cutaneous member of the *dendritic cell* (DC) family.

It is the exclusive DC population of the normal human *epidermis*. As with other DCs, they are capable of the initiation of *primary* and *secondary immune responses*. Of all DC subtypes, the LC is the most intensively investigated cell population. LCs are defined as epidermally located, nonlymphoid, dendritically shaped, *antigen-presenting cells* (APCs), which contain *Birbeck granules* and express *CD1* and *MHC class II molecules*. They are derived from the *bone marrow*.

Morphology

With their dendrites, LCs form a close network inside the upper epidermis, which may be regarded as the first barrier of the *immune system* toward the environment. All *antigens* that penetrate into the human body through the *epidermal barrier* have to pass this first immunological wall of defense. Routine light microscopic examination (formaline fixation, paraffin embedding, HE staining) shows the LC as a clear cell, which can be separated from surrounding *keratinocytes* due to a fixation artifact. These clear nonkeratinocytes include melanocytes (mostly basal), Merkel cells (very rare), but mostly LCs. LCs can also be directly identified by immunohistological staining of their *surface molecules HLA-DR* and *CD1a*. Using this technique, the dendrites of LCs are easily detected between keratinocytes. In normal human skin, LCs are homogenously distributed in a density of about 450/mm^2 along the entire body. Only palms and soles have lower cell densities of about 60/mm². In normal human skin, the LC frequency varies between 0.5 and 2% of all epidermal cells. The ultrastructural features of an LC include a clear cytoplasm, a lobulated nucleus, and the complete absence of desmosomes, melanosomes, or Merkel cell *granules*. Detection of the LC-specific, racket-shaped cytoplasmic LC, or Birbeck granules is the ultrastructural proof of an LC.

Immunophenotype

The surface antigen expression has been thoroughly investigated by *immunohistochemistry* and *flow cytometry*. The strength of immunohistochemistry lies in the preservation of the tissue architecture and the relative distribution patterns of the cells inside the skin, whereas the lack of quantitative analysis is its main weakness. In contrast, flow cytometric analysis allows for quantitative analysis, and has therefore become the state-of-the-art method for immunophenotyping of LCs. A variety of *immunoglobulin receptors*, *MHC class I* and class II molecules, and several *adhesion molecules* are hallmarks for the identification of normal LCs.

> CD1a, a nonclassical MHC class Ib molecule, is regarded as the most specific LC marker for normal human skin available at the moment.

Under inflammatory conditions, another CD1a⁺ cell is present in the skin that is called *inflammatory dendritic epidermal cell* (IDEC). Table 62 gives an overview of relevant markers expressed on LCs from normal human skin. The restriction to normal human skin is important, since the expression of surface molecules is regulated by inflammatory *mediators*.

TABLE 62
Immunophenotype of Normal Human Langerhans Cells

MHC Molecules	Immunoglobulin Receptors	Co-Stimulatory Molecules	Adhesion Molecules
CD1a⁺⁺⁺	FcεRI⁺	B7.1/CD80⁻	ICAM1⁺
CD1b⁻	FcεRII/CD23±	B7.2/CD86⁻	ICAM3⁺⁺
CD1c⁺	FcγRI/CD64⁻		LFA3/CD58⁺
MHC-class-I⁺⁺⁺	FcγRII/CD32⁺⁺		
MHC-class-II⁺⁺⁺	FcγRIII/ CD16⁻		

Antigen uptake and processing

LCs take up extracellular fluid by means of different processes: the fluid phase uptake, also known as *pinocytosis*, is an unsaturable permanent pathway of antigen uptake. This basic mechanism of filtration of extracellular fluid is based on the engulfment of extracellular space by the plasma membrane and subsequent translocation of the newly facturated vesicles, the endosomes, into the endocytic pathway of the cell. In receptor-mediated *endocytosis*, the cell takes up antigens, which bind to specific membrane-bound receptors such as the mannose receptor.

> Another structure with relevant receptor-mediated endocytotic function is the *high-affinity IgE receptor* (FcεRI), which facilitates antigen presentation of *aerollergens* toward autologous *T cells*.

This mechanism is assumed to play a central pathogenetic role in *IgE*-mediated atopic skin diseases, namely *atopic dermatitis*. LCs take up intact protein antigens, which enter the endocytotic pathway and are cleaved inside the cell by limited digestion into oligopeptides. These *antigenic peptides* are loaded onto MHC class II molecules for antigen presentation toward T cells. As a rule, extracellular proteins are presented in MHC class II complexes to *CD4+* T cells, whereas intracellularly generated proteins are presented by MHC class I molecules toward CD8+ T cells.

Antigen presentation

The oligopeptides are presented by LCs to T cells. This process of antigen presentation is a key event in the defense against pathogenic organisms and malignant tumor cells, as well as in the generation of unwanted *allergic inflammation*. Many cells from the human body are able to generate secondary immune responses toward antigens already known to the immune system. In contrast, DCs are the only APCs known today which are able to induce primary immune responses.

> The initiation of immune responses requires cell–cell interaction (see *cognate/noncognate interactions*).

Many cell surface molecules have been shown to contribute to a successful immune response. They may roughly be grouped into three categories: molecules involved in cell–cell adhesion (e.g., *ICAM-1/LFA-1*), molecules dealing with *peptide* presentation (e.g., MHC molecules and *T cell antigen receptors* [TCR]), and those molecules involved in *co-stimulation* (e.g., *CD80/CD86* and *CD28*). The peptides are presented after being loaded into the antigen-binding groove of the MHC molecules, with the TCR as a counterpart. The presence of co-stimulatory molecules is necessary to direct the immune system toward an immune response, but not *anergy*. However, normal human skin LCs do not express CD80 or CD86 molecules. The LCs acquire these molecules during *migration* and differentiation toward the mature DCs present within *lymph nodes*. Bacterial *superantigens*, such as SEA, SEB, or TSST from *Staphylococcus aureus* (S. aureus) circumvent the antigen specificity of LC–T-cell interactions. They attach to the MHC molecule outside of the peptide-binding groove and are able to directly stimulate entire Vβ-families of TCRs irrelevant of their antigen specificity. This mechanism might be of pathogenetic relevance for the exacerbation of atopic dermatitis due to staphylococcal superinfection.

Migration

Since there are almost no T cells inside the normal human epidermis, migration of LCs into T cell areas of lymph nodes is a prerequisite for initiation of immune responses by LC.

> LC migration is associated with a maturation process.

LCs develop from a good antigen-processing, but badly presenting cell, into a badly processing, but extremely well antigen-presenting cell. Isolation and short-term culture of LCs initiate a similar maturation cascade in vitro. Within the lymph nodes, the former LCs are called lymphoid DCs or *veiled cells*. The LCs migrate further into the cortex of the lymph node, and are then called *interdigitating reticular cells*. LCs may migrate out of the epidermis by application of contact *allergen* due to *IL-1* or *TNF-α* exposure. UV-B irradiation of the skin leads to LC emigration as well. However, mobilized cells may induce anergy instead of immune responses.

Involvement in skin disease

LCs are assumed to play a pathogenetic role in many different skin diseases. The defense against infectious diseases and cutaneous malignancies, the *T cell sensitization* and elicitation phase in allergic *contact dermatitis*, as well as the facilitated antigen presentation of aeroallergens and keratinocyte autoantigens in atopic dermatitis are only a selection of these skin diseases. Furthermore, LCs themselves may give rise to neoplasms of histiocytic cells. Histiocytosis X, also known as LC histiocytosis, is a pathogenic entity of three initially morphologically defined diseases: Abt–Letterer–Siewe disease, Hand–Schüller–Christian disease, and eosinophilic granuloma of the bone. However, the exact nature of the disease remains unclear.

LARYNGEAL WHEEZING

This condition should be considered in children thought to have *asthma*, whose wheezing (see *wheeze*) does not respond to anti-asthmatic medications (see *asthma treatment strategies*). Speech therapy has been demonstrated to be a successful treatment.

LATE-PHASE RESPONSE (LPR)

In many patients with *allergic diseases*, the *immediate hypersensitivity* reaction to *allergen challenge* is followed 4 to 8 hours later by persistent *leukocyte* infiltration, called *delayed hypersensitivity* reaction (see *Coombs and Gell classification*, type IV), which is associated with clinical symptoms termed LPR. LPRs may develop following *allergen*-specific *IgE*-dependent reactions in the respiratory tract, in the nose, in the conjunctiva, as well as in the skin. LPRs can also be seen following *skin tests*. The immediate response may evolve into late phase allergic reactions that are characterized by burning, *pruritus*, *erythema*, induration, and warmth. Cutaneous LPRs generally peak at 6 to 8 hours and may resolve by 24 hours. Pulmonary LPRs begin approximately 3 to 4 hours following exposure or challenge, *airway obstruction* reaches maximal intensity by 4 to 8 hours, and resolves after 12 to 24 hours.

> Experiments using *mast-cell*-deficient mice demonstrated that virtually all LPRs are mast-cell dependent.

LATEX ALLERGY

The latex *allergens* are found in the protein content of products made from natural latex, the milky sap of the rubber tree Hevia brasiliensis. Latex *antigen* exposure can occur by cutaneous, percutaneous, mucosal, and parenteral routes. The antigen can be transferred due to direct contact or *aerosol*. The clinical manifestations include *rhinitis*, *conjunctivitis*, *airway obstruction*, contact and systemic *urticaria*, and *anaphylaxis* due to an *immediate hypersensitivity* reaction (see *Coombs and Gell classification*, type I). There are also reports of *type IV reactions* to latex causing *contact dermatitis*. Risk groups for latex *allergy* are children with spina bifida or urogenital abnormalities, health care workers, and rubber industry workers, due to their higher exposure to the allergen.

> Health care workers have a 5 to 10% prevalence of latex allergy.

The risk for developing latex allergy appears to be higher in atopic than in nonatopic individuals. Skin *prick test* and latex-specific *IgE* measurements (see *RAST*, *Phadiatop*, and *CAP-system*) are recommended to establish the diagnosis. Some latex allergens are homologous to proteins that occur in fruits. Such *cross-reacting allergens* are responsible for the latex–fruit syndrome. Moreover, cross-reactivity to *fungal allergens* can occur (Mn-superoxide-dismutase or enolase).

LATEX–FRUIT SYNDROME

(See *latex allergy* and *cross-reacting allergens*.)

LEAD (Pb)

The major effect associated with lead is neurotoxicity and learning deficits associated with systemic absorption of inhaled lead. Other effects of lead include abnormalities of erythrocyte development. With the advent of unleaded fuels, this problem has decreased substantially. Moreover, and in contrast to *diesel exhaust*, no effect of lead on the initiation or maintenance of *allergic diseases* is known.

LEISHMANIASIS

Leishmania are dimorphic protozoa that cause *parasitic disease* in humans and other animals.

> Resistance to infection is associated with the detection of high levels of *IFN-γ* and induction of *delayed hypersensitivity*, whereas susceptibility is associated with a strong *Th2* response (high production of *IL-4* and *IL-5*).

In mice, this diversification is exemplified by strains, which mount a *Th1* response (C57BL/6, B10.D2, C3H/Hen) and are resistant to infection, whereas those which generate a Th2 response (Balb/c) cannot control the infection. The clearance of parasites is not attributed directly to the *cytokines* produced by *T cells*, but to their ability to activate *macrophages* for the efficient *antigen recognition, phagocytosis*, killing, and removal of infective parasites. In this respect, proinflammatory cytokines produced by *monocytes*, such as *IL-1, IL-6*, and *TNF-α*, may be important in direct parasite killing or initiating *inflammation*. *CD4+* T cells are thought to be the major subset of T cells involved in parasite recognition and subsequent disease outcome, but roles for *CD8+* T cells and *γ/δ T cells* have been identified, either in direct cytotoxicity or in primary *T cell sensitization*.

LEPIDOGLYPHUS

Genus of mite. These mites feed on decaying vegetation and are referred to as "storage mites." The primary species is L. destructor, which is associated with occupational *allergy* among farmers.

LEUKEMIA

Malignant *leukocytes* of lymphocytic, myelocytic, or monocytic origin circulate in blood. Both unrestrained proliferation and defective *apoptosis* may contribute to cell expansion. Malignant *T cells* may generate *cytokines* such as *IL-4* and *IL-5*, causing high *IgE* concentrations and *eosinophilia*.

LEUKOCYTE

White blood cell. Leukocytes include *lymphocytes, neutrophils, eosinophils, basophils*, and *monocytes*.

LEUKOCYTE ADHESION DEFICIENCY

Failure of *leukocytes* to express CD11a/CD18 (see *LFA-1*). This affects the ability of *neutrophils*, but not *eosinophils*, to enter sites of *inflammation*. This disease indicates that the *adhesion molecules* used by eosinophils and neutrophils are at least partially different.

LEUKOCYTE COMMON ANTIGEN

(See *CD45*.)

LEUKOCYTOSIS

Increased numbers of *leukocytes* in blood. It is commonly seen in acute infection, but also in other forms of *inflammation*. Moreover, *corticosteroid* therapy is often associated with leukocytosis due to increased numbers of *neutrophils*.

LEUKOCYTOTOXIC TEST

The leukocytotoxic test is a method used to diagnose patients with *allergic diseases*, and belongs to the *complementary procedures*.

LEUKOTRIENES (LTs)

LTs are primary products of the *5-lipoxygenase* (5-LO) pathway of *arachidonic acid* metabolism that are generated in *granulocytes*, *monocytes*, *mast cells*, *platelets*, and *macrophages* upon stimulation. Other cells, which do not express 5-LO, may be involved in later steps of LT synthesis (see below). The biologically active LTs were originally described as slow-reacting substances of *anaphylaxis* (SRS-A). The SRS-A is a mixture of compounds now known as LTC_4, and its metabolites LTD_4 and LTE_4.

LTs, as well as the *prostanoids*, are not preformed, but are synthesized upon cell activation.

Biosynthesis

The primary substrate for the synthesis of these *lipid mediators* is *arachidonic acid* (AA). 5-LO is the enzyme which metabolizes arachidonic acid to produce LTA_4 via *5-HPETE* (see Figure 32). LTA_4 is the substrate of two enzymes: (1) LTA_4 hydrolase generates LTB_4, and (2) *LTC_4 synthase* makes LTC_4. Whereas *neutrophils* and monocytes preferentially synthesize LTB_4, *eosinophils* appear to generate more LTC_4 (see Table 63), suggesting different expression and/or activities of these two enzymes in different cell types. Moreover, compared to the very restricted expression of 5-LO, LTC_4 synthase and LTA_4 hydrolase are widely distributed. Cells expressing these enzymes may take up LTA_4 from other cells, and generate LTC_4 and/or LTB_4. LTC_4 is further metabolized to LTD_4 and LTE_4 (see Figure 32). LTC_4, LTD_4 and LTE_4 are also called *cysteinyl LTs*.

It has been shown that LTs are present at increased concentrations in biological fluids from patients with *asthma* and *allergic rhinoconjunctivitis*, suggesting that they represent important *mediators* of *allergic inflammation*.

TABLE 63
LTB_4 and LTC_4 Generation in Peripheral Blood *Leukocytes* (10^6 Cells) upon Ionophore (A23187) Stimulation

	LTB_4	LTC_4
Neutrophils	50 ng	10 ng
Eosinophils	10 ng	40 ng
Monocytes	70 ng	30 ng

Biological activities

Besides increased generation of LTs in allergic inflammation, LTs exert several *receptor*-mediated effects (see *leukotriene receptors*) that also suggest a critical role in asthma and other *allergic diseases*. There are at least three effects of cysteinyl LTs which contribute to *airway obstruction* (Table 64).

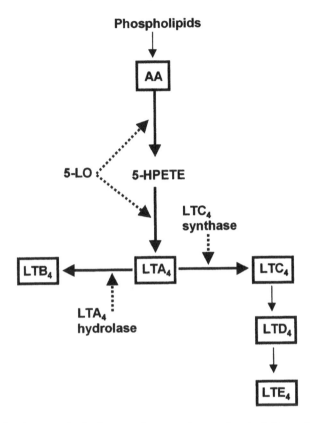

FIGURE 32 Leukotriene synthesis from nuclear membrane phospholipids and AA via the 5-LO pathway.

TABLE 64
Effects of Cysteinyl LTs that Mediate Asthmatic Symptoms

1. Bronchoconstriction due to *smooth muscle* contraction.
2. Mucosal *edema* due to extravasation of protein and water.
3. Increased *mucus* secretion.

Cysteinyl LTs are at least 100 times more potent than *histamine* in causing airway obstruction in *bronchial provocation tests*.

Moreover, LTB_4 (and to a lesser extent, LTD_4 and LTE_4) increases the *recruitment of inflammatory cells*, such as eosinophils and neutrophils.

In contrast, LT-mediated *chemotaxis* is not observed in the cases of *lymphocytes*, *plasma cells*, mast cells, or macrophages. Furthermore, following intradermal challenge (see *skin test*), cysteinyl LTs induce a prolonged wheal-and-flare reaction.

LEUKOTRIENE C$_4$ (LTC$_4$) SYNTHASE

An enzyme that catalyses the reaction between *leukotriene* A$_4$ (LTA$_4$) and glutathione to form LTC$_4$.

> LTC$_4$ is highly expressed in *eosinophils*, especially in patients with *aspirin-sensitive asthma*.

Gene expression is upregulated by *IL-3, IL-5* and *GM-CSF*, as well as vitamin D in responsive cells. Besides eosinophils, the enzyme is expressed in many other cell types. Interestingly, the LTC$_4$ synthase gene has been mapped to *chromosome* 5, but relatively far away from the *T helper (Th) 2 cytokine gene cluster*. For example, *endothelial cells* and bronchial *epithelial cells*, which do not express *5-lipoxygenase* (5-LO), can take up LTA$_4$ from cells that express this enzyme, and generate biologically active *cysteinyl leukotrienes*. LTC$_4$ synthase deficiency was reported to be associated with a fatal development syndrome, suggesting that LTC$_4$ (and, perhaps, other cysteinyl leukotrienes) acts as a neuromodulator in the central *nervous system* under physiological conditions.

LEUKOTRIENE E$_4$ (LTE$_4$) MEASUREMENTS

LTE$_4$ can be conveniently measured in urine by immunoassays or reverse phase-high performance liquid chromatography (RP-HPLC). Urinary LTE$_4$ has been found useful for evaluation of whole-body production of *cysteinyl leukotrienes*. Moreover, LTE$_4$ in the morning urine of patients with *aspirin-sensitive asthma* was found to be higher than in aspirin-tolerant asthmatics, suggesting an overproduction of cysteinyl leukotrienes in this subgroup of *asthma* patients. Increased urinary LTE$_4$ levels were also observed in patients with acute *airway obstruction* and *anaphylaxis*.

LEUKOTRIENE INHIBITORS

Since there is growing evidence for an important role of *leukotrienes* in the pathogenesis of *asthma* and other *allergic diseases*, several compounds have been developed to block their biological activities. Table 65 summarizes some of the general possibilities of how this can be achieved.

TABLE 65
Strategies to Inhibit Leukotrienes

1. Inhibition of leukotriene synthesis
   - *5-lipoxygenase (5-LO) inhibitors*
   - *5-lipoxygenase-activating protein (FLAP) inhibitors*
   - Inhibitors of *calcium mobilization*
2. *Leukotriene receptor antagonists*

LEUKOTRIENE RECEPTORS

The different main activities of *cysteinyl leukotrienes* and LTB$_4$ suggest that several *receptors* for *leukotrienes* (LTs) exist. Radioligand-binding studies and work with compounds that act as leukotriene antagonists revealed that there are at least three leukotriene receptors. The major effects that are mediated via these receptors are shown in Table 66.

The LTB$_4$ receptor has been cloned, and LTB$_4$ receptor *knockout mice* have been developed.

> LTB$_4$ receptor-deficient mice are unable to recruit *eosinophils* into the lungs following *allergen challenge*.

TABLE 66
Agonists and Biological Effects Mediated by Leukotriene Receptors

Receptor	Agonist	Effects
LTB$_4$ receptor	LTB$_4$	*Leukocyte* activation and *chemotaxis*
Cysteinyl leukotrienes receptor 1	LTC$_4$	*Bronchospasm*
	LTD$_4$	Plasma exudation
	LTE$_4$	Vasoconstriction
		Chemotaxis
		Mucus secretion
Cysteinyl leukotrienes receptor 2	LTC$_4$	Vasorelaxation and constriction
	LTD$_4$	*Smooth muscle* construction
	(LTE$_4$)	

The receptors of cysteinyl leukotrienes are not characterized at the molecular level yet, but it appears that they, like the LTB$_4$ receptor, may represent *G protein-coupled receptors*. Several *leukotriene receptor antagonists* have been introduced as a therapy for *asthma*.

LEUKOTRIENE RECEPTOR ANTAGONISTS

There have been several clinical studies with *leukotriene receptor* antagonists that block *receptor* 1 of *cysteinyl leukotrienes*. These antagonists block *airway obstruction* in patients with *asthma* induced by *allergen* (see *allergen challenge*), exercise (see *exercise-induced asthma*), or aspirin (see *aspirin-sensitive asthma*). Moreover, several studies have shown that these drugs have a *bronchodilator* effect on asthmatics, which appears to be additive to the effect mediated by *β2-agonists*.

Furthermore, leukotriene receptor antagonists appear to decrease *allergic inflammation*, and therefore it is often possible to reduce the dose of *corticosteroids*.

Since leukotriene receptor antagonists are given orally, it appears that the *compliance* of patients is greater compared to drugs with different application routes. In addition to their effectiveness in adult patients, these drugs also appear to be effective in children with asthma (see *childhood asthma*). In contrast to cysteinyl leukotriene antagonists, studies with an LTB$_4$ receptor antagonist showed no effect on *immediate* or *delayed hypersensitivity* reactions. From all compounds that somehow act as *leukotriene inhibitors*, most practitioners currently use cysteinyl leukotriene receptor antagonists.

LFA-1

(See *lymphocyte function-associated antigen-1*.)

LICHEN SIMPLEX CHRONICUS

A solitary lichenified, eczematous skin lesion (see *eczema*) resembling an *atopic dermatitis* lesion, but without underlying atopic dermatitis or *atopy* in general.

LICHEN VIDAL

(See *lichen simplex chronicus*.)

LICHENIFICATION

Lichenification is a chronic thickening of the *epidermis* with exaggeration of its normal markings, resembling an "elephant´s skin." This reactive hyperplasia of the epidermis is often a result of scratching or rubbing, and is frequently seen in *atopic dermatitis* patients.

LINEAGE-SPECIFIC MARKERS

Some *surface molecules* are specific for certain *leukocyte* populations. These molecules can be used to identify such cell populations in blood (see *flow cytometry*) and tissues (see *immunohistochemistry*) (see also *CD antigens, B cell surface markers, T cell surface markers*).

LINEAR EPITOPES

Most *T cell* interactions involving *antigen recognition* by the *T cell antigen receptor* (TCR) rely on the expression of linear *epitopes* being presented in the *major histocompatibility complex* (MHC) of *antigen-presenting cells* (APCs). Linear epitopes are contiguous *amino acid* sequences within an *antigen* or *allergen* that can be recognized by a T cell. Complementarity of structure and recognition by TCR and MHC mean that the same antigen may be presented to different T cells by different APCs. This may be a mechanism for functional phenotype switching following, for example, induced *anergy* of the *Th2 cell* by high-dose antigen (see *immunotherapy*) or failure of *co-stimulation*, and subsequent expansion of *Th1 cells* exhibiting, perhaps, a lower *affinity* for the antigen.

LINKAGE

Linked *genes* are located in close proximity on the same *chromosome*. Genes in linkage have a more than 50% expectancy of co-inheritance (see *linkage studies*).

LINKAGE DISEQUILIBRIUM

This is a nonrandom *association* of *alleles* at linked loci; the association of two linked alleles more frequently than would be expected by chance. For example, certain alleles of *human leukocyte antigen* loci (HLA-A, -B, -C, -DR, -DQ) occur together more frequently. In the case of several linked genes, *linkage* disequilibrium results in extended *haplotype*. In the caucasoid population, HLA-A1 (27%) and -B8 (16%) would have a predicted frequency of about 4% coinheritance. As the frequency of HLA-A1 plus HLA-B8 is 10%, this indicates linkage disequilibrium.

LINKAGE MAP

This is a map of the localization and definition of the order of *genes* based on *linkage disequilibrium* by linkage analysis.

LINKAGE STUDIES

The strategy of *linkage* studies to define *genes* important in the pathogenesis of *allergic diseases* (see *genetic predisposition*) had only limited success until a few years ago, when a region of *chromosome* 11q was thought to possibly be associated with *atopy*, but results in this area are equivocal at present. More recently, linkage studies have indicated that a *genetic locus* with strong influence on total serum *IgE levels* maps to chromosome 5q, a region with multiple *candidate genes* (see *Th2 cytokine gene cluster*), first and foremost the IgE-inducing *cytokines IL-4* and *IL-13*. However, it is clear that there is at least one additional *locus* — not identified to date — that accounts for the variability of total serum IgE and maps elsewhere in the *genome* (see *genome-wide screening studies*).

LIPID MEDIATORS

A subgroup of *mediators* that includes *leukotrienes* (LTs), *prostaglandins* (PGs), *thromboxane*, and *platelet-activating factor* (PAF), but excludes *cytokines*.

LIPOXINS

Lipoxins are generated from two main pathways: one involves the trancellular metabolism of 15-HETE by *5-lipoxygenase* (5-LO), and the other utilizes *leukotriene* A_4 (LTA$_4$), which is converted by either 12-LO or 15-LO. Lipoxins can be detected in *bronchoalveolar lavage* (BAL) fluids from patients with several *inflammatory lung diseases*.

Lipoxins inhibit the influx of effector cells such as *neutrophils*.

This might be achieved by mechanisms such as downregulation of *LFA-1*, reduced *TNF-α*-mediated *IL-8* release, and inhibition of LTB$_4$-mediated *chemotaxis*. They also stop vascular leakage, which is associated with *inflammation* and appears to modify the responses mediated by several *cytokines* (see *immunosuppressive mechanisms*). The effects of lipoxins are mediated via *G protein-coupled receptors*.

Lipoxins are triggered by *aspirin* and other *nonsteroidal antiinflammatory drugs* (NSAIDs).

5-LIPOXYGENASE (5-LO)

First committed enzyme within the *leukotriene* (LT) synthesis pathway. It catalysis two steps: (1) the generation of *5-HPETE* by oxygenation of *arachidonic acid* (AA) at carbon 5, and (2) the production of LTA$_4$ by dehydration of 5-HPETE. The enzyme depends on intracellular *calcium mobilization*, an event that is regularly observed following activation of *G protein-coupled receptors*. Activation of 5-LO is associated with a translocation from the cytosol (perhaps also from the nucleus) to the nuclear envelope where LT synthesis occurs. A variety of stimuli can activate or increase the cellular *gene* expression of 5-LO (see Table 67).

TABLE 67
Agents that Stimulate 5-LO Enzymatic Activity or 5-LO Gene Expression

Agents	Activation	Gene Expression
Zymosan	+	−
IgE	+	−
Aggregated *Ig*	+	−
fMLP	+	−
C5a	+	−
Plasmin	+	−
PAF	+	−
TNF-α	+	−
NGF	+	−
Vitamin D	−	+
GM-CSF	−	+
IL-3	−	+
TGF-β	−	+
Corticosteroids	−	+
LPS	−	+

5-LIPOXYGENASE-ACTIVATING PROTEIN (FLAP)

FLAP is an intracellular protein which is involved in the early phase of *leukotriene* generation. FLAP is an *arachidonic acid* (AA)-binding protein required for activation of *5-lipoxygenase*

(5-LO). FLAP is an integral membrane protein primarily located at the nuclear envelope. Specific antagonists of FLAP are in the process of development.

5-LIPOXYGENASE-ACTIVATING PROTEIN (FLAP) INHIBITORS

Similar to the *leukotriene receptor antagonists*, clinical studies with FLAP inhibitors revealed a significant inhibition of *immediate* and *delayed hypersensitivity* reactions following *allergen challenge*. In contrast to *leukotriene receptor* antagonists, FLAP inhibitors also block the biological activity of LTB_4, since its synthesis is reduced by these drugs. However, a general inhibition of *leukotrienes* is not necessarily an advantage, because these *mediators* may also have physiological functions. Therefore, the goal should be to develop selective *receptor* antagonists to be able to block only unwanted biological activities of leukotrienes.

5-LIPOXYGENASE INHIBITORS

General inhibitors of *leukotriene* synthesis. The clinical effects are similar to those described for *5-lipoxygenase-activating protein (FLAP) inhibitors*.

LOCAL (SEGMENTAL) ALLERGEN CHALLENGE

Instillation of *allergen* into an isolated lung segment in sensitized subjects has been used as a research technique to better characterize *allergic inflammation* associated with *late-phase responses* of patients with *asthma*.

> At 48 hours after segmental *allergen challenge*, the *bronchoalveolar lavage* (BAL) fluid reveals increased numbers of *eosinophils*, *neutrophils*, and *T helper* (*Th*) *cells*.

By 96 hours, neutrophil counts return to normal level, whereas eosinophils and *T cells* remain elevated. The BAL *eosinophilia* is associated with elevated levels of *eosinophil granule proteins* (MBP, ECP, EPO, EDN). It also correlates with *IL-5* concentrations measured in BAL. Other *Th2 cytokines* are also present in increased concentrations following segmental allergen challenge.

LOCUS

The precise location of a *gene* on a *chromosome*.

LOCUS HETEROGENEITY

Mutations in several different *genes* result in the same clinical *phenotype*.

lod SCORE

The lod score is a measure of the likelihood of genetic *linkage* between loci (see *locus*). The lod score is the logarithm of the odds favoring linkage (log odds ratio). A lod score of >+3 (1000:1 odds) is often taken as evidence of linkage, one that is <−2 (100:1 odds against) indicates no linkage.

LONG TERMINAL REPEAT (LTR)

This is a sequence directly repeated at both ends of a retroviral *DNA*. The LTR provides an efficient *promoter* and also carries an *enhancer* that can act on cellular as well as viral sequences. The mechanisms and nuclear proteins involved in both human and viral initiation of *RNA* synthesis are the same, including the usage of *RNA polymerase* II. This is the reason that integration of a retrovirus can lead to the activation of proto*oncogenes* by which a host cell may convert into a cancer cell.

LORATIDINE

This is a selective nonsedative H_1 *receptor* antagonist (see *antihistamines*). It effectively controls symptoms in *allergic rhinoconjunctivitis*.

LOW-AFFINITY IgE RECEPTOR (FcεRII, CD23)

FcεRII (CD23) is the low-affinity *receptor* for *IgE*. Compared to the *high-affinity IgE receptor*, it binds IgE with much lower *affinity* (10^{-7}M). FcεRII is expressed on *B cells*, *platelets*, *Langerhans cells*, and *monocytes/macrophages*.

> *T cell*-derived *IL-4* and *IL-13* are the principal inducers of FcεRII on monocytes and B cells.

Increased expression on the surface of B cells is found in *allergic asthma* and extrinsic *atopic dermatitis*, but not in *intrinsic asthma* or *intrinsic atopic dermatitis*. The FcεRII shows the characteristics of a membrane-bound molecule (transmembrane domain), but it lies "upside-down" in the cell membrane, the C-terminus being extracellular. Two forms (FcεRIIα and β) have been now identified, differing only in the N-terminal cytoplasmic region. FcεRII ligation enhances IgE *isotype* selection (see *immunoglobulin class switching*) induced by IL-4 by positive feedback mechanisms. Membrane FcεRII is susceptible to proteolysis, causing the release of several soluble fragments, the most important of which is a 25-kDa polypeptide (sCD23). Preventing release of sCD23 can inhibit IL-4-induced IgE production by B cells. The exact role of FcεRII is not understood, but membrane-bound FcεRII has a stimulatory capacity, facilitating adhesion between cells bearing FcεRII and B cells, whereas the soluble form probably acts as a co-factor for differentiation.

> *Allergen*-IgE complexes can be taken up by the FcεRII receptor, resulting in highly efficient *antigen presentation* by B cells and, perhaps, other *antigen-presenting cells* (APCs).

LTR

(See *long terminal repeat*.)

LUNG FIBROSIS

(See *cryptogenic fibrosing alveolitis*.)

LUNG FUNCTION TESTS

The purpose of the lung is to draw air in from the outside environment, distribute it evenly throughout the *gas exchange* units and allow oxygen (O_2) to diffuse in and carbon dioxide (CO_2) to diffuse out. This requires a bellows function and a gas exchange function. To do this, the lung has to expose a large surface area to the external environment (see *airway anatomy*). It therefore needs to protect itself (host defense function) and to conserve water.

> Standardized measurements of lung function are available to test the bellows function and the gas exchange function of the lung.

Dynamic lung function tests or *forced expiratory maneuvers* are most commonly used, as described by Tiffeneau. The *forced expiratory volume in first second* (FEV_1) provides an integrated measure of airways caliber, and the *forced vital capacity* (FVC) gives some indication of the lung size.

> In *asthma*, *emphysema*, and *chronic obstructive pulmonary disease* (COPD) the FEV_1/FVC ratio will be reduced, while in restrictive lung diseases both values will be reduced.

Other indices can be calculated from the forced expiratory maneuver, including the *mid-expiratory flow rate* (MEFR), which is regarded as a measure of small airways function, and the *peak expiratory flow rate* (PEFR), which is more closely related to large airways function. Assessments of airways resistance and compliance can be made using *body plethysmography*. This requires sophisticated machinery and good cooperation from the subject. Direct measurement of lung volumes can be made using helium dilution, and this is often combined with measurement of gas transfer function using a small concentration of *carbon monoxide*.

> The carbon monoxide transfer test is usually normal in asthma but reduced in emphysema.

This makes it a useful test for evaluating the underlying condition in older patients with *airway obstruction*. Carbon monoxide *transfer factor* is also reduced in certain *inflammatory lung diseases*, e.g., *sarcoidosis, extrinsic allergic alveolitis*, etc., reflecting the diminished capacity to transfer oxygen into the blood. Arterial *blood gas* measurements can also be useful indicators of lung function, reflecting gas transfer, *ventilation–perfusion mismatch*, and shunting.

LYELL SYNDROME

(See *dermatitis exfoliativa*.)

LYMPH NODE

Lymph nodes are small nodular structures of lymphoid tissue scattered along the human body. Skin, mucous membranes, and most organs are connected to the lymph system. *Antigens*, which enter the human body across epithelial or mucosal membranes, are likely to be drained by lymphatic vessels to the regional lymph nodes, with or without prior capture by *dendritic cells*. Many afferent lymphatic vessels lead into one single lymph node, but there is only one efferent vessel out of it. Each lymph node is surrounded by a fibrous capsule and consists of (1) a marginal outer cortex containing the follicles with germinal centers and mantle zone areas, and (2) a central *T cell*-rich region, the medulla. Antigen-stimulated *B cells* proliferate in the germinal centers of the cortex and produce *antibodies* of the various *isotypes*. T cells are mostly situated in the mantle zone between the follicles and in the cortex, also known as parafollicular areas. This is where *interdigitating reticular cells* present their antigens to the naive *T helper cells* (see *T cell sensitization*).

LYMPHOCYTES

Lymphocytes are *leukocytes* that have cell surface *receptors* for *antigen* (see *T cell antigen receptor*) that are encoded in rearranging *gene* segments (see *gene rearrangement*). There are two main classes of lymphocytes, *T cells* and *B cells*. Lymphocyte numbers in blood may be decreased (see *lymphopenia*) or elevated (see *lymphocytosis*).

LYMPHOCYTE CHEMOATTRACTANT FACTOR (LCF)

(See *IL-16*.)

LYMPHOCYTE FUNCTION-ASSOCIATED ANTIGEN-1 (LFA-1)

The 180-kDa *α-integrin* (CD11a, see *CD antigens*) associates with 95-kDa β2-integrin (CD18) to form the CD11a/CD18 complex, formerly referred to as gp 180/95 (gp = glycoprotein). LFA-1 is present on all *leukocytes* and is the functional ligand for *intercellular adhesion molecule-1* (ICAM-1; CD54). Other ligands are ICAM-2 (CD102) and ICAM-3 (CD50). LFA-1/ICAM-1 molecular interactions are important for firm adhesion (see *adhesion molecules*) of *eosinophils* to vascular *endothelial cells* in *allergic inflammation*.

LYMPHOCYTE TRANSFORMATION TEST (LTT)

In LTTs, *peripheral blood mononuclear cells* (PBMC) are isolated and then incubated with pan-*T cell* stimulators (e.g., anti-*CD3 antibodies*) or a supposed *antigen/allergen*. Thymidine incorporation assays with tritium-labeled thymidine are the most widely used readout systems. LTTs may be helpful in individual cases (e.g., to analyze the effects of *immunosuppressive drugs* or to diagnose *drug allergy*), but vary between laboratories because they are not easy to standardize. Therefore, LTTs are not widely used in routine diagnostics.

LYMPHOCYTOSIS

This term describes a situation of elevated *lymphocyte* numbers in blood. Lymphocytosis might be the consequence of infectious or lymphoproliferative diseases (see *T cell lymphoma*).

LYMPHOID DENDRITIC CELLS

Dendritic cells encountered in lymphatic vessels during their *migration* from the skin to the *lymph node* have been termed lymphoid dendritic cells. Due to the increasing knowledge on dendritic cell biology, many authors do not use this term any longer.

LYMPHOKINES

Lymphokines are *cytokines* that are produced by activated *T cells*. However, in most cases, lymphokines can also be produced by other cells. Therefore, the term "lymphokine" is not often used anymore.

LYMPHOPENIA

This term describes a situation of decreased *lymphocyte* numbers in blood. Lymphopenia might be the consequence of decreased production of lymphocytes in the *bone marrow*, increased *apoptosis* (see *acquired immunodeficiency syndrome*), or increased recruitment (see *recruitment of inflammatory cells*, e.g., *sarcoidosis*).

LYMPHOTOXIN (LT)

LT exists in two forms, LT-α (synonymous with *TNF-β*) and LT-β. LT-β is a 33-kDa trans-membrane glycoprotein, otherwise known as p33, that is not secreted and acts as an efficient *receptor* for LT-α. This receptor can mediate LT-α effects (see *TNF receptors*). The name "lymphotoxin" was given because LT-α is able to kill *lymphocyte*-derived (but also other) tumor cells (see *apoptosis*).

Lyn

This is an important *tyrosine kinase* of the *sarcoma (Src) tyrosine kinase* family and plays an important role in many *signal transduction* pathways, which are relevant for *allergic inflammation*.

LYONIZATION

One of the two X *chromosomes* in female *somatic cells* is randomly transcriptionally (see *transcription*) inactivated early in embryonic development. Therefore, a female is a mosaic of cells functionally hemizygous (see *hemizygote*) for one or the other X chromosome.

MACROPHAGE

Macrophages are large mononuclear phagocytic (see *phagocytosis*), inflammatory effector, and *antigen-presenting cells* (APCs) that participate in both innate and adaptive immune responses, and therefore play a critical role in host defense.

> In contrast to *dendritic cells*, uptake of *antigen* by macrophages during *primary immune responses* does not induce a marked humoral response.

However, antigen persistence in macrophage "reservoirs" can act as a "tick over" mechanism for antigen presentation, and may help explain the persistence of reactive *T cells* long after antigen exposure has ceased.

> During *secondary immune responses*, macrophage antigen presentation does provide the stimulus for a vigorous humoral response.

Interestingly, presentation of antigen by macrophages frequently leads to *Th2 cell* activation. The mechanisms of this are unclear. Moreover, macrophages also recognize and take up apoptotic cells (see *apoptosis*), a process that occurs continually, even under noninflammatory conditions. They are found in tissues throughout the body. A large population of specialized alveolar macrophages exists within the lung and constitutes the major resident cell population in *bronchoalveolar lavage* (BAL) fluids. Macrophages are migratory cells that develop from *monocytes*.

MACROSATELLITE

(See *tandem repeat*.)

MAJOR ALLERGEN

Pollen, animal dander, house-dust mite, and food (see *food allergy*) or latex (see *latex allergy*) *allergens* are composed of a number of proteins. Each single protein may function as an allergen. If more than 50% of sensitized individuals develop *IgE antibodies* against a specific allergen, it is called a major allergen. If less than 50% are affected, such an allergen is called a *minor allergen*.

MAJOR BASIC PROTEIN (MBP)

MBP is an important *eosinophil granule protein*. MBP has been shown to cause *epithelial damage* in the airways and may block M2 *muscarinic receptors*. Both mechanisms contribute to *airway hyperresponsiveness* in patients with *asthma*. MBP may form crystals (*Charcot–Leyden crystals*), which can be observed in the *sputum* of asthmatics.

MAJOR HISTOCOMPATIBILITY COMPLEX (MHC)

A cluster of *genes* on human *chromosome* 6 or mouse chromosome 17 that encodes MHC molecules that are involved in *antigen* presentation (see *antigen-presenting cells*).

> *MHC class I molecules* present *peptides* generated in cytosol to *CD8⁺ T cells*, whereas *MHC class II molecules* present peptides degraded in cellular vesicles to *CD4⁺ T cells*.

The MHC also encodes other proteins involved in antigen presentation and host defense. These class III genes encode diverse genes such as *complement system* molecules (C2, C4, factor B) and *TNF*. The MHC is the most polymorphic *gene* cluster in the human *genome*. Therefore, the MHC complex is an ideal marker for *linkage studies*. The *DNA* segment of the MHC is studied in greatest detail within the human genome. Because this *polymorphism* can often be detected using *antibodies* or specific T cells, the MHC molecules are also called major histocompatibility antigens.

MALARIA

Cerebral malaria is possibly the most important *parasitic disease* in which *CD4⁺ T cells* play an important pathologic role.

> The often lethal consequence of infection by Plasmodium falciparum is associated with dramatic elevations of serum *TNF-α* levels.

In certain strains of mice, similar findings are noted with infection by P. berghei, and the effects can be prevented with either anti-CD4 or anti-TNF-α *antibodies*. Treatment with anti-*IFN-γ*, anti-*IL-3*, or anti-*GM-CSF* antibodies also reduces pathology, and it is therefore suggested that a *Th1 cell* response is associated with disease susceptibility.

MALT

(See *mucosa-associated lymphoid tissue*.)

MANAGEMENT GUIDELINES OF ASTHMA

The vast majority of patients with *asthma* can be managed according to reasonably standard guidelines. Management guidelines crystallize existing clinical practice and provide guidance for patients and clinical staff in what is likely to be effective in the management of a particular patient's asthma. However, some individuals do not respond predictably to therapy, and adjustment may be necessary to ensure that patient *idiosyncrasies* are recognized.

> Most management guidelines are based on the use of regular *inhaled corticosteroids* (see *asthma treatment strategies*) as the mainstay of treatment, with an iterative process of increasing or reducing the dose according to response as measured by *peak expiratory flow rate* (PEFR).

Guidelines are useful for making decisions about drugs that are in current use, but do not offer any assistance in deciding where to place new therapies. Management guidelines work best when combined with self-management plans. This allows clinical staff to concentrate on patients who do not respond as expected or who are experiencing difficulties in their management, rather than spending their time on routine clinical care.

MAPK

(See *Mitogen-Activated Protein Kinases*.)

MARKER

(See *genetic marker*.)

MAST CELL

Mast cells are large cells (9 to 12 μm in diameter) found in connective tissues throughout the body, especially in submucosal tissues and the dermis. They store many *mediators* including *histamine* in their *granules*. On their surface, they express *high-affinity IgE receptors*, which bind *IgE*.

Allergens cross-link IgE *receptors* via IgE, leading to mediator release and consequent *immediate hypersensitivity* reactions (Figure 33).

Upon stimulation, they also generate *leukotrienes* (LTs) and *cytokines*, which contribute in *delayed hypersensitivity* reactions and maintain chronic *allergic inflammation*. Therefore, mast cells play a crucial role in *allergic diseases*. In contrast, less is known about their physiological role. However, it appears that they play a role in *immune responses* against Gram-negative bacteria and parasites (see *parasitic diseases*) as well as in *wound healing*. They may also have a protective role against cancer.

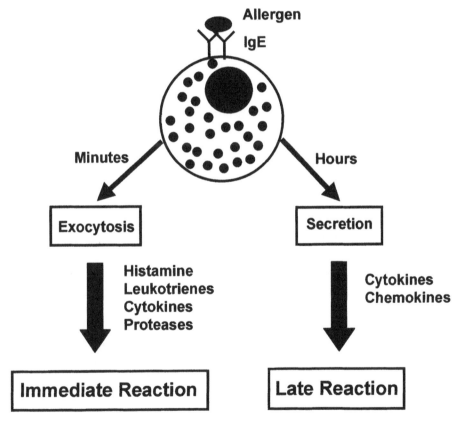

FIGURE 33   Release of inflammatory mediators from mast cells upon cross-linking of high-affinity IgE receptors.

Morphology

Mast cells were discovered by Paul Ehrlich in 1878. As with *eosinophils*, he also identified mast cells by a special staining technique. The intracellular *granules* appear purple when stained with aniline blue dyes. The color change, also called metachromasia, is due to the interaction of these dyes with the highly acidic *proteoglycans* contained within mast cell granules. Mature human mast cells are large cells and can be round, spindle-shaped, or spiderlike in shape in tissues. They are distinctive mononuclear cells. Mast cell nuclei are rather large unsegmented ovals, elliptically placed with partially condensed chromatin, and rarely show mitotic figures in tissue. Other features include variable amounts of intermediate filaments, nonmembrane-bound lipid bodies, and a small ribosomal complement, most of which are not bound to the endoplasmic reticulum. The secretory granules of human mast cells constitute most of the dry weight of the cell and half its volume. They have variable ultrastructural patterns. Mixtures of patterns augment the described complexities of these secretory organelles, but most of the granules consist of a predominant scroll pattern, a regular crystalline pattern, a particulate material, or mixtures of these patterns. Individual cells can contain granules with either a predominant substructural pattern or multiple subtypes. Human mast cells in different anatomic locations may display variations in the predominant granule patterns. In the human mast cells, some differences in granule morphology correspond to different protease compositions. For example, only granules with *chymase* exhibit a grating/lattice substructure, whereas cells that lack this protease exhibit a complete scroll pattern.

Development
Immature cells circulate as agranular precursors, which develop distinctive granules after leaving the blood vascular space. The general features of cellular immaturity include large nuclei with partially dispersed chromatin and large nucleoli. Moreover, immature mast cells have increased numbers of ribosomes and Golgi structures, and, if they are granulated secretory cells, evidence of Golgi-derived granulogenesis and the presence of immature granules. The study of mast cell development is notoriously difficult, because mast cells cannot be readily identified until they mature in the tissues and, as a consequence, contain their characteristic granules and express high-affinity IgE receptors.

> It is now believed that mast cells are derived from pluripotent hematopoietic stem cells in the *bone marrow*.

Via the blood, morphologically unidentifiable *mast cell progenitor cells* enter the connective or mucosal tissues, where they differentiate into phenotypically identifiable mature mast cells. A large number of in vitro studies have identified a number of mast cell growth factors, such as *IL-3*, *IL-4*, *IL-9*, and *SCF*.

High-affinity IgE receptors
Mast cells of various phenotypes express high-affinity IgE receptors, which bind IgE, and when aggregated by IgE-directed *antigens*, cause the release of preformed inflammatory mediators from granules, the synthesis of *arachidonic acid* (AA) metabolites and cytokines. The stimulation of mast cells via high-affinity IgE receptors is also called immunological activation. In immediate hypersensitivity reactions, this is mediated by allergens. In experiments, an immunological activation of mast cells can also be achieved using anti-IgE *antibodies*.

Other surface receptors
The presence of low-affinity *IgG*-binding receptors (FcγRII and FcγRIII) and receptors for the complement-derived *anaphylatoxins*, *C3a*, *C4a*, and *C5a*, also contributes to the reactivity of mast cells in *hypersensitivity* reactions. In addition, mast cells express SCF receptors (CD117). The receptor for SCF has been identified as the proto-oncogene c-kit. It is a receptor containing a *tyrosine kinase* domain, which is related to receptors for *platelet*-derived and epidermal growth factors. Mast cells also express *adhesion molecules* that bind to *extracellular matrix* glycoproteins. Such binding may initiate cytosolic signals to enhance, for example, high-affinity IgE receptor-mediated *degranulation*. *Adenosine* receptors are *G protein-coupled*

receptors also present on the mast cell surface. They may also increase mediator release from mast cells following immunological activation. Mast cells can also be activated by nonspecific stimuli, such as *ionophore* A23187, *compound 48/80*, *morphine*, codeine, desferrioxamine, *neuropeptides*, and *cytokines*. However, the responsiveness of different mast cell populations to individual stimuli varies.

Degranulation

Mast cells extrude membrane-free granules either into newly formed degranulation channels in the cytoplasm or individually through pores in plasma membrane to the exterior environment, when appropriately stimulated (see *exocytosis*). This process is associated with granule swelling. Moreover, human biopsies from multiple locations in a wide variety of pathologies have demonstrated that *piecemeal degranulation* of mast cells is another, frequently used way of secretion in vivo.

Mediators

The immunological activity of mast cells can, in principle, be explained by their mediators, which are released upon activation. The secretory granule of the human mast cell contains a crystalline complex of preformed inflammatory mediators, including histamine, proteases, and proteoglycans. Histamine effects such as vasodilation, increased vasopermeability, contraction of bronchial and intestinal *smooth muscle*, and increased *mucus* production are mediated via specific *histamine receptors*, and are normally of relatively short duration because of its rapid metabolism. The dominant proteoglycan in human mast cells is *heparin*. With their acidic sulfate groups of glycosaminoglycans, proteoglycans provide binding sites for other preformed mediators. Once released, heparin and, to a lesser extent, *chondroitin sulfate E*, may affect the stability or function of other mast cell mediators, such as *tryptase*. Besides histamine release, immunologic activation of mast cells induces the liberation of nuclear membrane-derived AA that is mainly metabolized by *cyclooxygenase* or by *5-lipoxygenase* (5-LO), leading to the formation of *prostaglandins* (PGs) and LTs. PGD_2 is a potent bronchoconstrictor that is rapidly degraded to another bronchoconstrictor, $PGF_{2\alpha}$. Both PGs are believed to cause *airway obstruction* by activation of their receptors. The effects of LTs include potent contraction of bronchial and vascular smooth muscle, enhanced permeability of postcapillary venules, increased bronchial mucus secretion, and eosinophil *chemotaxis*. In addition, mast cells produce small amounts of *platelet-activating factor* (PAF). Besides histamine and *lipid mediators*, it is well established that mast cells have the capacity to generate *Th2* cytokines such as IL-4, *IL-5, IL-6*, and *IL-13*. Human mast cells have also been reported to produce *IL-1, IL-2*, IL-3, *IL-8, IL-10, IFN-γ, GM-CSF*, but also *NGF* and *TNF-α*. At least in some cases, these cytokines can be rapidly released from preformed stores. Mast cell-derived IL-4 and IL-13 may help to facilitate *immunoglobulin class switching* for high IgE production. Moreover, IL-5 and GM-CSF may contribute to delayed *eosinophil apoptosis*. The mast-cell-derived TNF-α may be crucial for *recruitment of inflammatory cells*. Moreover, mast cells have also been reported to produce *CC chemokines*. A summary of important mast cell mediators and their pathophysiological role in *asthma* is given in Table 68.

Proteases

Mast cells exist as a heterogeneous family of effector cells (see *mast cell heterogeneity*). Therefore, there has been increasing awareness of the role of mast cell proteases in IgE-mediated *immune responses*. Immunohistochemical studies (see *immunohistochemistry*) have shown that human mast cells display two major different phenotypes distinguishable by their *neutral protease* content.

Whereas MC_T phenotype contains only tryptase, the MC_{TC} phenotype expresses both tryptase and chymase.

TABLE 68
Some Important Mast Cell Mediators and Their Role in Asthma

Mediator	Pathophysiological Role
IL-4	IgE production, *leukocyte* adhesion, *airway remodeling*, suppression of *Th1 cells*, development of Th2 cells
IL-5	*Eosinophilia*, enhanced eosinophil function
TNF-α	Leukocyte adhesion, activation of inflammatory cells
Histamine and PGD$_2$	Airway obstruction, nerve stimulation, *edema*, vasodilation, mucus secretion
Leukotrienes	Airway obstruction, nerve stimulation, edema, vasodilation, mucus secretion, chemotaxis
PAF	Airway obstruction, activation of inflammatory cells, chemotaxis

Initially, these respective subtypes were suggested to be the equivalent of the mucosal and the connective tissue previously described in rodents. It is now realized that variable amounts of both mast cell subtypes are present within any given tissue. Their relative abundance changes with disease (e.g., in *allergy* or *fibrosis*). However, some rules are becoming apparent.

> The MC$_T$ phenotypes appear to be immune-system-related with a primary role in host defense. In contrast, the MC$_{TC}$ phenotypes seem to be non-immune-system-related mast cells with functions in angiogenesis and tissue *remodeling* rather than immunologic protection.

Two other proteases, *carboxypeptidase* and *cathepsin G*, have been associated with the MC$_{TC}$ subset of human mast cells. Following activation of mast cells, chymase, carboxypeptidase, and cathepsin G are released together in a complex with proteoglycans, and are likely to act in concert with other enzymes to degrade proteins.

Role in diseases
The release of mast cell mediators by allergens has long been acknowledged to be responsible for immediate hypersensitivity reactions. This is supported by many studies showing increased levels of histamine and tryptase in *bronchoalveolar lavage* (BAL) fluid from patients with *allergic asthma*, in nasal washings and tears from patients with *allergic rhinoconjunctivitis*, and in blood during systemic *anaphylaxis*.

> Mast cells also play a major role in nonallergic diseases.

For instance, increased *mast cell numbers* can be found in scar tissue, especially in keloids, in callus tissue, in osteoporosis-linked diseases, and in various neuropathies. Mast cell participation has also been reported in various types of inflammatory reactions such as interstitial pneumonia, ulcerative colitis, intestinal helminthosis, and cases of ectodermal parasitosis (see *parasitic diseases*). A participation of mast cells is observed in connection with fibrotic disorders, such as Crohn's disease, peritoneal adhesions, idiopathic retroperitoneal fibrosis, *cryptogenic fibrosing alveolitis*, chronic *graft-versus-host disease* (GVHD), *wound healing*, *scleroderma*, and scleroderma-like diseases. They also have been shown to participate in the pathogenesis of certain tumors. Moreover, as mentioned above, mast cells play a critical protective role in bacterial infections (see *mast cells in innate immunity*).

MAST CELL ACTIVATION
Mast cells can be activated by immunological and non-immunological stimuli. Immunological activation means the interaction of an *allergen* with its specific *IgE antibody* attached to the cell membrane via the *high-affinity IgE receptor*. Besides allergens, lectins may also *cross-link*

receptor-bound IgE. Cross-linking of these receptors may also be induced by anti-IgE antibodies or antibodies against the IgE receptor (see *urticaria*). Non-immunological activation of mast cells can be achieved by *neuropeptides, complement factors, platelet-activating factor* (PAF), *chemokines* and *cytokines* (see *histamine-releasing factors*), *dextran, morphine, leukotrienes,* as well as *compound 48/80.*

MAST CELL ADHESION MOLECULES

Cell surface *integrins* detectable on *mast cells* are the β1 integrins CD29, CD49d, CD49e, and the vitronectin receptor (CD51/CD61). Mast cells lack significant amounts of β2 integrins. Other *adhesion molecules* on mast cells are *ICAM-1* (CD54), ICAM-2 (CD50), leukosialin (CD43), *CD44,* and CD58. Tissue mast cells lack *CD2,* CD22, CD31, and CD75. They also lack CD15, the thrombospondin *receptor* (CD36), and the *homing* molecule HML-1 (CD103) (see *CD antigens*).

MAST CELL APOPTOSIS

Apoptosis determines, besides other mechanisms, the *mast cell numbers* in tissues. It is regulated by *survival factors* such as *SCF* as well as *death factors* such as *Fas ligand. Corticosteroids* reduce *mast cell* numbers by the reduction of SCF *gene* expression (see *mast cells and corticosteroids*). Murine mast cells undergo apoptosis upon withdrawal of *IL-3.*

MAST CELL CYTOKINES

Mast cells are now recognized to be an important source of several *cytokines,* suggesting that these cells not only play an important role in *immediate,* but also in *delayed hypersensitivity* reactions and *allergic inflammation.* Human mast cells can express *TNF-α, IL-4, IL-5, IL-6,* and *IL-8.* IL-4 is preferentially expressed by MC_{TC} (see *mast cell heterogeneity*), whereas IL-5 appears to be restricted to the MC_T subset. Table 69 summarizes the data of several studies using primary human, mouse, and *rat mast cells,* as well as *HMC-1* cells.

MAST-CELL-DEFICIENT MICE

Mice with *mutations* at both copies of the W/c-kit locus (*SCF receptor*), such as $WBB6F_1$-W/W^v mice, or with mutations at the Sl/MGF (mast-cell growth factor; SCF) locus, such as Sl/Sl^d mice, are profoundly deficient in *mast cells.* Both types of mice are also anemic, lack melanocytes in the skin, and are sterile. They are considered useful models for studying the role of mast cells for physiologic or pathologic responses. For instance, *parasitic diseases* or bacterial infections induced in mast-cell-deficient mice are prolonged, indicating a role for *mast cells in innate immunity.*

MAST CELL DIFFERENTIATION

Mast cells commence their differentiation in the *bone marrow,* from which they are released into the circulation as committed precursors without any distinctive morphologic features. These circulating *mast cell progenitor cells* enter into tissues where they complete their differentiation and maturation. Human mast cells derive from CD34+ progenitor cells in the presence of *SCF,* but not *IL-3.* This is in contrast to murine mast cells that can differentiate under the influence of IL-3.

MAST CELL/FIBROBLAST CO-CULTURES

Mast cell/fibroblast co-cultures allow the study of long-term biochemical and functional characteristics of mast cells and their interactions with fibroblasts. Co-culture of rodent peritoneal *connective tissue mast cells* (CTMC) (see *rat mast cells*) with mouse embryonic

TABLE 69
Mast Cell-Derived Cytokines

mRNA	protein
IL-1∗ ♦i	IL-1∗
IL-2∗	IL-2∗
IL-3∗ ♦i	IL-3∗ ♦
IL-4∗ ∗∗ ♥i	IL-4∗ ∗∗ ♥
IL-5∗ ∗∗ ♥c	IL-5∗ ♥
IL-6∗ ∗∗ ♥♦i	IL-6∗ ♥
IL-8∗∗ i	IL-8∗∗
IL-10∗∗	*IL-16*∗∗
IL-12∗	
IL-13∗∗	
M-CSF∗∗c	
GM-CSF∗ ♦i	GM-CSF∗ ♦
IFN-γ ∗ ∗∗	IFN-γ∗
TNF-α∗ ∗∗♦ ♥c	TNF-α∗ ♥
TNF-β ♦i	
TGF-β∗ ♦c	TGF-β∗ ♦
PDGF-A ♦i	
SCF∗ ∗∗ ♦♥	SCF∗

∗ rodent

∗∗ human skin

♥ human lung

♦i HMC-1: inducible   ♦c HMC-1: constitutive

3T3 fibroblasts maintain CTMC viability, phenotype, and functional activity for more than a month. Similar data were obtained when human skin or lung mast cells were co-cultured with 3T3 cells or human lung/foreskin fibroblasts. Moreover, when *bone-marrow-derived mast cells* (BMMC) are cultured with 3T3 fibroblasts or *SCF*, they change their phenotype toward CTMC.

MAST CELL HETEROGENEITY

The concept of *mast cell* heterogeneity is based on evidence derived from studies in humans and animals that indicate that mast cells can vary in many aspects including morphology, histochemistry, *mediator* content, response to drugs, and stimuli of activation (see *mast cell activation*). For instance, *tryptase* is the only *neutral protease* present in a subpopulation of mast cells (MC$_T$), whereas other mast cells contain (besides tryptase) *chymase, carboxypeptidase*, and *cathepsin G* (MC$_{TC}$) (see Table 70). Moreover, the existence of an MC$_C$ subset (chymase alone) has been proposed as well. Initially, MC$_T$ and MC$_{TC}$ subtypes were suggested to be the equivalents of mucosal mast cells (MMC) and connective tissue mast cells (CTMC) described in rats (see *rat mast cells*), because of their tissue localization. MC$_T$ predominate in alveolar septa of the lung and small intestinal mucosa, whereas MC$_{TC}$ are preferentially located in skin and small intestine submucosa (see Table 70). However, *immunohistochemistry* studies have clearly demonstrated that both mast cell subtypes are present within any given tissue. Moreover, the relative abundance may change with disease (e.g., in *allergic diseases* or *fibrosis*).

> MC$_T$ appear to be "*immune-system*-related" mast cells with a primary role in host defense, whereas MC$_{TC}$ seem to be "non-immune-system-related" mast cells with functions in angiogenesis and tissue *remodeling* rather than immunologic protection.

Both phenotypes express *high-affinity IgE receptors* and participate in *IgE*-dependent allergic or *parasitic diseases*. Mast cells isolated from skin (MC$_{TC}$) release *histamine* in response to immunological (*allergen* and anti-IgE) as well as a wide variety of nonimmunological agents such as the calcium *ionophore* A23187, *compound 48/80, morphine* sulfate, *substance P*, and *anaphylatoxins*. In contrast, mast cells isolated from lung (MC$_T$) are activated by anti-IgE and calcium ionophore A23187, but not by any of the other agents listed above. Moreover, histamine release from MC$_T$ but not MC$_{TC}$ can be inhibited by sodium *cromoglycate*.

TABLE 70
Characteristics of Human Mast Cells

Characteristics	MC$_{TC}$	MC$_T$
Protease content	Tryptase	Tryptase
	Chymase	
	Carboxypeptidase	
	Cathepsin G	
Distribution		
Skin	99%	1%
Lung	7%	93%
Nasal mucosa	34%	66%
Tonsils	60%	40%
Small intestine mucosa	19%	81%
Small intestine submucosa	77%	23%
Increased numbers	Fibrosis	Allergic diseases
Decreased numbers	Unknown	AIDS
T cell dependence	No	Yes
Activation by		
IgE *cross-linking*	Yes	Yes
Compound 48/80	Yes	No
Substance P	Yes	No
Inhibition by cromoglycate	No	Yes

MAST CELL NUMBERS

In *allergic inflammation*, the numbers of *mast cells* are elevated. This has especially been demonstrated in allergic *conjunctivitis*. The responsible mechanisms may include increased generation of *mast cell progenitor cells* and inhibition of *mast cell apoptosis*. Clearly, *T cells* are involved in these processes. Elevated mast cell numbers have also been observed in *parasitic diseases*, tissue repair processes (see *wound healing* and *airway remodeling*), and *fibrosis*.

MAST CELL PROGENITOR CELLS

The study of *mast cell development* is notoriously difficult, because *mast cells* cannot be readily identified until they express *high-affinity IgE receptor*s and contain their characteristic *granules*. Many studies have been performed in murine systems. Mouse mast cell progenitor cells are present in the *bone marrow* as mononuclear cells mostly lacking high-affinity *IgE receptors*. However, they may be tentatively recognized by their expression of *SCF* and SCF receptor *mRNA*.

Reconstitution studies in normal irradiated mice and in *mast cell-deficient mice* strains, using mast cells with identifiable marker granules have provided a major breakthrough in the search for the origin and differentiation of mast cells. The results of these studies suggest that mast cells derive from pluripotent bone-marrow stem cell. Upon stimulation with *IL-3*, mast cell progenitor cells proliferate to produce immature cell colonies. The IL-3-dependent *bone-marrow-derived mast cells* (BMMC) were originally thought to represent an in vitro counterpart of *mucosal mast cells* (MMC) (see *rat mast cells*). However, these cells can acquire phenotypic features that are more similar to those of *connective tissue mast cells* (CTMC). Therefore, it is now believed that they represent an immature mast cell, which may be driven by appropriate microenvironmental signals to differentiate to either MMC or CTMC.

MAST CELL RECEPTORS

Immunoglobulin receptors

The group of *receptors* for *immunoglobulins* (Ig) are called *Fc receptors* by virtue of their capacity to interact with the Fc region of Ig. *Mast cells* express substantial amounts of *high-affinity IgE receptors* (FcεRI) and FcγRIII (*CD16*), which binds *IgG*. *Cross-linking* of FcεRI has been known for decades to induce rapid and extensive release of *mediators* from tissue mast cells and blood *basophils* (see *immediate hypersensitivity*). In rodent mast cells, CD16 activation can also trigger *histamine* release.

Cytokine receptors

Mature mast cells express *SCF* and *IL-4* receptors. They appear to lose other *cytokine receptors* (e.g., receptors for *IL-1*, *IL-3*, *GM-CSF*) during differentiation. Moreover, mast cells do not express receptors for *IL-2*, *IL-6*, and IL-7. This is in contrast to *HMC-1* cells, which express a wide range of *cytokine* receptors.

Complement factor receptors

Mast cells can express receptors for the *anaphylatoxins C3a*, *C4a*, and *C5a*. Human skin, but not lung mast cells, express C5a receptors. Activation of these *G protein-coupled receptors* leads to *histamine* release and can cause *anaphylaxis*.

MAST CELLS AND CORTICOSTEROIDS

> In spite of the clear efficacy of *corticosteroids* in *allergic diseases*, *allergen challenge* reactions are not influenced by corticosteroid treatment.

This includes the *immediate hypersensitivity* reactions in *skin tests*, as well as nasal and *bronchial provocation tests*, suggesting that *mast cells* may not be affected by these drugs. Moreover, human mast cells are also insensitive to 1- to 2-day exposures to corticosteroids in in vitro test systems. For instance, *dexamethasone* does not inhibit the *IgE*-dependent release of *histamine, prostaglandin* D_2, or *leukotriene* C_4 in purified human lung, skin, or gut mast cells.

> Corticosteroids have been shown to downregulate *SCF* expression in resident cells such as *fibroblasts*.

Since SCF is an important *survival factor* for mast cells, corticosteroid therapy is associated with a reduction of *mast cell numbers*, probably due to the induction of *mast cell apoptosis*. Moreover, corticosteroids reduce the expression of *cytokines* such as *TNF-α* and *IL-5* in mast cells.

MAST CELLS AND IgE SYNTHESIS

Mast cells from patients with *allergic diseases* are able to provide all essential factors to directly stimulate *IgE* synthesis.

> Mast cell-derived *IL-4* and *IL-13* are able to initiate *immunoglobulin class switching* in *B cells* independent of *T cells*.

A second signal needed to generate mature IgE *mRNA* is initiated by *CD40 ligand*, which can also be delivered by mast cells. Therefore, mast cells may play a critical role in the initiation, amplification, and maintenance of IgE-mediated *allergic inflammation*.

MAST CELLS AND PARASITIC DISEASES

Mast cells participate in adaptive immunological responses against parasites. Infections with helmintic parasites (see *parasitic diseases*) are associated with increased *mast cell numbers* and levels of parasite-specific *IgE*. Moreover, the ability of worm *antigens* to cause *degranulation* of mast cells obtained from parasite-infected animals as well as the toxic properties of some mast cell *mediators* on these parasites are well documented.

MAST CELLS IN INNATE IMMUNITY

Mast cells appear to orchestrate life-saving host responses against bacterial infections. *Mast-cell-deficient mice* are unable to clear efficiently either an intranasal or intraperitoneal Klebsiella pneumonia infection. This defect was correlated with an impaired ability to generate *TNF-α* and recruit *neutrophils* to the site of infection. Reconstitution of the mast-cell-deficient mice with purified mast cells from normal mice brought the bacterial clearance rates back to normal levels and restored the production of early high levels of TNF-α as well as the recruitment of neutrophils into the site of infection.

MAST CELLS IN THE CENTRAL NERVOUS SYSTEM

Mast cells have been identified in the brain of rats. *Histamine* can be released from hypothalamic slices by *compound 48/80* and from thalamic/hypothalamic mast cells in response to somatostatin, *substance P*, and neurotrophic factors, such as *nerve growth factor* (NGF), brain-derived neurotrophic factor (BDNF), and ciliary neurotrophic factor (CNTF).

MAST CELL STABILIZERS

Cromones are considered to be *mast cell* stabilizers, and they have been used for the prevention of symptoms in *allergic diseases*. Despite intense efforts to understand the mechanism(s) by which cromones inhibit *histamine* release from mast cells, this is still unclear. It has been proposed that these drugs may inhibit histamine release by suppressing both calcium uptake from external milieu and *calcium mobilization* from intracellular stores. Other theories on the mode of action of cromones involve changes in protein *phosphorylation*. Finally, recent studies suggest that cromones would block chloride channels that provide the driving force for calcium influx during *mast cell activation*.

MASTOCYTOSIS

This disease is characterized by an accumulation of *mast cells* at different sites of the body, in which the skin is almost always involved. The extent ranges from a solitary mastocytoma, through the spontaneously resolving lesions of childhood *urticaria* pigmentosa and the more progressive adult forms which lead to accumulation of mast cells in the viscera, bones, and *bone marrow*, to the very rare mast cell leukemia. Systemic symptoms are flushing, headache, *wheeze*, diarrhea, and syncope. Mast cells from patients with mastocytosis are larger with larger *granules* and nuclei compared to normal mast cells, but retain normal functional integrity and *surface molecules*.

MATRIX

(See *extracellular matrix* and *nuclear matrix*.)

MATRIX ATTACHMENT SITE

This is a *DNA* sequence with the property to bind to the *nuclear matrix* in vitro. It defines transcriptional active regions in vivo (see *transcription*).

MBP

Abbreviation for both *major basic protein* and myelin basic protein (see *multiple sclerosis*).

M CELL

Specialized epithelial cells of the gut that act as *antigen-presenting cells* (APCs) (see *gut-associated lymphoid tissue*).

MCP-1

(See *monocyte chemotactic protein-1*.)

MCP-2

(See *monocyte chemotactic protein-2*.)

MCP-3

(See *monocyte chemotactic protein-3*.)

MDI

(See *metered dose inhalers*.)

MEDIATOR

Substances that are released by inflammatory cells, such as *mast cells*, *eosinophils*, *neutrophils*, *basophils*, and *macrophages*, in response to *allergen* or other challenges and which act on other cells to induce the clinical features of *allergic disease*. The key mediators of mast cells and basophils are spasmogens, activators, and *chemotactic factors* (including *chemokines*). Some mediators are preformed and stored within *granules* (e.g., *histamine* in mast cells and *eosinophil cationic protein* in eosinophils), and are released upon *receptor* activation. Other mediators are newly synthesized, such as *arachidonic acid* (AA) metabolites, including *prostaglandins* (PGs) and *leukotrienes* (LTs), *platelet activating factor* (PAF), and many *cytokines*. These mediators are responsible for both the *immediate* as well as the *delayed hypersensitivity* reactions in *IgE*-mediated allergic diseases.

MEIOSIS

This is a special type of cell division in the germ cells of sexually reproducing organisms by which gametes with *haploid* sets of *chromosomes* are produced from *diploid* cells. In the development of the germ cells, two meiotic cell divisions occur. The reduction from diploid to haploid chromosome sets occurs in the first meiotic division (meiosis I).

MEMBRANE CHANNEL

Cell membranes have different types of ion channels, e.g., calcium, chloride, and *potassium channels*. The driving force for calcium influx can be modified by chloride or potassium channels, which set the membrane potential of cells. For instance, blocking of potassium channels leads to *histamine* release from *mast cells*. Moreover, chloride channels may play a role in volume regulation following *degranulation*.

MEMORY B CELL

Secondary responses to most *antigens* are characterized by high-*affinity IgG* and IgA *antibodies*. They are elicited by lower antigen doses recognized by memory *B cells*. IgA is produced mainly by memory B cells residing in mucosal tissues. After immunization, virgin B cells (see *naive lymphocytes*) interact with *T cells* in the T cell areas of lymphatic organs (spleen and *lymph nodes*) and proliferate. Some B cells develop into antibody-secreting *plasma cells*. *IL-4* and *IL-13*, produced by T cells, stimulate B cells to express CD23, the *low-affinity IgE receptor*. Activated B cells are then directed into follicules to proliferate and form new germinal centers. Germinal centers are the primary sites for the formation of memory B cells. Germinal centers contain follicular *dendritic cells*, which play a major role in B cell memory. Follicular dendritic cells are nonphagocytic (see *phagocytosis*), and express high levels of *Fc* and *complement factor receptors*. During differentiation in germinal centers, B cells acquire the memory cell phenotype, which is characterized by the expression of high levels of *MHC class II molecules*, CD21, CD22 (see *CD antigens*), *CD45*, and all five *isotypes* of surface *immunoglobulins*.

MEMORY T CELL

Downregulation of the *primary immune response* leads to the clearance of many *CD4+ T cells* (see *T cell apoptosis*), but a population of long-lived memory T cells (CD4+CD45RA−, CD45RB+) remains which are able to respond rapidly to secondary or subsequent exposure to their specific *antigen*. Together with activation of *memory B cells,* a more rapid, heightened, and sustained response to *antigen* can be mounted.

MENDELIAN PATTERN OF INHERITANCE

A trait inherited in a simple Mendelian fashion means that a certain *phenotype* depends on the presence or absence of a specific *genotype* at a single *locus*.

MESSENGER RNA (mRNA)

These are *RNA* molecules that encode polypeptides or proteins. mRNA is commonly transcribed (see *transcription*) as precursor molecules that are spliced (removal of *intron* sequences) and modified at the 5′-(cap) and 3′-(poly A tail, see *polyadenylation*) ends, exported from the nucleus, and they can be translated (see *translation*) at the ribosomes.

METALLIC SALTS

Metallic salts such as chromium, *nickel*, platinum, palladium, zinc, and cobalt may cause *asthma*. In some cases, *IgE*-mediated reactions have been demonstrated for these metals. Metallic salts readily dissociate, and metal ions are transported into the lungs. The prevalence of *occupational asthma* due to chromium, zinc, nickel, and cobalt is rare and relatively high in the platinum industry. In addition to allergic reactions, exposure to metal fumes can cause *bronchitis*, *emphysema*, or metal fume fever. Pneumoconiosis due to hard metals has also been reported.

METALLOPROTEASE

A metalloprotease is an enzyme that degrades *extracellular matrix* proteins. *Fibroblasts* and *phagocytes* are important sources of several metalloproteases, such as *collagenase*. Released *proteases*, together with reactive *oxygen metabolites*, lead to tissue damage and contribute to *remodeling*. Metalloproteases are inhibited by *tissue inhibitors of metalloproteases* (TIMPs). The interactions between metalloproteases and TIMPs in *asthma* and other chronic *allergic diseases* is not very well understood.

METERED DOSE INHALER (MDI)

A medical *aerosol* device that delivers a fixed dose of a drug in a spray form upon activation. Historically they have used *CFC propellants*, but these are now being replaced by *HFA propellants* or *dry powder inhalers*. MDI may be activated by the patient or may be breath-activated. Lung delivery may be improved by using a *spacer device*.

METHACHOLINE

Methacholine is a cholinergic agonist that causes *airway obstruction* by direct action on airway smooth muscle cells. It is used as an alternative to *histamine* in *bronchial provocation tests* of *airway hyperresponsiveness*.

METHOTREXATE

Methotrexate is an antimetabolite that is a useful *immunosuppressive drug*, also used in *asthma*.

METHYLPREDNISOLONE

Methylprednisolone is a *corticosteroid*. It is sometimes used intravenously in high doses to treat various forms of acute *allergic inflammation* and *anaphylaxis*.

METHYLXANTHINE

Methylxanthine is a *phosphodiesterase inhibitor*.

MHC CLASS II COMPARTMENTS

Inside the cytoplasm of *antigen presenting cells* (APCs) there are *major histocompatibility complex* (MHC) class II compartments, also known as MHC class II vesicles, filled with newly synthesized *MHC class II molecules*. The MHC class II compartments are fused with the early *endosomes* during *endocytosis*. Inside these MHC class II compartments, the MHC class II molecules are associated to the *invariant chain* and bind *antigenic peptide* before migrating to the surface of the cell (see *antigen processing* and *antigen recognition*).

MHC CLASS I MOLECULES

The presentation of *antigenic peptides* in *major histocompatibility complex* (MHC) molecules on the cell surface, the *antigen* presentation, is done by MHC class I and *MHC class II molecules. Human leukocyte antigen* (HLA) class I molecules are classified from A to F. MHC class I is a heterodimer of a membrane-anchored 43-kDa α-chain, which is folded into the α1, α2, and α3-domains, and a second, non-covalently associated, 12-kDa β2-microglobulin protein. Binding of the antigenic *peptides* takes place inside the groove which is formed between the α1 and α2 domains. The size of the peptides bound to MHC class I ranges from 8 to 10 *amino acids*. Peptides cleaved from proteins originating from the cytoplasm of the cell are presented to *CD8+ T cells*.

MHC CLASS II MOLECULES

MHC class II is a complex of two membrane-anchored glycoproteins, the 34-kDa α-chain and 29-kDa β-chain. MHC class II molecules are encoded by *genes* of the *major histocompatibility complex* (MHC). *Human leukocyte antigen* (HLA) class-II molecules classified as DR, DP, DQ molecules are responsible for presentation of exogenous *antigens* (soluble) to *CD4+ T cells* (see *antigen recognition, genetic predisposition*, and *MHC restriction*). In MHC class II molecules, *peptide* binding takes place inside the groove between the α1 and β1 domains. In contrast to MHC class I molecules, the antigen-binding groove of MHC class II molecules is open at both ends. As a consequence, the size of *antigenic peptides* bound to MHC class II molecules ranges from 10 to 30 *amino acids*. Newly synthesized MHC class II molecules are associated to an *invariant chain*.

> The *transcription* of MHC class II molecules is regulated by *cytokines*, especially by *IFN-γ*.

Therefore, IFN-γ-deficient mice (see *knockout mice*) demonstrate decreased expression of these molecules. Moreover, drug-induced or other immunosuppressions are associated with decreased expression of MHC class II molecules.

> In *asthma*, high doses of *corticosteroids* reduce their expression on *monocytes*, indicating a possible drug-induced immunodeficiency.

The protein that activates transcription of MHC class II *genes*, the MHC class II transactivator, is defective in the disease *bare lymphocyte syndrome*.

MHC RESTRICTION

Antigen recognition by *T cells* is *major histocompatibility complex* (MHC)-restricted.

> MHC restriction means that a given T cell will recognize *antigen* only when its *peptide* fragments are bound to a particular MHC molecule.

Therefore, in *allergic diseases*, recognition of allergenic peptides (see *antigenic peptides*) by *CD4+ T cells*, resulting in *T cell antigen receptor* activation and development of effector function, is dependent on presentation of the *allergen* by *MHC class II molecules* of *antigen-presenting cells* (APCs). In humans, the MHC antigens are known as *human leukocyte antigens* (HLA). Somatic recombination permits a highly polymorphic (see *genetic polymorphism*) and diverse repertoire of antigen presenting capability by the HLA molecules, which take up processed peptides (see *antigen processing*) and present them on the cell surface. The HLA-restricted responses have been studied in allergic patients, e.g., by inhibiting T cell proliferative responses (usually *T cell clones*; see *T cell proliferation*) to define allergenic peptides with *monoclonal antibodies* directed toward different HLA structural or framework regions associated with peptide binding. In this way, T cell dependence on specific HLA haplotypes can be assessed. In addition, methods using T cell proliferative responses to allergens using HLA-typed Epstein–Barr virus (EBV)-transformed *B cells* as APCs have been used, as have more sophisticated techniques involving transfection of APCs with specific HLA *genes*. Earlier studies involved examining other immunological endpoints such as *IgE* production in *peripheral blood mononuclear cell* (PBMC) cultures to specific allergen exposure of HLA-typed individuals (see *genetic predisposition*).

MICROSATELLITE

This is a small repeat block of multiple copies of a specific *DNA* sequence, often less than 0.1 kb. Length variations in the population and their detection by *polymerase chain reaction* (PCR) make microsatellites useful *markers* for *linkage* analyses in genetic studies and for forensic medicine (see also *tandem repeat*).

MID-EXPIRATORY FLOW RATE (MEFR)

The MEFR is a more sensitive indicator of small *airway obstruction* than the *peak expiratory flow rate* (PEFR), which is affected by large and small airway obstruction. The MEFR is measured from the *flow volume loop*, and is most useful in patients with mild airflow obstruction with near-normal *lung function tests*.

MIGRATION

The process of inflammatory cell movement into tissues following firm attachment on *endothelial cells* is usually called migration. The movement is controlled by *adhesion molecules* and *chemotactic factors*. Some chemotactic factors are specific for inflammatory cells. For instance, *IL-8* may only cause *neutrophil* migration, whereas *eotaxin* may selectively attract *eosinophils*. For *T cell* migration, *RANTES* and other *chemokines* play an important role (see *T cell trafficking*).

MILK

(See *cow's milk allergy*.)

MILK CRUST

(See *milk scurf*.)

MILK SCURF

Milk scurf is a morphologically distinct reaction pattern of atopic skin (see *atopy*), resembling the crust of cooked milk. Almost exclusively present in young children, milk scurf (Lat.: crusta lactea) is frequently the first manifestation of an *atopic dermatitis*.

MINERALOCORTICOSTEROIDS

Mineralocorticosteroids are steroids whose principal action is on salt balance as opposed to carbohydrate metabolism.

MINISATELLITE

(See *tandem repeat*.)

MINOR ALLERGEN

Minor *allergens* are proteins within *pollen*, *animal dander*, *house-dust mite*, and other allergens against which less than 50% of sensitized individuals develop *IgE antibodies* (see *major allergens*).

MIP-1

(See *monocyte inhibitory protein-1*.)

MISSENSE MUTATION

This is a single *base pair* (bp) *mutation*, leading to a *codon* specifying another *amino acid*.

MITE

(See *house-dust mite*.)

MITOGEN-ACTIVATED PROTEIN KINASES (MAPKs)

MAPKs represent a family of 40- to 46-kDa serine/threonine *kinases* which are activated via many *cytokine receptors*, members of the *TNF receptor superfamily*, *antigen receptors*, and *G protein-coupled receptors*. The central pathway is a *signaling* cascade, which requires activation of *Ras*. Ras activates *Raf*, which is a serine/threonine kinase. Raf activates MAPK kinase (MEK). MEK phosphorylates MAPK on both tyrosine and threonine residues, leading to full activation of MAPK (now called ERK). ERK translocates from the cytosol to the nucleus, where it activates *transcription factors*. ERK activation has also been associated with *granulocyte priming*. In addition to the classical pathway, which is especially important for the transduction of proliferation and differentiation signals, two alternative pathways are known. They are important for stress-induced *signal transduction* in *inflammation* and *apoptosis* (e.g., *IL-1*, *TNF-α*, *UV light*, etc.). These pathways involve *Jun-N-terminal kinase* (JNK) and p38 activation (see Figure 34).

MITOSIS

Mitosis is the process of nuclear and cell division during *somatic cell* division.

MODIFIED ALLERGEN VACCINES

In order to improve the safety of *immunotherapy* schedules, many attempts have been made to reduce the *IgE*-binding properties of *allergen extracts* while retaining their effect on *T cells*. Formaldehyde inactivation cross-links the proteins and blocks the sites recognized by IgE *antibodies*. The *peptide* sequence is retained and can be seen by T cells (see *linear epitopes*) after digestion in *antigen-presenting cells* (APCs) (see also *peptide vaccines*).

MODULATION OF T CELL RESPONSES

> The balance between activation and suppression of an *immune response* is often mediated by *T cells*.

In this respect, models *of allergic diseases* offer a valuable insight into the mechanisms of control of activation and suppression of the *immune system* when it is presented with, or exposed to, different *antigens* or different amounts of the same antigen. Activation of immune responses by T cells is mediated by direct contact between T cells and other immune effector cells, or indirectly via *cytokines* (see *cognate/noncognate interactions*).

> Suppression of immune responses was once thought to be mediated by specific suppressor T cells that resided mainly in the *CD8+* T cell population.

However, it was recognized that CD8+ T cells could be functionally active in other ways, such as cytotoxicity, and hence the term "suppressor/cytotoxic T cell" became synonymous

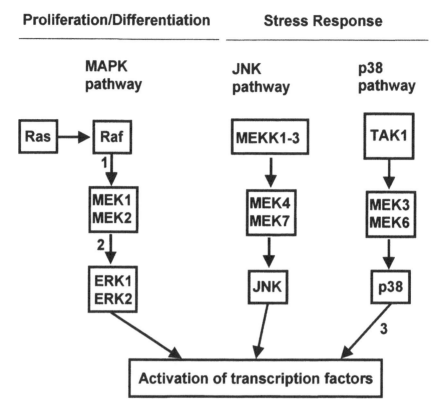

FIGURE 34 Besides the classical MAPK cascade, two alternative MAPK pathways are known. The kinase cascades can be inhibited by pharmacological compounds, which are used in signal transduction research. (1) PD098059 blocks Raf activity; (2) U0126 blocks MEK1 and MEK2 activity; (3) SB203580 is a p38 blocker.

with CD8+ T cell. This nomenclature has persisted, although it is now recognized that specific functionality is not restricted by CD8 or *CD4* phenotype, other than the important dichotomy of class I and class II *MHC restriction*.

> It is clear that the two antagonistic *Th1* and *Th2 cell* subsets have "suppressor" activity related to the function of the other subset.

Similar relationships exist within CD8+ T cells and between reactions to antigens by CD4+ and CD8+ T cells. T cells play a major role in providing help for *B cell activation* and *antibody* production, activating and expanding *eosinophils*, producing cytokines that enhance *mast cell* reactivity, and recruiting various immune effector cells to the sites of *inflammation*. They are also involved in the mechanism of *sensitization* and activation of professional *phagocytes* by the production of *IFN-γ*. Likewise, under different circumstances they can induce *isotype* selection in *B cells,* which may enhance or suppress an ongoing immune response.

> T cells may downregulate effector cell function by direct contact or cytokine secretion and remove inflammatory cells and pathogens by direct cytotoxicity (see *immunosuppressive mechanisms*).

Activation and suppression of T cells are mediated by a combination of mechanisms that achieve a dynamic balance in vivo. T cells are principally activated by engagement of the *T cell antigen receptor* (TCR) with antigen/*major histocompatibility complexes* (MHC) with co-receptor ligation (CD4 or CD8) and synergistic *co-stimulation*. They also have other *receptors* that can contribute to activation, including those for cytokines and *adhesion molecules*.

In contrast, suppression of T cell responses can be achieved by anergic (see *anergy*) and apoptotic (see *apoptosis*) mechanisms or by competitive inhibition of receptor binding.

MOLD ALLERGENS

(See *fungal allergens* and *molds*.)

MOLDS

True allergic reactivity to mold spores and hyphae results in *IgE*-mediated *allergic disease*. Mold spores, including those of species of Penicillium, Cladosporium, Alternaria, *Aspergillus*, and Candida are important *fungal allergens* and have been identified as causative agents for *allergic asthma*. For example, IgE *antibodies* to Candida albicans can be detected in some atopic subjects, being associated with severe *atopic dermatitis* and *asthma*. The IgE response is associated with a *Th2 cytokine* response. In mice, protection from invasive candidiasis was associated with a *Th1* response (*IFN-γ* production), whereas susceptibility was associated with the production of *IL-4* or was enhanced by treatment with anti-IFN-γ antibodies. Therefore, besides *immediate hypersensitivity* reactions, molds may also cause *delayed hypersensitivity* reactions (see *Coombs and Gell classification*, type IV).

MOLECULAR EPIDEMIOLOGY

Epidemiological research using molecular genetic and biochemical methods.

MOLECULAR GENETICS

Molecular genetics is a research field in which the physicochemical properties of *genes* with regard to inheritance are studied.

MONKEYS

Monkeys are a useful model for studying *asthma*, because they have been shown to display both *airway obstruction* and *airway hyperresponsiveness*. Large numbers of *mast cells* are obtained by *bronchoalveolar lavage* (BAL) of Macaco arctoides monkeys infected with the nematode Ascaris suum. These mast cells release *histamine*, *leukotriene* C_4 (LTC$_4$), and *prostaglandin* D_2 (PGD$_2$) when challenged with Ascaris *antigen* or *antibody* to human *IgE*, but not with *compound 48/80*. *Nedocromil* sodium, but not *cromoglycate*, inhibited the *mediator* release from these cells.

MONOCLONAL ANTIBODY (mAb)

A mAb is an *antibody* derived from a population of cells originating from a single *B cell*. B cells, which ordinarily would only live for a few days in culture, are fused with a non-*immunoglobulin*-secreting myeloma cell line to produce immortal hybridomas. These cells generate immunoglobulin with the same specificity as the original.

MAbs are now used routinely in a wide range of diagnostic tests including *ELISAs*, *immunohistochemistry*, and *flow cytometry*.

Moreover, recent developments have allowed the humanization of mouse mAbs, thus avoiding anti-mouse immunoglobulin responses in patients. Such mAbs are used for in vivo treatment against *cytokines* such as *TNF-α* and against cell surface *receptors* (see *antibody therapy* and *anticytokine therapy*).

MONOCYTE

Monocytes occupy a compartment of the myeloid cell ontogeny.

> Monocytes are principally found in the peripheral circulation, and their main role is as *antigen-presenting cells* (APCs).

They have limited phagocytic capability, which is considerably enhanced in *macrophages*. There is still uncertainty as to whether all monocytes have the potential to differentiate into macrophages when recruited to tissue sites, but there is considerable overlap in function and expression of *surface markers* between these cell types. Under appropriate conditions, monocytes produce large amounts of *cytokines* (see *monokines*), including *TNF-α, IL-1β,* and *IL-6* (also known as proinflammatory *cytokines*), as well as *IL-12*, an important cytokine in *Th cell* subset regulation (IL-12 up-regulates *IFN-γ* and other *Th1* cytokines). Monocytes and macrophages are activated for effective intracellular killing of bacteria and upregulation of *major histocompatibility complex* (MHC) molecules by IFN-γ.

MONOCYTE CHEMOTACTIC PROTEIN-1 (MCP-1)

MCP-1 is a *chemokine* of the *CC chemokine* subgroup that is induced by a variety of proinflammatory stimuli. It is highly effective as an inducer of *histamine* release in *basophils*, but not necessarily in *mast cells*. In contrast, MCP-1 is only a weak *chemotactic factor*.

MONOCYTE CHEMOTACTIC PROTEIN-2 (MCP-2)

MCP-2 is a *chemokine* of the *CC chemokine* subgroup that is important in *allergic diseases*, since it inhibits, under certain experimental conditions, the action of the more effective *MCP-3* analog. Thus, MCP-2, which is inducibly expressed by the *Th1 cytokine IFN-γ*, may have an inhibitory effect in allergic diseases in vivo.

MONOCYTE CHEMOTACTIC PROTEIN-3 (MCP-3)

MCP-3 is a *chemokine* of the *CC chemokine* subgroup that is important in *allergic diseases*, since it strongly attracts and activates all allergic effector cells (*eosinophils, basophils, T cells,* and *monocytes*).

MONOCYTE INHIBITORY PROTEIN-1 (MIP-1)

MIP-1α and MIP-1β are *CC chemokines* important in the *migration* of *lymphocytes* (see *T cell trafficking*). MIP-1α attracts *CD8+* cytotoxic *T cells* and *B cells*, whereas MIP-1β selectively attracts naive *CD4+/CD45*RA+ T cells (see *naive lymphocytes*). During induction of T cell *anergy* in the presence of high concentrations of specific *antigen* (see *immunotherapy*), MIP-1 is overexpressed, whereas *RANTES* production declines.

MONOKINES

Cytokines that are produced by *monocytes* and *macrophages*. However, in most cases, monokines can also be produced by other cells. Therefore, the term "monokine" is not much used anymore.

MONOSENSITIZATION

This term is used for patients who only show *skin test* reactions to a single *allergen*.

MONTELUKAST

Montelukast is a potent *leukotriene receptor antagonist*.

MORPHINE

Narcotics such as morphine represent examples of pharmacological agents that can induce *mediator* release from *mast cells* in a non-immunological manner (see *idiosyncrasy*). Since morphine predominantly activates skin mast cells (see *mast cell heterogeneity*), it appears that cutaneous mast cell activation alone is sufficient to induce systemic responses (see *anaphylactoid reactions*).

mRNA

(See *messenger RNA*.)

MUCOCILIARY CLEARANCE

The tracheobronchial tree is lined by ciliated (see *cilia*) *epithelial cells,* which propel a thin layer of *mucus* upward from the lungs to the throat, where it is swallowed. In normal health, people are not aware of this process, but if there is excessive mucus production, the patient will *cough* up *sputum*. Mucociliary clearance removes the majority of particles that are inhaled and impact on the airways. In the case of chronic persistent cough, measuring of mucociliary clearance using radio-*aerosols* is a helpful diagnostic tool. The mucociliary clearance is reduced in patients with *asthma* due to *epithelial damage*.

MUCOSA-ASSOCIATED LYMPHOID TISSUE (MALT)

MALT is a collection of lymphoid tissues in the submucosa that play an important role in the defense of mucosal body surfaces against exogenous pathogens.

MUCOSAL MAST CELL (MMC)

MMC are *mast cells* within the mucosa of different organs with special functional characteristics that differ from those of *connective tissue mast cells* (CTMC) (see *rat mast cells*).

MUCUS

Respiratory mucus is the thin viscoelastic fluid layer lining the upper and lower airways. Its functions include providing protection against physicochemical insults and invading microorganisms, serving as a medium for the transport and removal of entrapped inhaled particles, humidifying inspired air, and providing a detoxifying surface. It is produced by *epithelial cells* and cells of the submucosal glands. Mucus is a complex mixture composed of about 95% water, 1% proteins, 0.9% carbohydrates, and 0.8% lipids. The proteins include serum proteins such as albumin, α1-antitrypsin, α2-macroglobulin, haptoglobin, transferrin, IgA, *IgG*, and IgM, as well as locally produced proteins such as lysozyme, lactoferrin, IgA, and *IgE*. The mucus glycoproteins (MGP) mediate the viscosity and elasticity. The volume of tracheobronchial secretion is estimated to range from 10 to 100 ml per day. Increased mucus secretion is seen with stimulation of the autonomous *nervous system* as well as by inflammatory *mediators* (e.g., *leukotrienes*), cellular products from the airways, serum proteins and by exogenous environmental substances, particulates, and gases (see *air pollution*). In *asthma*, the mucus is particularly thick and difficult to *cough* up.

MUCUS PLUGGING

Obstruction of small airways by plugs of inspissated *mucus* and *eosinophil* debris. A characteristic feature of *death from asthma* and *asthma exacerbations*.

MUGWORT ALLERGENS

Like other *weed pollen*, mugwort *pollen* is wind-pollinated and may cause *IgE*-mediated *allergic rhinoconjunctivitis*. The pollen season peaks in July and August. Mugwort *allergens* contain *profilin*. Mugwort-allergic patients may therefore also respond with allergic symptoms following contact with various fruits and vegetables (see *cross-reacting allergens* and *oral allergy syndrome*).

MULTIFACTORIAL INHERITANCE

This form of inheritance is due to the interplay of multiple *genes* at different loci (polygenic) with multiple environmental factors. Multifactorial traits may be discontinuous with distinct *phenotypes* (e.g., diabetes mellitus) or continuous with a lack of distinct phenotypes (e.g., weight). The common diseases (including *allergic diseases*) have multifactorial inheritance, whereby an *allele* or alleles at different loci predispose individuals to particular environmental agents (see *genetic predisposition*). Twin and family studies confirm a genetic contribution to disease susceptibility; they do not identify the number and the function of the genes involved. The genes responsible can be localized and identified through population *association* studies, sib pair analysis, and *linkage* analysis. In allergic and autoimmune diseases (see *autoimmunity*), the genetic constitution leads to disease susceptibility. Several contributing loci have been identified that are involved in the regulation of the *immune response*: specific *antigen* presentation and recognition (see *antigen-presenting cells*), immune activation and immunoregulation (see *T helper cell differentiation*), and environmental triggers have been recognized (i.e., viruses, *pollutants*).

MULTIGENIC DISEASE

(See *multifactorial inheritance*.)

MULTIPLE CHEMICAL SENSITIVITY (MCS)

An ill-defined condition in which patients report a variety of nonspecific symptoms upon exposure to a wide variety of chemicals. Symptoms may include headaches, tiredness, muscle ache, as well as joint pains, bowel disturbance, loss of concentration, irritability, sleep disturbance, weight loss, skin rashes, anxiety, etc. Most patients who believe that they have this condition attribute their problems to exposure to household chemicals, insecticides, aldehydes, traffic fumes, etc. Many conventional allergists dispute the existence of MCS, but the condition has been championed by practitioners of clinical ecology. It is usually impossible to demonstrate a specific *sensitization* against the suspected chemicals by standard laboratory tests.

MULTIPLE SCLEROSIS (MS)

MS is a human autoimmune disease (see *autoimmunity*), associated with a strong *Th1* cell response toward myelin basic protein (MBP). The induction of or therapy with *Th2 cytokines* might be beneficial. *Experimental allergic encephalomyelitis* (EAE) serves as a model for pathophysiologic and therapeutic studies of this disease.

MUSCARINIC RECEPTORS

Muscarinic *receptors* are a subtype of *acetylcholine* receptors found on airway *smooth muscle* cells.

Acetylcholine, which is released from nerves, causes *airway obstruction* by stimulating M_3 muscarinic receptors.

They are so called because the actions of these receptors are mimicked by the alkaloid muscarine, and are different from those stimulated by nicotinic cholinergic receptors found in autonomic ganglia and at neuromuscular junctions (see *nervous system*).

> *Atropine* and other *anticholinergic drugs* such as *oxitropium* and *ipratropium* block the muscarinic, but not the nicotinic, effects of acetylcholine.

Moreover, neuronal M_2 muscarinic receptors which, under normal conditions, inhibit the release of acetylcholine, might be inhibited by *major basic protein* (MBP) released by *eosinophils* in *asthma*. This mechanism has been shown to cause *airway hyperresponsiveness* in *allergen*-challenged guinea pigs. Airway hyperresponsiveness is not due to alterations in the function of M_3 muscarinic receptors.

MUTATION

This is an alteration of the genomic *DNA* sequence, which is permanently heritable.

MYELOPEROXIDASE

This is a *mediator* derived from *neutrophils* and *monocytes* (see *peroxidase*).

MYOFIBROBLAST

Myofibroblasts are specialized *fibroblasts*, found in the airways and gut, that possess some properties of *smooth muscle* as well as characteristic fibroblast behavior. Myofibroblasts are thought to be responsible for the *collagen* deposition that occurs beneath the basement membrane in *asthma* (see *subepithelial fibrosis*), and contributes to *airway remodeling*. Although bronchial myofibroblasts cannot respond to specific *allergens*, the allergen-induced release of *cytokines* from cells bearing *allergen receptors* may stimulate these cells. Besides the production of *extracellular matrix* components, myofibroblasts are themselves able to produce cytokines, which may lead to the perpetuation of the process of *inflammation* in *allergic diseases*.

N

N-ACETYLCYSTEINE

N-Acetylcysteine is a precursor of *glutathione* biosynthesis and is used for *antioxidant* therapy, e.g., in *cryptogenic fibrosing alveolitis*.

NADPH OXIDASE

This enzyme generates, together with other components such as cytochrome b558 and several GTP-binding proteins, reactive *oxygen metabolites*. This multicomponent enzyme forms an electron-transport chain, using NADPH as a donor to reduce oxygen to *superoxide anion* (O_2^-), which is then dismuted to *hydrogen peroxide* (H_2O_2), and thereafter metabolized to hydroxyl radicals (OH^-). Defective cytochrome b558 results in a disease with severe infections (X-linked chronic granulomatous disease).

NAIVE LYMPHOCYTES

These are *lymphocytes* that, in contrast to *memory T cells* or *memory B cells*, have never been activated via their *antigen receptors*. All *T cells* that leave the *thymus* and all *B cells*, which leave the *bone marrow*, are naive lymphocytes (for identification, see *CD45*).

NARCOTICS

Some narcotics, such as *morphine* and meperidine, may induce *histamine* release from *mast cells*, especially in the skin, resulting in rash, *pruritus*, or hypotension (see *idiosyncrasy*). However, *IgE*-mediated *immediate hypersensitivity* reactions have also been reported due to these substances (see also *anesthetic allergy* and *drug allergy*).

NASAL LAVAGE (NAL)

Nasal *epithelial cells* are exposed to *pollutants*, *allergens*, and other agents, because the nasal passages are the first site of contact of the respiratory tract with the inhaled air.

> NAL is a noninvasive technique for sampling *mediators* and inflammatory cells in the nose.

Extracellular components include *cytokines* such as *IL-6, IL-8, TNF-α, antioxidants, eicosanoids, neuropeptides*, nasal glandular products, increased vascular permeability products, and other products from cells, such as *eosinophils* (e.g., *eosinophilic cationic protein*), *neutrophils*, and *mast cells*. In the classic NAL technique, a buffer solution is introduced in each nostril while the subject tilts the head back, retaining the solution in the nose for 10 seconds, after which it is expelled into a receptacle. After processing, the cells yielded from this technique can be identified by type and cultured for in vitro studies. Another method allows a prolonged NAL, which avoids contamination from the nasopharynx. In this technique, one of the subject's nostrils is occluded and then the subject retains saline solution in the other nostril, while leaning forward, for a period of up to 10 minutes. Another variant of the classic technique involves the patient administering the solution to himself using a nasal sprayer several times in each nostril. NAL is frequently performed following *allergen challenge* or exposure to *pollutants* (see *pollutants and nasal lavage*).

NASAL POLYPS

Nasal polyps are hypertrophic enlargements of the mucous membrane of the nose that form a projection from the wall of the nasal cavity or the nasal *sinuses*. They protrude into the nasal cavity from the middle meatus, resulting in nasal blockage and abolished airflow to the olfactory region. Nasal polyps can cause local infection due to deranged drainage of *mucus* secretions. Nasal polyps are strongly associated with *aspirin* intolerance (see *aspirin-sensitive asthma*) (see Table 71).

> Many of the features of *allergic inflammation* in *asthma* can also be detected in nasal polyp tissues.

For example, nasal polyps are strongly infiltrated by *eosinophils*, *mast cells*, *T cells*, *B cells*, and *NK cells*. Therefore, and because they are easily accessible, they represent a suitable model for immunological studies. For instance, the mechanism of delayed *eosinophil apoptosis* contributing to the development of tissue *eosinophilia* has been directly demonstrated in nasal polyps. *Corticosteroids* are the only type of drug with a proven effect on symptoms and signs of nasal polyposis.

TABLE 71
Prevalence of Nasal Polyposis
in Different Patient Groups

Aspirin intolerance	36–72%
Asthma	7%
Extrinsic	5%
Intrinsic	13%
Chronic *sinusitis*	2%
IgE-mediated	1%
Non-IgE-mediated	5%
Childhood asthma/sinusitis	0.1%
Cystic fibrosis	
Children	10%
Adults	50%
Allergic fungal sinusitis	66–100%
Primary ciliary dyskinesia	40%

NASAL PROVOCATION

(See *allergen challenge*.)

NATURAL KILLER CELL

(See *NK cell*.)

NEBULIZER

A nebulizer is a device that produces an *aerosol* by physical or ultrasonic dispersion of a liquid. Nebulizers are widely used to treat chronic severe *asthma* and *asthma exacerbations*. They are also used for long-term *bronchodilator* treatment of *chronic bronchitis* and *emphysema* as well as to administer *antibiotics* to patients with *cystic fibrosis*, bronchiectasis, or *acquired immunodeficiency syndrome* (AIDS).

NECROSIS

Necrosis is an accidental cell death characterized by overall cell and organelle swelling, with subsequent early loss of membrane integrity followed by cell and organelle lysis.

> Unlike *apoptosis*, necrosis is accompanied by a strong inflammatory response (see *inflammation*) in vivo.

In *allergic inflammation*, *eosinophils* are sometimes strongly activated and release high amounts of toxic *eosinophil granule proteins* and reactive *oxygen metabolites* into their microenvironment, resulting in necrosis (e.g., *epithelial damage* or *eosinophil cytolysis*).

NEDOCROMIL

Belongs to the *cromones*. Sodium *cromoglycate* and nedocromil have similar effects on *IgE*-mediated and *mast-cell*-dependent reactions. In contrast to sodium cromoglycate, nedocromil may have additional effects on *eosinophils*. For instance, it has been described as blocking functional eosinophil effects upon stimulation with *mediators,* such as *platelet-activating factor* (PAF) or *leukotrienes* (LTs). In addition, it may inhibit *airway hyperresponsiveness* when given before *allergen challenge.*

> Nedocromil is beneficial in mild *asthma*, especially in children and young adults.

It can also be given in addition to *β2-agonists* to control *exercise-induced asthma.* Moreover, nedocromil is effective in treating *allergic rhinoconjunctivitis.*

NEGATIVE REGULATORY SEQUENCE

(See *repressor.*)

NEMATODE INFECTIONS

Susceptibility to nematode infection in mice is associated with a functional *Th2* response to nematode *antigens*, with subsequent *IgE* production and *eosinophilia*. In an *IL-4 knockout mouse* model, infection with Nippostrogylus brasiliensis was shown to reduce *IL-5* levels and inhibit the development of eosinophilia. Moreover, increased *IFN-γ* production was detected in these mice. Impaired Th2 *cytokine* production did not diminish *B cell* help, but induced an *isotype* switch from IgE and *IgG*1 to IgG2 and IgG3 production (see *parasitic diseases*).

NERVE GROWTH FACTOR (NGF)

NGF is a *mediator* that functions on both immune and nerve cells. It upregulates the expression of *neuropeptides* in sensory neurons. *Monocytes*, *T cells*, *B cells*, and *mast cells* express NGF *receptors* (see *TNF receptor superfamily*), suggesting that NGF modulates at least some functions of these cells. NGF concentrations are increased in *allergic inflammation*. Sources of NGF are T cells, *macrophages*, nerve cells (*see nervous system*), *fibroblasts*, mast cells, and *eosinophils*.

> NGF may augment *Th2 cell* differentiation and appears to contribute to the development of *airway hyperresponsiveness.*

NERVOUS SYSTEM

Neural control of lower airway function and *inflammation* is dependent upon a balance between the excitatory (cholinergic and noncholinergic) and the inhibitory (adrenergic and nonadrenergic) nervous system.

Acetylcholine, substance P, neurokinin A (NKA), NKB, NKK, and *calcitonin-gene-related peptide* (CGRP) are the neurotransmitters of the excitatory nervous system and may cause *smooth muscle* contraction.

In contrast, *adrenaline, noradrenaline, vasoactive intestinal polypeptide* (VIP), *peptide* histidine methionine (PHM), and *nitric oxide* (NO) belong to the inhibitory nervous system and act as anti-asthmatics.

Excitatory and inhibitory neurotransmitters can be localized in the same nerve. Thus, stimulation of a given nerve can result in release of different neurotransmitters with synergistic and/or antagonistic biologic effects.

The postganglionic parasympathetic nerves directly innervate bronchial smooth muscle and *mucus* glands (see *airway tone*).

In *asthma*, the abnormalities of the cholinergic excitatory system are due to increased local acetylcholine concentrations and an enhanced sensitivity or responsiveness of smooth muscle to acetylcholine (see *bronchial provocation tests*). Treatment with nonspecific muscarine antagonists (see *antimuscarinic agents*), such as *ipratropium*, improves airflow. The neurotransmitters of the noncholinergic excitatory nervous system (e.g., the *neuropeptides* substance P, NKA, CGRP) can be released by either mechanical or chemical stimulation of nonmyelinated afferent nerves in and around airway *epithelial cells*. Observed effects are *airway obstruction*, increased submucosal gland secretion, and increased vascular permeability. Moreover, these neurotransmitters may directly activate inflammatory cells including *eosinophils, macrophages*, and *B cells*.

The neural elements of the adrenergic inhibitory system are the efferent sympathetic nerves that innervate submucosal glands, bronchial arteries, and airway ganglia, but not airway smooth muscle.

The neurotransmitter is *noradrenaline*. Since the sympathetic innervation of the lower airways is only marginal in humans, *adrenaline*, which is produced in the adrenal medulla, is suggested to be the major ligand for *adrenergic receptors*.

The biological response of adrenaline and noradrenaline depends on the *receptor* expression of the target organ.

Potential abnormalities that could lead to asthma symptoms include a reduction of adrenaline secretion, an increased α1-receptor responsiveness, or a reduced α2- or β2-receptor responsiveness. Stimulation of α1-receptors causes airway obstruction, increase in mucus secretion, and enhanced *mast cell degranulation*. Activation of α2-receptors inhibits both cholinergic and noncholinergic neurotransmission.

β2-Receptor stimulation (see *β2-agonists*) causes *bronchodilation*, and reduces mast cell degranulation and cholinergic-nerve activity.

The neurotransmitters of the nonadrenergic inhibitory nervous system, VIP and PHM, are co-localized with acetylcholine in the parasympathetic efferent nerves. VIP receptors can be found on pulmonary vascular smooth muscle, smooth muscle of the large airways, airway epithelium and ganglia, submucosal glands, and alveolar walls.

VIP and PHM are potent *bronchodilators* and exhibit antiinflammatory effects.

NETHERTON'S SYNDROME

Netherton's syndrome is an autosomal recessive disease, consisting of an atopic constitution (see *atopy*), ichthyosis linearis circumflexa (Comél), and trichorrhexis invaginata.

NEUROGENIC INFLAMMATION

Sensory peptidergic nerve stimulation with resultant antidromic *neuropeptide* release participates in mucosal inflammatory reactions.

The inflammatory response triggered by neuropeptides has been termed "neurogenic *inflammation*."

Neuropeptides are involved in the dilation of arterioles, capillaries, and venules. Moreover, they regulate increased permeability and blood flow with consequent exudation of fluid and plasma proteins. Neurogenic inflammation has been described in many organs and tissues, and the contribution of the *nervous system* to the pathophysiology of local inflammatory responses is now a widely accepted concept.

NEUROKININS

The neurokinins A and B are *neuropeptides* and belong to the family of *tachykinins*, which also includes *substance P*. The two neurokinins may contribute to *airway obstruction* and *mucus* production in *asthma*.

NEUROPEPTIDES

Neuropeptides are low-molecular-weight *peptides* that mediate a number of airway responses. The initial description of activity later ascribed to neuropeptides was made in the gastrointestinal tract, leading to the hypothesis that a distinct neural pathway, comprised of inhibitory *nonadrenergic noncholinergic (iNANC) nerves*, was present in mucosal tissues. Similar observations were made in airway tissues as well. A number of small peptides have been identified that can induce bronchoconstriction (see *airway obstruction*), *bronchodilation*, vasodilation, and vasoconstriction. Immunohistochemical techniques have shown that these peptides are localized in afferent parasympathetic fibers, sympathetic fibers, and unmyelinated sensory nerves (see *nervous system*).

Neuropeptides such as *substance P* (SP), *vasoactive intestinal peptide* (VIP), *neurokinins*, somatostatin (SOM), and *calcitonin-gene-related peptide* (CGRP) play a role in initiation, modulation, and perpetuation of *allergic inflammation*.

Immune cells, e.g., *mast cells, eosinophils*, and *B cells*, are microanatomically associated with autonomic and peptidergic nerve fibers. Moreover, a variety of inflammatory cell populations express specific *receptors* for neuropeptides. For instance, substance P stimulates the release of *histamine* from mast cells. In addition, electrical stimulation of nerves induces *degranulation* of mast cells, clearly demonstrating a role for mast cells in *neurogenic inflammation*.

NEUROTRANSMITTERS

Neurotransmitters are *neuropeptides* released from nerves (see *nervous system*). They also play a role in local inflammatory responses, and therefore they may contribute to *allergic inflammation* (see *neurogenic inflammation*).

NEUTRAL PROTEASES

These *proteases* belong, like *histamine*, to the preformed *mast cell mediators*. The expression of the proteases differs between the two mast cell subtypes MC_T and MC_{TC} (see *mast cell heterogeneity*). Table 72 shows the distribution pattern of neutral proteases.

TABLE 72
Distribution of Neutral Proteases in Mast Cell Subtypes

MC_T	MC_{TC}
Tryptase	*Tryptase*
	Chymase
	Carboxypeptidase
	Cathepsin G

NEUTROPHIL

Neutrophils are terminally differentiated white blood cells which rapidly migrate into tissues in response to invading pathogens. They are inflammatory effector cells that perform *phago-cytosis* and kill bacteria. Killing is done via the generation of reactive *oxygen metabolites* and the release of lytic enzymes stored in *granules*. Neutrophil growth and survival (see *neutrophil apoptosis*) is regulated by *G-CSF*, but also by *IL-3* and *GM-CSF*. Neutrophil recruitment (see *recruitment of inflammatory cells*) is mediated through the *intercellular adhesion molecule-1* (ICAM-1) and a variety of *chemokines*, including *IL-8*. Neutrophils may play a role in *IgE*-mediated *allergic diseases* since they are recruited into allergic inflammatory sites in the early phase following *allergen challenge*. Like *eosinophils*, neutrophils have the capacity to generate a large panel of *cytokines*.

NEUTROPHIL APOPTOSIS

Neutrophils are short-lived cells. The physiologic cell death of these cells is *apoptosis*. Under inflammatory conditions, neutrophil apoptosis can be inhibited by *cytokines* such as *G-CSF* and *GM-CSF*. (For more comprehensive information about factors that influence neutrophil apoptosis, see Table 39 in *eosinophil apoptosis*.)

It has been demonstrated that delayed neutrophil apoptosis is an important mechanism to accumulate these inflammatory effector cells during bacterial infections.

One important intracellular mechanism is the downregulation of the pro-apoptotic Bax molecule (see *Bcl-2 family*). Similar observations can be made in eosinophilic *inflammation* (see *allergic inflammation*), where delayed eosinophil apoptosis contributes to tissue *eosinophilia*, although the responsible *survival factors* are different.

Taken together, it appears that delayed apoptosis is a general and important mechanism to expand inflammatory cells.

NEUTROPHIL CHEMOTACTIC FACTOR (NCF)

NCF exists in two different forms: (1) heat-stable and high-molecular-weight (600 kDa) NCF, and (2) heat-sensitive and low-molecular-weight (60 kDa) NCF. During both *immediate* and *delayed hypersensitivity* reactions, increased *neutrophil* chemotactic activity has been detected in serum (see *chemotaxis*).

NEUTROPHIL SURFACE MOLECULES

Neutrophils express a large number of known *surface molecules*. Many of them are listed within the *CD antigen* classification. *Cross-linking* of many *receptors* induces functional responses, such as *degranulation, respiratory burst, cytokine* and *leukotriene* generation, or *delayed apoptosis*. Whereas most of the surface molecules are shared with other cells, *G-CSF* and *IL-8* receptors are almost selectively found on neutrophils. Many of the neutrophil surface molecules are also expressed by *eosinophils* (see Table 43 in *eosinophil surface molecules*).

NF-AT

(See *nuclear factor of activated T cells*.)

NF-κB

(See *nuclear factor κB*.)

NGF

(See *nerve growth factor*.)

NICKEL

> Nickel is a common *allergen* causing allergic *contact dermatitis*.

The high prevalence of nickel *allergy* (about 30% in women) is thought to be due to ear piercing and the wearing of nickel earrings. In sensitized persons, *dermatitis* results at any site of direct contact with nickel (earrings, watch, jeans), but also at secondary sites such as neck, eyelids, elbow flexures, hands, and thighs. Occasionally, there may be skin reactions from implanted nickel or after oral provocation. Moreover, a few cases of *occupational asthma* due to nickel have been reported. Exposure to nickel occurs during milling, smelting, and refining, as well as in electroplating industries or nickel catalyst production.

NITRIC OXIDE (NO)

NO is an endogenous relaxant of arterial *smooth muscle*. It was first identified as endothelial-derived relaxant factor (EDRF). NO is generated in the airways by inducible *NO synthase* (iNOS). iNOS is induced by a wide variety of inflammatory triggers.

> NO synthesis can be considered an indicator of airways *allergic inflammation*.

Large amounts of NO are generated in the nose, so if one wishes to measure synthesis from the lower airways, it is important to avoid contamination from the upper airway when making measurements.

> NO acts as a *bronchodilator*.

However, it remains unclear whether the effects of NO in *asthma* are primarily beneficial or deleterious, because NO may also perpetuate the inflammatory state through increased plasma leakage from postcapillary venules. Moreover, it can directly induce *epithelial damage* by interacting with *superoxide anion* (O_2^-) to generate toxic peroxynitrite (see *oxygen metabolites*).

> NO has effects on inflammatory cells.

It has been reported to favor the development of *Th2 cells*. Moreover, NO blocks *Fas receptor*-mediated *apoptosis* in *eosinophils*, a mechanism that may contribute to delayed *eosinophil apoptosis* and therefore to *eosinophilia*. These data suggest that NO is a proinflammatory molecule in asthma. However, it is clear that much more work is required to understand the many and diverse roles of NO in human biology.

NITRIC OXIDE SYNTHASE (NOS)

Nitric oxide (NO) is synthesized in mammalian cells by a family of three NO synthases (NOS). In neuronal and *endothelial cells* two *isoforms* are constitutively expressed and are called nNOS and eNOS, respectively. In inflammatory cells, another isoform can be induced by certain inflammatory *mediators*. This isoform has been termed iNOS, and this is the enzyme that is highly expressed in *allergic inflammation*. The overall *amino acid* sequence identity for the three human NOS isoforms is 55%, with a particularly strong *homology* within the catalytic regions. All NOSs use L-arginine as a substrate to form NO plus L-citrulline.

NITROGEN DIOXIDE (NO$_2$)

This irritant gas (see *irritants*) is a result of petroleum use in automobiles (see *pollution*). NO$_2$ has been shown to cause increased nonspecific *airway hyperresponsiveness* in patients with *asthma*. While not thought to be a very potent proinflammatory *mediator*, high levels of this gas do cause airway *inflammation* in normal subjects. Increased bronchial reactivity to inhaled *allergen* has also been reported following experimental challenge of asthmatics with this agent (see *bronchial provocation tests*). Animal studies have shown that NO$_2$ exposure causes increased susceptibility to bacterial infection.

NK CELL

NK cells are *lymphocytes* that do not express *antigen receptors*. They are important in innate immunity to viruses and other intracellular pathogens as well as in *antibody*-dependent cell-mediated cytotoxicity (ADCC). NK cells can also kill tumor cells. Under normal conditions, the cytotoxic activity of NK cells is inhibited by *receptors* that contain *ITIM* motifs. Moreover, under inflammatory conditions (see *inflammation*), NK cells can generate *IL-12* and *IFN-γ* and may therefore favor *Th1 cell* differentiation.

NMR

(See *nuclear magnetic resonance spectroscopy.*)

NO

(See *nitric oxide.*)

NO SYNTHASE

(See *nitric oxide synthase.*)

NOCTURNAL ASTHMA

Asthma is characteristically most marked in the early hours of the morning. This is an exaggeration of the normal diurnal variation in airway caliber.

> Patients who wake at night with asthma usually have marked variability of their *peak expiratory flow rate* (PEFR).

The presence of nocturnal asthma is taken as an indication of poorly controlled airway *inflammation*; this usually responds to an increase in regular antiinflammatory treatment such as inhaled *corticosteroids*. Nocturnal asthma may also respond to long-acting agents such as *theophylline, leukotriene receptor antagonists,* or long-acting *β2-agonists.* Recently, reduced *corticosteroid receptor* binding affinity associated with decreased steroid responsiveness has been observed at night in these patients.

NONADRENERGIC NONCHOLINERGIC (NANC) NERVES

NANC autonomic nerves are sometimes referred to as the third autonomic *nervous system.* A wide variety of *neuropeptides* are involved, including *substance P, neurokinins,* and *vasoactive intestinal peptide* (VIP). NANC nerves are implicated in a variety of local inflammatory responses, which are sometimes called *"neurogenic inflammation."*

NONCOGNATE INTERACTIONS

(See *cognate/noncognate interactions.*)

NONIMMUNOLOGICAL ACTIVATION

This is a general term for mechanisms of cell activation that does not involve *antigen receptors* (e.g., *T cell antigen receptor, B cell antigen receptor,* and *high-affinity IgE receptor*). The term can be used for both *receptor*-mediated (e.g., receptors for *complement factors, platelet-activating factor, leukotrienes, cytokines,* etc.) and non-receptor-mediated forms (*compound 48/80, calcium ionophore* A 23187, etc.) of cell activation.

NONSENSE MUTATION

This is a *mutation* in a triplet, leading to a translational *stop codon.*

NONSPECIFIC BRONCHIAL RESPONSIVENESS

(See *airway hyperresponsiveness.*)

NONSTEROIDAL ANTIINFLAMMATORY DRUGS (NSAIDs)

NSAIDs include compounds such as *aspirin,* ibuprofen, and naproxen.

> NSAIDs are effective in many acute and chronic inflammatory diseases, including arthritis, tendinitis, and pericarditis.

In addition, low doses are effective in preventing heart disease and stroke in high-risk patients. Side effects associated with their use include gastric ulcers, acute renal failure, and headache.

> The principal mechanism of action of NSAIDs is the inhibition of *prostaglandin* synthesis through the inhibition of *cyclooxygenase* (COX).

By reducing prostaglandin production they reduce pain and *inflammation.* However, NSAIDS can trigger *aspirin-sensitive asthma.* Several members of the cyclooxygenase family have been identified, including COX-1, constitutively expressed, and COX-2, induced at sites of *inflammation.* NSAIDs inhibit both molecules; COX-1 inhibition leads to side effects of the drug, while COX-2 inhibition results in clinical efficacy (see *cyclooxygenase-2 inhibitors*). Recently published work suggests that NSAIDs are also blockers of *nuclear factor-κB* (NF-κB) and inducers of *lipoxins.*

NOON UNIT

The Noon unit has been used for standardization of *allergen extracts* and is defined as the extract from 1 μg of *allergen*; the allergen content is given in Noon units per milliliter. An alternative unit represents the *protein nitrogen unit* (PNU).

NORADRENALINE

Noradrenaline is a *neurotransmitter* of the sympathetic *nervous system.*

NO SYNTHASE

(See *nitric oxide synthase.*)

NSAIDs

(See *nonsteroidal antiinflammatory drugs.*)

NUCLEAR FACTOR OF ACTIVATED T CELLS (NF-AT)

NF-AT is a family of *transcription factors* that influences the *transcription* of *genes* involved in *allergic inflammation*. NF-ATs are expressed in *T cells*, *B cells*, *mast cells*, and *NK cells.*

> NF-AT binding sites are in the *promoter* regions of genes encoding *Th1* and *Th2 cytokines.*

NF-AT nuclear translocation is controlled by *calcineurin*, which depends on intracellular *calcium mobilization*, and is blocked by immunosuppressive drugs such as *cyclosporin A* (CsA) and *FK506*. There are multiple *isoforms* of NF-AT that are differentially expressed in resting and activated *T cells*. There are currently four NF-AT genes: NF-ATp (NF-ATc2, NF-AT1), NF-ATc (NF-ATc1, NF-AT2), NF-AT3 (NF-ATc4), and NF-AT4 (NF-ATc3, NF-ATx). NF-ATc *knockout mice* have a selective decrease in *IL-4* production, suggesting that NF-ATc is a positive regulator of the *immune system*. In contrast, NF-ATp knockout mice demonstrate a dramatic and selective increase in IL-4 and *IL-5* production associated with increased levels of IgE and eosinophils.

> The differentiation of Th1 and Th2 cells might be regulated by a critical balance among NF-AT family members.

NUCLEAR FACTOR (NF)-κB

NF-κB is an important *transcription factor* in the cellular response to environmental changes. NF-κB is a member of the Rel family of transcription factors, which share a common motif important for *DNA* binding and dimerization. There are several different NF-κB proteins. The classical form is a heterodimer of a 65-kDa protein (Rel A) and a 50-kDa subunit (Rel B).

> Under resting conditions, NF-κB is found in the cytosol associated with an inhibitory protein called *inhibitory factor of κB* (IκB).

IκB is phosphorylated and, as a consequence, NF-κB is released and translocates to the nucleus to initiate *transcription* (see Figure 35). Rel A is important for transcription, whereas Rel B lacks a transactivating domain. Important activators of NF-κB are *allergens* and other *antigens* as well as *cytokines,* such as *TNF* and *IL-1*. In contrast, antiinflammatory drugs such as *corticosteroids*, *aspirin*, and *cyclosporin A* inhibit NF-κB activation (Table 73).

NUCLEAR MAGNETIC RESONANCE (NMR) SPECTROSCOPY

NMR spectroscopy is a technique used to determine the atomic structure of macromolecules in solution. NMR is based on the intrinsic magnetic character of certain atomic nuclei such as hydrogen, carbon, and nitrogen. When an external magnetic field is applied to a charged proton such as H, a resonance frequency results. NMR structures are built by assigning the resonance frequencies of all the hydrogens of a protein and connecting the resonances

---

TABLE 73
Inhibitors of NF-κB

- Corticosteroids
- Cytokines (*IL-4, IL-10*)
- *Cyclooxygenase* and *5-lipoxygenase* inhibitors
- Antiinflammatory drugs (aspirin, sodium salicylate)
- Immunosuppressive drugs (*cyclosporin A, tacrolimus*)

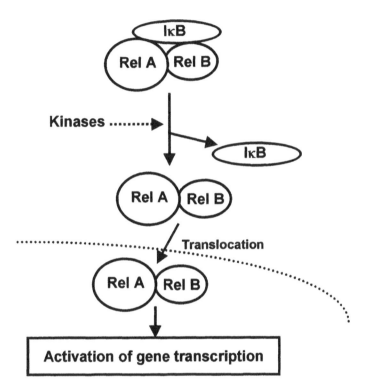

FIGURE 35   Mechanism of NF-κB activation. Following the release of phosphorylated IκB, NF-κB is translocated into the nucleus to induce gene transcription.

sequentially through the peptide bond. Multiple NMR experiments using ^{13}C and ^{14}N-labeled proteins for determining torsional angles and inter-proton distances are required for refining the final structure. NMR spectroscopy is limited to proteins of 30 kDa or less due to the complexity of sorting the resonances of such a large number of protons.

NUCLEAR MATRIX

The nuclear matrix is a non-*DNA* structure within the cell nucleus stabilizing the nucleus.

NUCLEOSOME

A nucleosome is the basic structural unit of *chromatin*. Complexes are formed by 146 bp of *DNA* wrapped around a core of eight *histone* proteins. *DNA fragmentation* during *apoptosis* occurs between nucleosomes.

NUCLEOTIDE

Basic repeated unit of a *DNA* strand containing a sugar with an attached base and phosphate group (see also *DNA sequencing*).

NUMMULAR ECZEMA

(See *discoid eczema*.)

OBSTRUCTIVE SLEEP APNEA

A condition found most often in overweight men, in whom the pharynx collapses at night, causing obstruction of the upper airway. In mild cases this causes snoring, but in more severe cases the respiratory muscles become fatigued, and the patient develops pulmonary hypertension and respiratory failure associated with daytime somnolence. A characteristic feature is respiratory failure with relatively normal daytime lung function (see *lung function tests*). Treatment is by weight loss or by surgical revision of the uvula and soft palate.

OCCUPATIONAL AGENTS

A range of substances in occupational environments can initiate the development of *asthma*. These range from soldering fumes to proteins from animals and pharmaceuticals to organic dusts from trees and plants. Common agents that cause *occupational asthma* include *isocyanates* (see *isocyanate-induced asthma*), acid anhydrides, epoxy resins, organic dusts, *metallic salts*, flour, aldehydes, latex (see *latex allergy*), and various drugs (see *drug allergy*). In addition, hard metals, platinum, Western red cedar (see *wood dust*), and synthetic metals are often associated with occupational asthma.

Both *allergens* and *irritants* can cause an occupational disease.

The mechanisms by which irritants exert their effect is not entirely understood. Many of these compounds do not induce an *IgE* response. Toluene diisocyanate is an example of a small molecule that clearly causes occupational asthma, yet is not always associated with development of an IgE-mediated response. Phthalic anhydride may induce IgE-mediated reactions by acting as a *hapten*, with complete immunologic recognition being dependent on binding to albumin. Even minute quantities of these substances can cause asthma symptoms and even death in sensitized asthmatics (see *death from asthma*).

OCCUPATIONAL ASTHMA

Occupational asthma refers to *asthma* that is associated with exposure to agents in the workplace. These *occupational agents* may exert their effect through *IgE*-dependent (see Table 74) or nonimmunologic mechanisms (see *idiosyncrasy*).

Diagnosis

An approach to occupational asthma includes getting an appropriate history to identify potential *allergen* or *irritant* exposures. If this reveals a likely causative allergen, *skin tests* for IgE-mediated responses may be feasible.

Skin testing with irritants is not useful.

Moreover, interpretation of occupational *allergen challenge* tests can be difficult, especially when the patient has been removed from the workplace. Measurement of airflow pre- and post-workshift as well as comparison of nonspecific *bronchial provocation tests* before and after a vacation or weekend may identify increased *airway hyperresponsiveness* due to occupational exposures. Such assessment is important, as this serves to document the occupational nature of the asthma episode, which may be important in maintaining (or receiving) unemployment compensation.

Therapy

After a diagnosis of occupational asthma has been made, mild symptoms may be managed with pharmacologic therapy (see *asthma treatment strategies*). Industrial hygiene techniques in which an assessment of the workplace exposure is made may lead to improved methods to minimize exposure to the offending irritant. Occasionally, complete avoidance (see *allergen avoidance*) may be necessary to prevent severe *asthma exacerbation*. However, many patients with occupational asthma will continue to experience symptoms even after leaving the workplace. This does not mean that their asthma is not occupational in origin. Rather, it is considered that they became sensitized (see *sensitization*) in the workplace and the asthmatic process has now become self-perpetuating.

Economic impact

Most countries have workers' compensation schemes that have well-established rules for judging whether an individual has occupational asthma. The economic impact of occupational asthma is large, and most individuals who are diagnosed with occupational asthma suffer considerable financial loss due to having to change jobs.

Prevention

In recent years, protective legislation has been introduced in many countries that excludes certain individuals from employment in industries that are at high risk of inducing occupational asthma.

> Atopic individuals (see *atopy*) are at greater risk of becoming sensitized to certain occupational allergens, but this is not universally true.

In some instances, e.g., *isocyanate-induced asthma*, the risk of sensitization is greatest in those who are atopic and who also smoke cigarettes (see *smoking*). Individuals with a history of asthma are usually advised to avoid occupations that have a high rate of occupational asthma.

TABLE 74

Allergens and Professions that Are Frequently Associated with Occupational Asthma

Allergens	Professions
1. Laboratory animal allergens (see *rodent allergy*)	Research workers
2. Avian antigens	Bird fanciers, poultry workers
3. Insect antigens	Mites: grain workers; river fly: power company workers
4. Plant antigens	Latex: health care workers; hops: brewery workers, castor bean and tea industry workers, cabinet-makers
5. Invertebrate seafood antigens	Snow crab, prawn fishermen
6. Detergent enzymes	Papain, pepsin-pharmaceutical workers

OCCUPATIONAL DERMATITIS

The skin may respond to external agents either by immunological reactions (allergic *contact dermatitis*) or directly by release of inflammatory *mediators* following injury of cells in the *epidermis* or dermis (irritant contact dermatitis). Studies have shown that 13 to 34% of all cases of occupational diseases are due to skin diseases, predominantly contact dermatitis.

> Wet work exposure to chemicals such as alkalis or acids, cutting oils, detergents, and solvents are the main causes of irritant dermatitis.

Occupations with a high risk of developing irritant dermatitis include hairdressing, catering, health care, engineering, and construction industries. The spectrum of symptoms in irritant contact dermatitis is wider than that of allergic contact dermatitis. Following acute and severe damage, chemical burns and ulcerations are seen. Less severe injury may result in *erythema*, weakening, sensations of burning, or *dermatitis*. However, chronic or repetitive injury leads to *dry skin*, *scales*, and *eczema*. The clinical feature of allergic contact dermatitis is eczema due to a *delayed hypersensitivity*. Common occupational *allergens* include plants, biocides, chromate, resins, rubber chemicals, *nickel*, and essential oils. *IgE*-mediated *urticaria* may occur in chefs following contact with foods (see *food allergy*), or in health care workers sensitized to latex (see *latex allergy*). The diagnosis is mainly based on the clinical history, work-related symptoms, and *skin tests*.

OCCUPATIONAL RHINITIS

The causes of occupational *rhinitis* seem to be similar to those of *occupational asthma*. Organic *allergens* include laboratory animals (see *animal dander*), grain, *wood dust*, and latex (see *latex allergy*). But inorganic substances such as platinum and acid anhydrites may also cause rhinitis. The history of work-related symptoms, *prick tests*, allergen-specific *IgE* (see *RAST*, *Phadiatop*, *CAP-system*) and nasal challenge tests (see *allergen challenge*) may confirm the diagnosis.

OCULAR ALLERGY

(See *allergic keratoconjunctivitis* and *allergic rhinoconjunctivitis*.)

OLIGONUCLEOTIDE

A small single-stranded nucleic acid molecule containing fewer than 100 *nucleotides* (see *antisense* and *primers*).

OLIVE POLLEN

Although olive trees are insect pollinated, large amounts of *pollen* can become airborne (see *aeroallergens*). Olive pollen is a very common cause of seasonal *allergic rhinoconjunctivitis* in Mediterranean regions. Cross-reactivity (see *cross-reacting allergens*) to other Oleaceae species, such as ash, privet, and lilac, has been shown by the presence of a shared *major allergen*.

ONCOGENE

Oncogenes are *genes* that have the ability to transform (immortalize) eukaryotic cells in vitro or induce tumors in vivo. The physiological function of these genes is often related to the control of cell growth. Oncogenes are mutated copies of cellular genes (protooncogene) regulating cell proliferation. The *mutations* act dominantly and result either in an overexpression of the gene or a mutated gene product that escapes negative regulation.

OPEN READING FRAME (ORF)

(See *reading frame*.)

OPSONIZATION

The process of binding of proteins of the *complement system* to microbial or particle surfaces is called opsonization. Opsonization is largely mediated by the proteolytic fragment C3b. *Phagocytes* express C3b *receptors*. Thus, opsonization promotes *phagocytosis*.

ORAL ALLERGY SYNDROME (OAS)

Many patients with *hay fever* report local symptoms in and around the mouth after eating fresh fruit, especially apples, pears, cherries, plums, peaches, and apricots. However, they do not have symptoms when they eat cooked fruit.

OAS is a form of *contact urticaria*.

Rapid onset of *pruritus* and an *angioedema* of the lips, tongue, palate, and throat represent the typical symptoms. This condition is usually associated with *allergy* to *tree pollens* and is attributable to *sensitization* to heat-labile proteins found in a wide range of fruit (for complete list, see *cross-reacting allergens*). Two common proteins have been implicated: the major birch *allergen* Bet v I and *profilin*. The OAS rarely progresses to *anaphylaxis*, and it is usually safe for patients to eat jams, fruit juice, cooked fruit, etc. Skin *prick tests* with commercial *allergen extracts* may be negative, but the patient will usually give a positive wheal to fresh fruit by a "prick–prick" technique in which the lancet is pricked into the fruit first and then straightaway into the patient. Management is by avoidance of the suspect fruit (see *allergy diet*). Some improvement has been reported in patients who have been desensitized to tree pollen (see *immunotherapy*).

OTITIS MEDIA

Otitis media is an acute or chronic *inflammation* of the middle ear. It occurs mostly in children under the age of 4 years.

Bacterial infection is the main cause of otitis media.

In addition, *IgE*-mediated reactions have been suggested in the pathogenesis of otitis media. However, there is no clear evidence that the middle ear mucosa may function as a target organ in *allergy*. Otitis media in association with *allergic rhinitis* may be due to a swelling of the Eustachian tube, obstruction of the nose and nasopharynx, and a reflux or aspiration of bacterial-laden secretion from the nasopharynx into the middle ear.

OUTDOOR AIR POLLUTANTS

Most *pollutant* exposure results from burning of fossil fuels associated with operation of motor vehicles (see *air pollution*). Areas in which air inversions occur frequently and which are rimmed by mountains are at particular risk for increases in ambient air pollutants (see *smog*). Municipal approaches to this problem center on decreasing motor vehicle use with mass transit or direct limitation of vehicle usage (e.g., limiting car use to a given day of the week based on license tag number). Use of alternate fuels, more efficient gasoline engines, or electric vehicles may also be employed.

OUTDOOR ALLERGENS

(See *pollen* and *fungal allergens*.)

OVALBUMIN

Ovalbumin is one of the egg-white proteins and has been identified as a *major allergen* (Gal d 2) in *egg allergy*.

OXITROPIUM

Oxitropium belongs to the group of *anticholinergic agents*. Anticholinergic drugs provide effective protection against spasmogens and are potent *bronchodilators* in *asthma* and *chronic obstructive pulmonary disease* (COPD).

OXYGEN METABOLITES

Macrophages, eosinophils, and *neutrophils* are major sources of reactive oxygen metabolites. Such *respiratory burst* occurs when the cells receive both *priming* and triggering (e.g., *PAF, C5a*) signals. These metabolites include *superoxide anion* (O$_2^-$), *hydrogen peroxide* (H$_2$O$_2$), and hydroxyl radicals (OH$^-$). O$_2^-$ is generated from oxygen by *NADPH oxidase*. H$_2$O$_2$ is generated from O$_2^-$ by *superoxide dismutase*. These molecules are important in the damage of bacteria by *phagocytes*.

Reactive oxygen metabolites also have the potential to injure local tissues.

For instance, oxygen radicals alone or in combination with *eosinophil granule proteins* cause *epithelial damage* in chronic *allergic inflammation*.

OXYGEN RADICALS

(See *oxygen metabolites*.)

OZONE (O$_3$)

Ozone is a secondary *pollutant* produced by the action of *ultraviolet* (*UV*) *light* on *nitrogen dioxide* (NO$_2$) (see *air pollution*).

As an *irritant*, ozone is known to cause both a transient restrictive defect in lung function (see *lung function tests*) as well as to induce *inflammation* in both upper and lower airways.

Interestingly, these two effects are not correlated with each other. The effect on lung function is likely mediated by sensory neurons (see *nervous system*). In contrast, ozone-mediated inflammation appears to occur via activation of *nuclear factor* (*NF*)-*κB*, resulting in the induction of many *cytokine genes*, including *IL-6* and *IL-8*. Ozone clearly exerts an effect in both normal subjects and patients with *asthma*. Epidemiologic studies have revealed ozone-induced *asthma exacerbations*.

In experimental challenge of asthmatics, ozone causes *airway obstruction*, *epithelial damage*, as well as infiltration of *eosinophils* and *neutrophils*.

The degree of *granulocyte* influx is greater in asthmatics than in normal subjects. This gas also enhances both *immediate* and *delayed hypersensitivity* reactions after *allergen challenge*. Ozone also blunts *macrophage* function and has been shown in animal studies to increase susceptibility to bacterial infection (see *pollution and infectious diseases*).

P

p_aCO_2

The arterial gas tension of carbon dioxide. Normal range 4.5 to 6.3 kilopascals (kPa). Low values indicate *hyperventilation*, whereas high values indicate alveolar hypoventilation.

PAF

(See *platelet-activating factor.*)

PAF-ACETYLHYDROLASE

Platelet-activating factor (PAF) acetylhydrolase catalyzes the degradation of PAF and related phospholipids, which have proinflammatory, allergic, and prothrombotic properties. Deficiency of plasma PAF acetylhydrolase is an autosomal (see *autosome*) *recessive* disorder that has been associated with severe *asthma* in Japanese children. Acquired deficiency has been described in several human diseases usually associated with severe *inflammation.*

PAF RECEPTOR ANTAGONIST

Platelet-activating factor (PAF) *receptor* antagonists were originally developed as therapeutic agents. However, they proved to be ineffective in *asthma*. Today, they are used as research tools to specifically block PAF-mediated effects in experimental systems.

PALINDROME

This is a stretch of *DNA* that contains the same 5′ to 3′ sequence on both strands, e.g., the DNA-binding motif of the immunoregulatory *transcription factor nuclear factor-κB* (NF-κB) of *HLA* class I *genes* has the following sequence: 5′-GGGGATTCCCC-3′ and 3′-CCCCT-TAGGGG-5′. *Restriction enzymes* and transcription factors often bind palindromic *DNA* sequences due to the formation of a certain DNA epitope recognized by the DNA-binding domain of the protein.

p_aO_2

The arterial gas tension of oxygen; normal range 12 to 15 kilopascals (kPa). The p_aO_2 is reduced by *ventilation–perfusion mismatch*. Due to the sigmoid shape of the hemoglobin–oxygen dissociation curve, the p_aO_2 can fall to 7.6 kPa before the oxygen saturation (s_aO_2) drops significantly.

PAPAIN

Papain is a plant-derived enzyme widely used in the food, cosmetic, and pharmaceutical industries. It is used as a baking additive. It may cause *occupational asthma* (see *Baker's asthma*).

PAPILLOMATOSIS

Papillomatosis is the formation of multiple, aggregated, nipple-like skin protrusions forming a dense plaque or tumor, as frequently seen in vulgar warts or in chronic stasis *dermatitis.*

PARASITIC DISEASES

Mast cells, eosinophils, and *IgE* are important components in the defense against many parasites
(see *filariasis, nematode infections, schistosomiasis*).

The immunological mechanisms in parasitic diseases are similar to those observed in *allergic
inflammation*, including *Th2 cell* differentiation, *immunoglobulin class switching*, *eosinophilia*, and *mast cell activation*. Several studies have shown that animals lacking eosinophils,
mast cells, or IgE are deficient in their capacities to resolve parasitic infections. Parasitic
antigens can directly or indirectly activate mast cells and eosinophils, causing the generation
of *oxygen metabolites* as well as the release of *eosinophil granule proteins* and inflammatory
mediators. In contrast to most parasitic diseases, *malaria* and *leishmaniasis* are associated
with *Th1* responses.

PARASYMPATHOLYTICS

(See *anticholinergic agents*.)

PARATOPE

A paratope is the part of an *antibody* that binds to an *antigen*.

PARTICULATE MATTER

(See *PM-10*.)

PASSIVE CUTANEOUS ANAPHYLAXIS (PCA)

PCA can be caused in animals that have been immunized by specific *IgE* treatment (see
passive immunization). A subsequent *allergen challenge* causes an *immediate hypersensitivity*
reaction without previous *allergen-induced immune responses*. For instance, rats are injected
intradermally with serum containing IgE *antibodies* to *antigens*. After a latent period of 24 to
72 hours to permit IgE binding on *high-affinity IgE receptors* of the cutaneous *mast cells*,
the animal is injected intravenously with a mixture of antigen and marker dye. The animal
is subsequently killed and the dorsal skin deflected to reveal the undersurface. Mast-cell-
derived *mediators* (e.g., *histamine*) have produced a local increase in capillary permeability,
which can be detected by extravasation of the dye. Measurement of this response provides
an estimate of the intensity of the cutaneous *anaphylactic reaction*. The IgE-mediated PCA
reaction in the rat was one of the first in vivo models for the screening of *anti-allergic/anti-
asthmatic drugs* (see also *Prausnitz–Küstner reaction*).

PASSIVE IMMUNIZATION

Passive immunization is the administration of *antibodies* (e.g., from immunized individuals),
causing specific immunity. For instance, passive immunization against snake venoms is a
life-saving treatment for potentially lethal snake bites.

PATCH TEST

The patch test or epicutaneous test is a bioassay for *contact dermatitis*.

The test is based on the epicutaneous application of *allergens* to induce an eczematous reaction
(see *eczema*) on a patient's skin. Patch testing was established by Jadassohn about 100 years
ago and further developed during the following decades. Allergens are applied for 24 to 48 h

in aluminium finn chambers on the patient's back, and results are read at 24 h, 48 h, and 72 h by a dermatologist. Irritative/toxic reactions (see *irritants*) tend to decrease in strength from 24 to 72 h, whereas truly allergic reactions are stable or even increase in strength. Some allergens require reading at later time points. For instance, *antibiotics* and *corticosteroids* tend to become positive at day 7, whereas reactions at day 3 are often read negative.

> Patch testing should be undertaken only if necessary, since there is a low risk of inducing a contact *allergy*.

For quality assurance, reliability, and reproducibility of the reactions, selection of the proper vehicle (petrolatum, saline) and the allergen concentration are crucial. Many centers use a common standard test series for all patients, which includes the most frequent allergens, and add some standardized series of allergens for different topics (e.g., ointment bases, disinfectants, fragrances) or for some professions with common *occupational dermatitis* (e.g., hairdressers, dentists) as needed. Some structurally related substances show cross-reactivity (see *cross-reacting allergens*), leading to the definition of allergen groups. *T cell sensitization* against a whole group is frequently caused by contact with a single substance only, whereas elicitation of an allergic reaction is possible by contact with many of the group substances.

Patch test results are given in a semiquantitative scale and are usually read in three grades (see Table 75). In addition, toxic/irritative reactions and questionable results are documented.

TABLE 75
Semiquantitative Scale of Patch Test Results

+	*Erythema* and minimal palpable infiltration
++	Erythema and papulation
+++	Erythema, papulation, and blister formation

To avoid false negative results, the discontinuation times must be considered (see Table 76).

TABLE 76
Recommended Discontinuation Times for *Anti-Allergic Drugs* before Patch Testing

Corticosteroid ointments (at test site)	1 week
Corticosteroid ointments (elsewhere)	None
High-dose systemic steroids (long-term use)	3 weeks
High-dose systemic steroids (short-term use)	1 week
Low-dose systemic steroids (long-term use)	3 weeks
Low-dose systemic steroids (short-term use)	3 days
Oral *antihistamines*	None
Intensive sun exposure	3 weeks

To avoid false positive results, patch tests should not be applied if there are eczematous skin lesions elsewhere on the body. This frequently leads to multiple nonspecific test reactions, which cannot be repeated if retested. This has led to the definition of the "angry back," when the test results must be discarded. If positive test reactions toward five allergen groups are observed, an "angry back" is diagnosed (see also *photopatch test*).

Pb

(See *lead.*)

PC₂₀

Concentration of *allergen*, *histamine*, or *methacholine* that produces a 20% fall in *forced expiratory volume in first second* (FEV$_1$) (see *bronchial provocation test*).

PCR

(See *polymerase chain reaction.*)

PD₂₀

Dose of *allergen*, *histamine*, or *methacholine* that produces a 20% fall in *forced expiratory volume in first second* (FEV$_1$) (see *bronchial provocation test*).

PEACH ALLERGEN

Oral allergy syndrome after ingestion of peach may occur in patients allergic to *birch pollen* and fresh apple (see *apple allergen*). Cross-reactivity (see *cross-reacting allergens*) to several fruits of the Prunoideae family, such as apricot, cherry, and plum, is very common.

PEAK EXPIRATORY FLOW RATE (PEFR)

The maximum rate achieved during a *forced expiratory maneuver*. PEFR reflects *airway obstruction* in the small and large airways (see *lung function tests*).

PEAK FLOW METER

A hand-held device that measures the *peak expiratory flow rate* (PEFR). Peak flow meters are useful in the serial monitoring of *asthma* and provide valuable information in monitoring the disease (see *asthma treatment strategies*).

PEANUT ALLERGY

Peanut is one of the most allergenic foods known (see *food allergy*). *IgE*-mediated allergic reactions are often acute and severe. Peanut *allergy* is seldom outgrown. The peanut belongs to the family of leguminosae. A large number of peanut constituents are relevant to allergy and are either proteins or glycoproteins belonging to the arachin and conarachin fraction. Some of them, such as peanut-1, concavalin A-reactive glycoprotein (CARG), Ara h 1, and Ara h 2, have been isolated.

PEFR

(See *peak expiratory flow rate.*)

PENETRANCE

This is the frequency of expression of a *genotype*.

PENICILLIN

Penicillin is an *antibiotic* drug that often causes *allergy*. Penicillin *hypersensitivity* is the most frequent cause of *anaphylaxis* (see *drug allergy*). Allergic reactions to penicillin are observed in 0.7 to 10% of treatment courses; 42% of the allergic reactions are *IgE*-mediated *immediate hypersensitivity* reactions.

PENICILLIUM

(See *fungal allergens*.)

PEPTIDE

Peptides are single chains of *amino acids* joined together. Two amino acids joined together form a dipeptide, three form a tripeptide, and so on. A chain of up to 100 amino acids is called a polypeptide. If more than 100 amino acids are involved, the molecule is called a protein.

PEPTIDE EPITOPES

Peptide epitopes are usually contiguous sequences within, or derived from, *allergen* sequences. They represent the particular *amino acid* sequence that is recognized by a *T cell* when presented in the *major histocompatibility complex* (MHC) binding groove of an *antigen-presenting cell* (APC). Allergen sequences can be epitope mapped, and synthetic peptides representing dominant epitopes manufactured or expressed using recombination technology (see *recombinant allergen*).

> Identification of peptide *T cell epitopes* has been used as a rational approach to allergen *immunotherapy*.

Studies using peptides derived from the major *cat allergen* Fel d I and *bee venom phospholipase A₂* (PLA₂) administered to allergic subjects has demonstrated the potential usefulness of this approach (see *peptide immunotherapy*).

PEPTIDE IMMUNOTHERAPY

Peptide immunotherapy involves the use of purified, or more often synthesized, peptide fragments of a particular *allergen* in place of the whole allergen or mixture of allergens during specific immunotherapy. A sequenced allergen can contain several short subsequences or peptide *epitopes* that are preferentially recognized by *T cells*, but not *B cells* or *IgE antibodies*. Identification of major *T cell epitopes* and their use in peptide immunotherapy is thought to enhance the likelihood of successful desensitization.

> Fractionation of allergen polypeptides often destroys the *tertiary structure* of IgE-binding portions of that allergen, thus theoretically avoiding potential IgE-mediated *immediate hypersensitivity* reactions such as *anaphylaxis* during immunotherapy.

Problems current with this approach relate to epitope selection and efficacy, the requirement or not for *antigen processing*, and the requirement or not for IgE-mediated interactions in inducing long-term desensitization. A new variant of this treatment is the *altered peptide ligands* (APL) immunotherapy.

PEPTIDE VACCINES

(See *recombinant peptide vaccines*.)

PERENNIAL RHINITIS

Allergic rhinitis can be subdivided into seasonal and perennial rhinitis. While seasonal *rhinitis* is frequently triggered by *pollen* and outdoor *mold* spores (see *seasonal allergens*), perennial rhinitis can be attributed to *house-dust mite*, *animal dander*, and mold spores (see *fungal allergens*). Nasal blockage due to *edema* of the mucosa is the predominant symptom. In addition, 20% of patients with perennial rhinitis develop *asthma*. In contrast to seasonal rhinitis, the cellular infiltration of the mucosa is more prominent in perennial rhinitis, suggesting an important role of *late-phase responses*.

Numbers and activation of *mast cells*, *eosinophils*, and *Th2 cells* are increased in the inflamed nasal mucosa (see *allergic inflammation*).

However, blood *eosinophilia* is only an inconsistent finding. Intranasal *corticosteroids* have proved to be effective in the treatment of perennial allergic rhinitis and may have beneficial effects on *airway hyperresponsiveness* or asthma. *Antihistamines* and *cromones* demonstrate only minimal benefit. *Immunotherapy* with extracts of Dermatophagoides pteronyssimus can be tried in patients who are allergic to house-dust mites, and may reduce symptoms and make possible a decrease in medication.

PERIPHERAL BLOOD MONONUCLEAR CELLS (PBMC)

This term is frequently used for a mixed cell population containing both *lymphocytes* and *monocytes*. PBMC can be easily purified from peripheral blood and used for diagnostic tests or research.

PERIPLANETA

Periplaneta is a genus of cockroach (order Cursoria, class Hexapoda; see *cockroach allergens*). The primary species associated with respiratory *allergy* is *Periplaneta americana*, the American cockroach.

PERIPLANETA AMERICANA

American cockroach (see *cockroach allergens*). Periplaneta americana is a large cockroach, approximately 2 inches in length, that infests houses, schools, hospitals, and other large buildings. American cockroaches have less fecundity than German cockroaches and require higher temperatures (~80°C) and humidity for optimal population growth.

PEROXIDASE

Peroxidase is, like *catalase*, a heme enzyme, which catalyzes the dismutation of *hydrogen peroxide* (H_2O_2) (see *oxygen metabolites*). H_2O_2 is reduced to water by a reductant (AH_2).

$$H_2O_2 + AH_2 \rightarrow 2\ H_2O + A$$

Peroxidase has been identified with the secretory *granules* of inflammatory cells, such as *mast cells* and *eosinophils*.

Peroxidase activity in cells can be used to detect mast cells and eosinophils in tissues.

PERTUSSIS TOXIN

Pertussis toxin is used to block *signal transduction* via *G protein-coupled receptors*.

PESTICIDES

Pesticides can be used to decrease *cockroach allergen* and *house-dust mite* exposures (see *allergen avoidance*). Chlorpyrifos, diazinon *aerosol* sprays, boric acid powder, or bait stations containing hydramethylnon are recommended for treating cockroaches. Benzyl benzoate and pirimiphosmethyl have been shown to kill mites in carpets. Benzyl tannate, a complex of benzyl alcohol and tannate, has not only *acaricide* effects, but it may also denature mite *allergens*.

PEYER'S PATCHES

Peyer's patches are aggregates of lymphoid follicles throughout the intestinal mucosa. They belong to the *gut-associated lymphoid tissue* (GALT).

PHADIATOP

Phadiatop is an in vitro test to measure *IgE antibodies* concentrations against the most *common allergens* (*grass pollen*, rye *pollen*, *birch pollen*, artemisia pollen, *house-dust mite*, *cat allergen*, *dog allergen*, and *cladosporium*) in serum. The intention of this test is to provide information on the atopic state (see *atopy*) of an individual. Results are given as positive or negative (see also *RAST* and *CAP-system*).

PHAGE

Phages can be used as *vectors*. They are useful in *DNA cloning* procedures (see *cloning of allergens*).

PHAGOCYTE

A phagocyte is a cell that is able to take up and digest pathogens (e.g., bacteria) and apoptotic cells (see *apoptosis* and *phagocytosis*).

PHAGOCYTOSIS

Phagocytes such as *macrophages* and *granulocytes* remove pathogens and apoptotic cells (see *apoptosis*) by phagocytosis (compare *endocytosis*). Following phagocytosis, the particles are found in vesicles (phagosomes), which fuse with lysosomes. The ingested material is destroyed by lysosomal enzymes and degraded into small molecules.

Efficient phagocytosis is mediated via *Fc receptors* on the cell surface following *antibody* recognition of the *antigen*. Moreover, bacterial wall components or apoptotic cells may also be bound directly or indirectly by *CD14*.

PHENOCOPY

A phenocopy is an environmentally induced mimic of a genetic disease.

PHENOTYPE

The phenotype is the observable expression of a particular *gene* or genes. It is usually the result of interaction between *genotype* and environmental factors. The phenotype can also be defined as the observable characteristics of an individual.

PHORBOL ESTER

A phorbol ester is a compound that bypasses *receptor*-mediated early *signal transduction* events, resulting in direct intracellular *protein kinase C* (PKC) activation. Several compounds are known and used, alone or together with a *calcium ionophore*, to nonspecifically activate cells.

PHOSPHATASE

Phosphatases are enzymes that dephosphorylate target proteins within cells. They play important roles in *signal transduction* (see also *tyrosine phosphatase*). In contrast, *phosphorylation* is performed by *kinases*.

PHOSPHATIDIC ACID (PA)

PA is the major product generated by *phospholipase D* (PLD).

PHOSPHATIDYLINOSITOL-4,5-BISPHOSPHATE (PIP₂)

All *isozymes* of *phospholipase C* (PLC) use PIP₂ as a substrate to generate *inositol-1,4,5-triphosphate* (IP₃) and *diacylglycerol* (DAG) (see *inositol polyphosphate cascade*). PIP₂ is also known to be a substrate for *phosphatidylinositol-3-kinase* (PI3-kinase).

PHOSPHATIDYLINOSITOL-3-KINASE (PI3-KINASE)

PI3-kinase is responsible for the conversion of *phosphatidylinositol-4,5-biphosphate* (PIP₂) to phosphatidylinositol-3,4,5-triphosphate (Figure 36). This lipid is a signaling molecule that mediates a number of cell functions in different cells. For instance, in *eosinophils* and *neutrophils*, this pathway appears to be important for the generation of reactive *oxygen metabolites*. Moreover, PI3-kinase activation is important in *co-stimulation* of *T cells* via *CD28*.

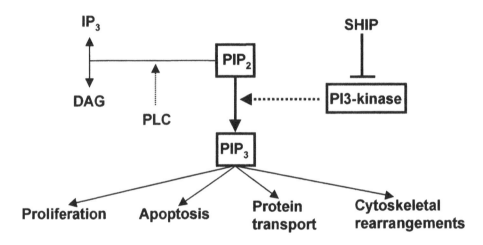

FIGURE 36 PI3-kinase uses PIP₂ as a substrate to generate the second messenger PIP₃, which is involved in a number of host responses. Note that PIP₂ is also a substrate for *phospholipase C* (PLC). PI3-kinase is blocked by the *tyrosine phosphatase* SHIP.

PHOSPHATIDYLSERINE (PS)

Apoptotic cells are removed by *phagocytosis* by neighboring cells, while retaining their intact plasma membrane. Several kinds of structural changes of the plasma membrane have been identified that lead to *phagocyte* recognition. PS is one example of how apoptotic cells are recognized by phagocytes. PS expression can be easily monitored using fluorescence-conjugated annexin V and *flow cytometry*, and therefore represents a frequently used marker to define *apoptosis*.

PHOSPHODIESTERASES

> Phosphodiesterases are intracellular enzymes that degrade *cAMP* and *cGMP*.

Many different isoenzymes exist, differing not only in their primary *amino acid* sequence and cellular expression, but also in substrate specificity, kinetic properties, and susceptibility to inhibition by various compounds (see *phosphodiesterase inhibitors*). The phosphodiesterases can be subdivided into seven families (see Table 77). The different isoenzymes are derived from different *genes* or the consequence of *alternative splicing*. All phosphodiesterases share a highly conserved catalytic domain.

TABLE 77
Expression and Characteristics of the Phosphodiesterase Families

Family	Expression	Characteristics
1	*Mast cells, neutrophils, monocytes, macrophages, platelets, epithelial cells*	Calcium- and calmodulin-dependent, variable affinity for cAMP and cGMP
2	Mast cells, macrophages, *T cells*, platelets, *endothelial cells*, epithelial cells	cGMP stimulated, low affinity for cAMP and cGMP
3	Mast cells, *basophils*, monocytes, macrophages, T cells, platelets, endothelial cells, epithelial cells	cGMP inhibited, high affinity for cAMP and cGMP
4	Mast cells, basophils, *eosinophils*, neutrophils, monocytes, macrophages, T cells, endothelial cells, epithelial cells	cAMP specific
5	Mast cells, basophils, macrophages, T cells, platelets, endothelial cells, epithelial cells	cGMP specific
6	Retina cells	cGMP specific
7	T cells	cAMP specific

PHOSPHODIESTERASE (PDE) INHIBITORS

Cyclic AMP (cAMP) is an important second messenger in most inflammatory cells. Moreover, increased *IL-4* production in *allergic diseases* is associated with increased cAMP *phosphodiesterase* activity. Therefore, PDE inhibitors may be beneficial in diseases associated with *allergic inflammation.*

> Nonselective PDE inhibitors include *theophylline*, which has been used to treat *asthma.*

However, their use is limited by toxic side effects. Selective PDE inhibitors, such as rolipram and Ro 20-1724, inhibit IL-4-induced *IgE* production in *peripheral blood mononuclear cells* (PBMC), but not purified *B cells.* Type IV PDE inhibitors seem to be the most important isoenzymes in regulation of cAMP levels in *mast cells, eosinophils,* and *basophils.* In contrast, type III PDE inhibitors, such as SK&F 95654, and type V PDE inhibitors, such as zaprinast, have no effect on these allergic inflammatory cells.

PHOSPHOLIPASE A$_1$ (PLA$_1$)

The vespid phospholipase is approximately twice the size of *bee venom phospholipase A$_2$* (PLA$_2$). It consists of 300 *amino acids* and has a molecular weight of 35 kDa. Although the pharmacological effects of both wasp and bee venom phospholipases are similar, they do not represent *cross-reacting allergens.* Comparison of their sequences confirms that the enzymes are immunochemically distinct proteins. PLA$_1$ together with *hyaluronidase* and antigen 5 are important *allergens* of wasp venoms (see *hymenoptera allergy*).

PHOSPHOLIPASE A$_2$ (PLA$_2$)

Following intracellular *calcium mobilization* upon cell activation, PLA$_2$ is translocated to the nuclear envelope, where it initiates *leukotriene* (LT) and *prostaglandin* (PG) synthesis by catalyzing the hydrolysis *arachidonic acid* (AA) from nuclear membrane phospholipids (Figure 37). Although there are multiple *isoforms* of PLA$_2$, *cytosolic PLA$_2$* appears to be most important for this function. Other isoforms include a secreted isoform, which may also initiate *eicosanoid* generation, and another PLA$_2$ molecule that specifically hydrolyzes *phosphatidylserine* (PS). AA is then the substrate of *5-lipoxygenase* (5-LO) to generate *5-HPETE* and

LTA$_4$ or of *cyclooxygenase* (COX) to synthesize PGs and *thromboxane*. *Cytokines* that are responsible for *granulocyte priming* may do so by serine 505 *phosphorylation* of PLA$_2$ (for PLA$_2$ as a *major allergen* in bee venom, see *bee venom phospholipase A$_2$*).

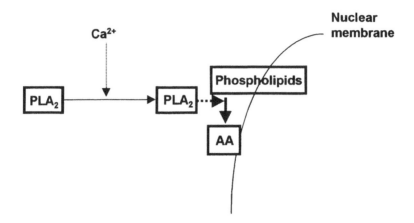

FIGURE 37   Cytosolic PLA$_2$ generates arachidonic acid (AA) from nuclear membrane phospholipids.

PHOSPHOLIPASE C (PLC)

PLC is a central molecule within *signal transduction* pathways initiated via many cell surface *receptors*.

Several *isoforms* exist. Surface receptors often activate only one isoform upon activation. For instance, *T cell antigen receptor cross-linking* leads to activation of PLCγ1, whereas *platelet-activating factor* (PAF) receptor stimulates PLCβ. In *B cells*, PLCγ2 plays an important role in *antigen receptor signaling*. The different PLC isoforms are activated by *tyrosine kinases* and/or *G proteins*. PLC activation results in the hydrolysis of *phosphatidylinositol-4,5-bis-phosphate* (PIP$_2$) to *inositol-1,4,5-trisphosphate* (IP$_3$) and *diacylglycerol* (DAG). IP$_3$ generation leads to intracellular *calcium mobilization*, while DAG promotes the activation of *protein kinase C* (PKC).

PHOSPHOLIPASE D (PLD)

Leukotrienes, *C5a*, and *PAF* stimulate PLD in inflammatory effector cells. Three pathways have been discussed in PLD activation: (1) via *G proteins*, (2) via *phospholipase C* (PLC) and *calcium mobilization*, or (3) via *tyrosine kinases*. PLD mediates the cleavage of phos-phatidylcholine to generate phosphatidic acid (PA). PA is then the substrate of phosphatidate phosphohydrolase to generate *diacylglycerol* (DAG). PLD activation appears to be important for ligand-mediated *degranulation* of *mast cells*, *basophils*, *eosinophils*, and *neutrophils*. PLD is negatively regulated by *cAMP* (see *immunosuppressive mechanisms*).

PHOSPHORYLATION

Several proteins receive phosphate groups on tyrosine, serine, or threonine residues (see *amino acids*) in the process of *signal transduction*. Such enzymatic reactions are mediated by *kinases* and usually result in activation of the target protein.

PHOTOALLERGY

In photoallergic skin diseases, proallergens are modified/metabolized in vivo inside the cutaneous compartment by *ultraviolet (UV) light* or visible light to form the relevant *allergen* for a *delayed hypersensitivity* reaction (see *Coombs and Gell classification*, type IV).

> The diagnosis of a photoallergy is based on clinical grounds, but confirmation of diagnosis and identification of the relevant allergen require a *photopatch test.*

Two identical patch test series are applied to the patient's back. One of them is removed after 24 h, and a dose of UV-light is applied. *Skin test* reactions of the two identical test series are read after 48 and 72 h. A photoallergy is diagnosed if test reactions occur in the UV-treated test series, but not in the identical, UV-untreated series.

PHOTOCHEMICAL POLLUTION

(See *smog.*)

PHOTOPATCH TEST

The photopatch test (see *patch test*) is a standard diagnostic procedure for photoallergic reactions (see *photoallergy*).

PICHIA PASTORIS

> The Pichia system has been used successfully to express several *recombinant allergens* (see Table 78).

Pichia pastoris is a methylotrophic yeast capable of utilizing methanol as its sole carbon source through the use of alcohol oxidase (AOX), an enzyme involved in the first step of the methanol utilization pathway. Under culture conditions, where cells derive carbon sources from glucose, glycerol, or ethanol, alcohol oxidase is undetectable. However, when cells are grown in methanol, alcohol oxidase may comprise up to 30% of the soluble protein produced by the cell. *Transcription* of alcohol oxidase *mRNA* is tightly regulated by the AOX1 *promoter.* The Pichia pastoris expression system was designed to take advantage of this by incorporating the highly inducible promoter into expression vectors used with Pichia. The *gene* of interest is cloned behind the promoter, and after integration of the *vector* construct into the Pichia genome, high-level expression of *allergen* is induced using methanol. The protein can be expressed intracellularly or targeted into the media using a secretion signal sequence.

> Since Pichia itself secretes relatively few proteins, secretion of recombinant *allergen* serves as an initial purification step.

In addition to producing large quantities of biologically active material, other advantages of the Pichia system include the use of *antibiotic*-resistant vectors that aid in the selection of high copy, high expression transformants, and the ease with which production can be scaled up to fermentor level using inexpensive media. In addition, the eukaryotic yeast system offers the advantage of processing, folding, and possibly glycosylation of recombinant allergens as they pass through the secretory pathway. However, glycosylation may not be desirable if the allergen is not glycosylated in the native state, and the oligosaccharide structure will differ from mammalian glycoproteins.

TABLE 78
**Expression of Allergens Using
the Pichia System**

Allergen	Vector	Expression Level
Cockroach		
Bla g 2	pPIC9	14 mg/l
Bla g 4	pPIC9	50 mg/l
Per a 1	pPIC9	10 mg/l
Mouse		
MUP	pHIL-D2	270 mg/l
Pollen		
Cyn d 1	pHIL-S1	1.5 g/l
Fungal		
Alt a 1	pPIC9	10 mg/l
Tri t 4	pPICZαA	20 mg/l

PIECEMEAL DEGRANULATION (PMD)

PMD is an alternative route for the secretion of *mediators* (e.g., *histamine* or *eosinophil granule proteins*) from inflammatory cells such as *mast cells*, *basophils*, *eosinophils*, and *neutrophils*. PMD represents a mechanism for slow release of *granule* contents, and thus differs from the much more rapid secretion seen in *receptor*-mediated *exocytosis* (e.g., *immediate hypersensitivity* reaction following *high-affinity IgE receptor* activation in mast cells). Human skin mast cells present in *wound healing* and human heart *fibrosis* can display signs of PMD.

PIGEON FANCIER'S LUNG

This is a form of *extrinsic allergic alveolitis* (EAA) that occurs in 10 to 20% of sensitized individuals after a variable period of regular exposure to pigeons. Pigeon droppings, blooms, and mucin are considered to be the major sources of the sensitizing *allergen*.

PINOCYTOSIS

Pinocytosis is an unsaturable permanent pathway to uptake extracellular fluid. It is based on the engulfment of extracellular space by the plasma membrane, forming *endosomes*.

Pinocytosis can be considered as non-*receptor*-mediated *endocytosis*.

Basically, all cells are able to perform pinocytosis. *Antigen-presenting cells* (APCs) take up *antigens* for *antigen processing* and presentation by pinocytosis, in addition to receptor-mediated endocytosis.

PIRBUTEROL

This is a *β2-agonist*.

PITYRIASIS ALBA

Pityriasis alba represents an almost invisible, white scaling of mostly *dry skin* usually seen in atopic individuals. It is more a skin condition than a skin disease (see *atopy stigmata*).

PITYROSPORUM OVALE

(See *fungal allergens*.)

PLANT DERMATITIS

All types of allergic, toxic, photoallergic, and phototoxic *dermatitis* caused by contact with plant substances are summarized as plant dermatitis. The so-called rhus dermatitis, an acute allergic plant *contact dermatitis* due to the urushiol of poison oak and poison ivy (both members of the Anacardiaceae family) is very common in North America. The phototoxic dermatitis pratensis due to the furocoumarines from heracleum species (members of the Umbelliferae family) are a frequent cause of phytophotodermatitis (see also *photoallergy*).

PLASMA CELL

Antibody-producing *B cells* often differentiate into specialized forms called plasma cells. They are found only in lymphoid organs and at sites of *immune responses*. They do not circulate in blood under normal conditions. Plasma cells are, like mature *granulocytes*, terminally differentiated cells with no capacity for mitotic division.

PLASMID

A plasmid is an independently replicating, extrachromosomal (see *chromosome*) circular *DNA* molecule often carrying *antibiotic* resistance *genes* and propagated in bacteria. They have been engineered to become vehicles or "*vectors*" for manipulating genes and gene fragments *in vitro*. Because plasmid DNA is much smaller than the bacterial chromosome, it can be easily isolated, manipulated in the laboratory, and reintroduced into bacteria (e.g., for the production of *recombinant allergens*). Plasmid DNA can also be used for *DNA vaccination*.

PLATELET

Platelets are specialized cells without a nucleus, responsible for the initiation of tissue repair after injury. In addition, platelets are believed to play an important role in *allergic diseases*, especially in *asthma*. Platelets release a variety of inflammatory *mediators* that contribute to *allergic inflammation* (see Table 79).

TABLE 79
Mediators Released from Platelets and Their Possible Effects in Asthma

Mediators	Effects
Adenosine	*Airway obstruction*
Histamine	Airway obstruction, vasodilatation, vascular permeability
RANTES	*Chemotaxis*
PAF	Airway obstruction, *airway hyperresponsiveness,* chemotaxis, *mucus* secretion, vascular permeability
PDGF	*Smooth muscle* proliferation, chemotaxis
TGF-β	Smooth muscle proliferation, chemotaxis
Platelet factor 4	Airway hyperresponsiveness, chemotaxis
12-HPETE	*Leukotriene* synthesis by *leukocytes*
Thromboxane A$_2$	Airway obstruction, vasoconstriction
Arachidonic acid	Leukotriene synthesis by leukocytes
Leukotrienes (following uptake of LTA$_4$)	Airway obstruction, mucus secretion, chemotaxis
Cationic proteins	Tissue damage
Oxygen metabolites	Tissue damage

PLATELET-ACTIVATING FACTOR (PAF)

PAF (1-alkyl-2-acetyl-sn-glycero-3-phosphocholine) is a short-lived *lipid mediator* that aggregates *platelets*. It is generated from its precursor lyso-PAF by acetylation. One way to generate lyso-PAF is from *arachidonic acid* (AA), which is generated by activated cytosolic *phospholipase A2* (PLA_2). Therefore, *eicosanoids* and PAF may be produced together under inflammatory conditions. *Granulocytes, fibroblasts,* and *endothelial cells,* but not *lymphocytes,* are able to synthesize PAF.

> Besides its action on platelets, PAF is a *chemotactic factor* and potent activator of granulocytes.

Inhalation of PAF causes *airway obstruction,* mucosal *edema, mucus* secretion, and increased *airway hyperresponsiveness.* In addition, PAF stimulates the synthesis of *cysteinyl leukotrienes* and *thromboxane A2.* In general, PAF *receptors* are expressed by cells that are able to generate PAF. *T cells* and *B cells* do not express PAF receptors. Although PAF appears to be an important mediator in *allergic inflammation,* specific *PAF receptor antagonists* are ineffective in *asthma* (see *asthma treatment strategies*).

PLATELET-DERIVED HISTAMINE RELEASING FACTOR (PDHRF)

Platelets activated with thrombin, *collagen,* or *platelet-activating factor* (PAF) liberate PDHRF, which stimulates *histamine* release from *mast cells* and *basophils.* PDHRF has also been shown to be a *chemotactic factor* for *eosinophils.*

PLEIOTROPISM

Property of almost all *cytokines* that act on many different cell types.

PM-10

Particulate matter <10 μm in size is of particular concern. A number of chemicals (including transition metals, silica, polyaromatic hydrocarbons) and biological agents (endotoxins and glucans) may contribute to the action of respirable particles. Epidemiologic studies suggest two significant at-risk populations: *asthma* patients and the elderly. Medication use, symptoms, and need for medical attention are increased in asthmatics following increases in ambient levels of PM-10. More notable is the increase in deaths observed in elderly persons with preexisting cardiac or pulmonary disease associated with increases in PM-10. Animal studies in dogs suggest that PM-10 exposure may induce arrhythmias. Other animal studies and in vitro experiments suggest that these PM-10 particles induce *inflammation* and, like *ozone,* activate *NF-κB* and *cytokine* secretion. To date, the only human challenges with PM-10 are *nasal provocations* with *diesel exhaust* particles (DEP). These studies indicate that DEPs enhance production of *IgE* and increase cytokine and cell influx associated with specific *allergen challenge.*

POINT MUTATION

This form of *mutation* defines an alteration of a *DNA* sequence affecting one single *base pair* (bp).

POISON IVY

Contact dermatitis due to the woodland plant poison ivy represents the most frequently encountered *delayed hypersensitivity* reaction in the United States. It is caused by a highly reactive, lipid-like molecule of the leaves, called pentadecacatechol, which functions as a *hapten* (see *plant dermatitis*).

POISON OAK

(See *plant dermatitis.*)

POLLENS

Pollen grains from many species have been found to be allergenic (see *aeroallergens*). Due to their small size, abundant production, and ubiquitous distribution, pollens represent a significant cause of seasonal *allergic disease,* such as *hay fever.* The reason pollens, as opposed to other particles of similar size, are often allergenic is not fully understood, but the innate enzymatic activity of the major pollen *allergens* may be responsible, causing direct release of preformed *IL-4* from bronchial *mast cells* by local cellular disruption (see *cytotoxicity of allergens*). Examples of allergenic pollens include those of various grasses and reeds, olive, birch (see *birch pollen*), hazel, alder (*alder pollen*), ragweed (see *ragweed pollen*), and oil seed rape (see *grass* and *tree pollen*). Allergens from many pollens have been purified, sequenced (see *DNA sequencing*), *epitope* mapped, and produced as *peptide* fragments or whole allergens by recombinant expression (see *recombinant allergens*). Major purified pollen allergens include those from rye grass (Lol p 1-4), orchard grass (Dac g 1-5), timothy grass (Phl p 4-7), birch pollen (Bet v 1), and ragweed (Amb a 1-6).

POLLEN COUNTING

For the routine monitoring of airborne concentrations of *pollen* and *fungal allergens*, two techniques are applied most frequently. One is the rotorod system, which is widely used in the U.S. It consists of a rotating impact sampler that collects particles on the surfaces of two upright metal arms, rotating at about 2500 rpm. The rotorod system provides information on average concentrations over the duration of sampling time. Another technique is used throughout Europe. Volumetric traps are made for continuous isokinetic sampling. Air is sucked into the trap at a rate of 10 l/minute. It flows over a rotating drum, which moves past the orifice at 2 mm/hour and is covered with a tape coated in adhesive. The pollen traps are usually situated on rooftops. The counts should be considered as a guide to the conditions in the surrounding area. Pollen concentrations can vary greatly during the day, even when the weather does not change. On rainy days the average pollen count may be low.

POLLENOSIS

(See *allergic rhinoconjunctivitis* and *hay fever.*)

POLLUTANTS

The role of *air pollution* in the causation and exacerbation of *asthma* has been widely disputed. Ambient concentrations of traditional pollutants such as black smoke and *sulfur dioxide* (SO_2) have declined dramatically in the Western world following the introduction of clean air legislation. This period has coincided with a marked increase in the prevalence of asthma and other *allergic diseases.*

> Traditional pollution might protect against asthma; certainly there is no evidence that it causes asthma, whereas it undoubtedly does have an adverse effect on *chronic bronchitis*, *cough*, and *COPD*.

Newer forms of pollution including photochemical smogs (principally *ozone*), oxides of nitrogen (due to combustion of fossil fuels, see *nitrogen dioxide*), and fine particulate pollution (see *PM-10*) have increased in the last 30 to 40 years, especially in areas with high levels of motor vehicle traffic. Ozone causes a reduction in maximal inspiratory capacity and hence a reduction in *forced expiratory volume in first second* (FEV_1).

> Ozone affects both normal individuals and those with asthma.

Patients with asthma are more sensitive to the effects of ozone, because they start from a lower baseline. In contrast, oxides of nitrogen do not have any measurable effect on normal healthy subjects, but can potentiate the effects of *allergen challenge*. This mechanism may contribute to the frequent complaint by those with asthma that they are affected by traffic fumes. Fine particulate pollution has been associated with increased respiratory and cardio-vascular morbidity. In developed countries, the principal source of fine particulate pollution is diesel-powered vehicles.

> *Diesel exhaust* particles activate *macrophages* and other inflammatory cells and can be shown to induce acute *inflammation* in healthy human airways.

However, the significance of these acute inflammatory events in relation to the causation of asthma remains to be determined.

> While it is hard to argue that pollution is good for people, there is at present relatively little evidence that current levels of air pollution in Western nations have any direct influence on the increased prevalence of asthma.

POLLUTANTS AND BRONCHOALVEOLAR LAVAGE

Bronchoalveolar lavage (BAL) fluid has been used in research demonstrating that even low concentrations of *ozone* (O_3) are associated with the influx of both *eosinophils* and *neutrophils* into the lung. Other changes observed include increased proteins, which suggest potential for *edema*, the presence of enzymes, which suggest *epithelial damage*, and other BAL fluid constituents with potential inflammatory properties, including *complement factors*, *fibronectin*, *IgG*, and *IL-6*. The *mast cell* marker *tryptase* has been observed in BAL fluid from nonasthmatic subjects exposed to ozone, suggesting that ozone-induced *inflammation* may share features with the response of subjects with *allergic rhinitis* after *allergen challenge*. Other studies using BAL have found similar markers of lung injury and inflammation in subjects exposed to *nitrogen dioxide* (NO_2), *sulfur dioxide* (SO_2), and *diesel exhaust* (see *air pollution*).

POLLUTANTS AND NASAL LAVAGE

Nasal lavage (NAL) can be used for *allergen challenge* and other controlled exposure studies using real-world *pollutant* mixtures (see *air pollution*).

> Experimental and epidemiological studies of *ozone* (O_3) exposure have revealed, via NAL, a positive association between O_3 exposure and an increased number of *granulocytes* and *lymphocytes*, as well as nasal congestion and increased levels of *histamine*.

In *sulfur dioxide* (SO_2) exposure studies, the levels of S-sulfonate measured in NALs are effective short-term markers of exposure to SO_2. NAL has also been used to explore other endpoints in relation to air pollutants, including the *antioxidant* content of respiratory tract lining fluids, which provide an initial defense against environmental toxins. Uric acid in NAL samples is scavenged by O_3 in a dose- and time-dependent manner. Exposure of the nasal *epithelial cells* to mutagens and carcinogens could give rise to *DNA* adducts, which could be used as markers of exposure. A study of fuel oil ash exposure in boilermakers and utility workers (see *occupational agents*) showed a significant increase in NAL *neutrophils* in nonsmokers, but not in smokers.

> *Diesel exhaust* particle exposure has been associated with increased nasal *cytokine* expression with concomitant enhanced local *IgE* production.

Studies in Mexico City showed that children had abnormal nasal cytology with decreased numbers of ciliated cells, abnormal ciliated cells with shortened *cilia*, and deciliated areas (see *epithelial damage*), in addition to squamous metaplastic cells and neutrophils. In a controlled exposure study of volatile organic compounds (VOCs), subjects exposed to a mixture of VOCs also showed a significant increase in neutrophils in NAL.

POLLUTION

Areas in which large amounts of automobile exhaust remain trapped in the atmosphere and are acted upon by *ultraviolet* (*UV*) *light* will likely have elevated levels of *ozone* (O_3) and *nitrogen dioxide* (NO_2). This is especially likely in valleys in which air inversions are possible. In areas such as Los Angeles, peak ozone levels are reported in the late morning through the afternoon. Areas in which coal-burning industries are prevalent, usually found in large metropolitan areas in the northeastern regions of the U.S., are more likely to have increased levels of *sulfur dioxide* (SO_2) and particulate matter (see also *air pollution* and *pollutants*).

POLLUTION AND INFECTIOUS DISEASES

Air pollution, e.g., *ozone* (O_3) and *nitrogen dioxide* (NO_2), has been shown to exert effects on alveolar *macrophages*.

> Epidemiologic studies also indicate that increased frequency of respiratory infection occurs in concert with increased levels of ozone.

In vitro studies of *macrophages* recovered from both humans and animals following ozone exposure reveal decreased phagocytic activity (see *phagocytosis*), oxidative metabolism (see *oxygen metabolites*), and *cytokine* release of these cells following stimulation. Likewise, direct exposure of alveolar macrophages recovered after clean air exposure to ozone also have diminished phagocytic activity. In addition to a direct effect of ozone on macrophage function, *mediators* released during ozone exposure may also adversely alter macrophage function. This is supported by in vivo studies in rodents in which inhibition of *prostaglandin* E_2 (PGE_2) secretion with *cyclooxygenase* inhibitors preserves macrophage function following ozone exposure. Similar results have been observed in rodent studies with NO_2 as well. Another way in which air *pollutants* may alter host defense is the impairment of *mucociliary clearance*. This has been observed in both humans and animals as a result of exposure to *sulfur dioxide* (SO_2) and sulfates.

> Persistent exposure to sulfates induces a long-term impairment of ciliary clearance, which is associated with both hypertrophy and hyperplasia of airway secretory cells.

To date, only a few controlled exposure studies of humans have been performed. However, decreased macrophage function and mucociliary clearance following ozone exposure have been confirmed in humans. These findings suggest that pollutant exposure could blunt host defense such that increased frequency or severity of infection could occur.

POLLUTION-RELATED THERAPY

For those persons unavoidably exposed to *air pollution*, optimal treatment of chronic respiratory diseases such as *asthma* is important (see *asthma treatment strategies*).

> If possible, exercise should be avoided when conditions favorable for increased ambient *pollutant* exposure are present.

When pollutant avoidance is not possible, certain currently available medications may be useful in preventing adverse effects on *lung function*.

> *Anticholinergic agents* may be useful in mitigating the effects of *ozone* (O_3), and *β2-agonists*, anticholinergics, and *cromones* have been shown to attenuate the effects of *sulfur dioxide* (SO_2) in asthmatics.

Of note, *corticosteroids* have not been shown to specifically protect against the effects of either O_3 or SO_2 in either asthmatics or nonasthmatics. However, use of such medications should not be discontinued when used for other indications, including treatment of moderate or severe chronic asthma or a marked *asthma exacerbation*. Lack of understanding of the mechanisms by which other pollutants (*acid aerosols, particulate matter,* or *nitrogen dioxide* (NO_2) influence lung function (see *lung function tests*) precludes any rational recommendation for prophylactic intervention strategies other than avoidance of these agents.

POLYADENYLATION (poly-A) SITE

Upon termination of *mRNA* synthesis (see *transcription*), a sequence of about 200 *adenosine* residues is added at the 3' end. The poly-A tail is involved in the transport of the mRNA out of the nucleus and in mRNA stability.

POLYGENIC DISEASE

These are diseases that are determined by multiple *genes* at different loci (see *locus*), each with a relatively minor but additive effect (see *multifactorial inheritance*). *Allergic diseases* appear to be polygenic diseases.

POLYMERASE CHAIN REACTION (PCR)

PCR was developed in the mid-1980s as a method of generating many copies of a specific segment of *DNA*. The technique is used in place of the more time-consuming approach of *gene* cloning (see *DNA cloning*), and especially for the identification of rare sequences within a large genome. PCR employs the fundamental aspects of DNA replication; *DNA polymerase* initiates DNA synthesis using a single-strand DNA template and generates the *complementary* strand. This synthesis is targeted to specific DNA sequences by specific *primers* that are short *oligonucleotides* designed to anneal to the region of interest. Single-stranded DNA templates are generated by heating double-stranded DNA to 95°C (*denaturation*); a controlled cooling allows the oligonucleotide primers to preferentially anneal (*hybridization*); and synthesis is initiated at 72°C by a heat-stable DNA polymerase in the presence of free *nucleotide* triphosphates (elongation). The cycle is repeated, heating to 95°C to denature the double-stranded DNA, cooling to allow the primer to anneal, and heating to 72°C for efficient and accurate DNA synthesis (Figure 38). After 30 cycles, as many as 10^9 copies of the target sequence may be generated. PCR has many applications, including the diagnosis of human inherited disorders, forensic analyses, *DNA cloning*, gene expression studies, and *in vitro mutagenesis*.

POLYMORPHISM

(See *genetic polymorphism*.)

POLYMORPHONUCLEAR LEUKOCYTE

(See *neutrophil*.)

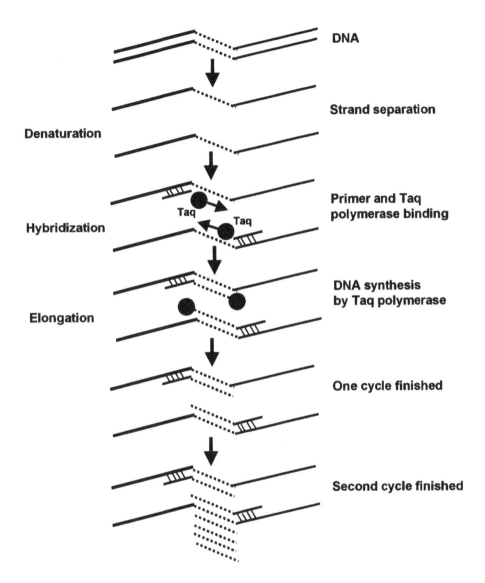

FIGURE 38 Basic principle of the polymerase chain reaction (PCR). Note that after one PCR cycle, the amount of target DNA (dashed) is doubled. After two cycles, the DNA of interest is again doubled. The flanking DNA is not amplified.

POLYMORPHOUS LIGHT ERUPTION

The term "polymorphous light eruption" describes a group of heterogenous, idiopathic, acquired, acute recurrent photodermatoses. They are characterized by delayed abnormal skin reactions to *ultraviolet (UV) light*. The morphologic types include papules, papulovesicules, erythematous macules, plaques, and vesicles. However, in each individual patient, the type of lesion is consistently monomorphous. Skin lesions tend to reappear in spring with the first intensive sun exposure of the year.

POLYMORPHISM

(See *genetic polymorphism*.)

POLYPOSIS

(See *nasal polyps*.)

POLYSENSITIZATION

Patients who show multiple positive *skin tests* to several different *aeroallergens* are said to be polysensitized. In general, polysensitized patients are less likely to improve with *allergen avoidance* measures or specific *immunotherapy*, as compared to those who are monosensitized.

POMPHOLYX

A unique, clinically defined reaction pattern of the skin with vesicules and blisters underneath a thickened stratum corneum on the palms (cheiropompholyx) and soles (podopompholyx).

POPULATION ASSOCIATION STUDY

Such a study compares the frequency of *polymorphisms* of *genes* (*alleles*) of interest between affected patients and unaffected individuals.

POTASSIUM CHANNELS

4-Aminopyridine, a potassium channel blocker, induces *histamine* release from *mast cells*. It appears that blocking of potassium channels opens up calcium channels (see *calcium mobilization*) eliciting *mediator* release. Therefore, potassium channel openers may be beneficial in the treatment of *allergic diseases* (see *β2-agonists*)

POTATO

Patients with *birch pollen allergy* may develop *contact urticaria* after peeling a potato or *oral allergy syndrome* (OAS) after ingestion of raw potatoes. These individuals often tolerate cooked potatoes without difficulties. The responsible *allergen* is *profilin*.

POWDER INHALER

(See *dry powder inhaler*.)

PRANLUKAST

(See *leukotriene receptor antagonists*.)

PRAUSNITZ–KÜSTNER REACTION

In 1921, Carl Prausnitz injected himself with the serum of his fish-allergic colleague Küstner. A local application of the fish-*allergen* at the site of injection resulted in a positive *skin test* reaction (see *immediate hypersensitivity*). This reaction indicated that an allergic reactivity is transferred with serum proteins. About 50 years later, the responsible protein was identified and is now called "allergen-specific *IgE*." Due to a high risk of infection, the Prausnitz–Küstner test has been completely abandoned in clinical *allergy* treatment (see *passive cutaneous anaphylaxis*).

PREDNISOLONE

This is an oral *corticosteroid* that requires metabolism in the liver before it is biologically active.

PREDNISONE

The biologically active form of *prednisolone*, also available as an oral tablet. Prednisolone is preferred in Europe, while prednisone is usually the standard oral *corticosteroid* in the U.S.

PREMENSTRUAL ASTHMA

Approximately 30% of women complain of somatic or psychologic symptoms shortly before or during their menstruation, which may include *asthma exacerbation*. Although the underlying mechanism is unclear, a marked increase of *airway hyperresponsiveness* and a decrease of *peak expiratory flow rates* (PEFR) can be demonstrated in some cases.

PREVALENCE

The proportion of individuals in a community who have a disease at any given time.

PRICK TEST

The prick test is a bioassay for *immediate hypersensitivity*, and is performed at the volar surface of the forearm or the back. The principle of this *skin test* is to apply a drop of the supposed *allergen* in saline solution to the skin and to disturb the *epidermal barrier* by manipulation with a prick lancet. This procedure should not draw blood. About 15 to 20 minutes later, a wheal and flare reaction appears at the positive test site.

> Prick test results (see Table 80) correlate with the amount of specific *IgE* to the tested allergen.

In general, *aeroallergens* tend to give stronger results than food allergens (see *food allergy*). There is a low, but significant, risk for induction of systemic *anaphylactic reactions* by prick tests. Therefore, only physicians experienced in the management of anaphylactic reactions and adequately equipped for shock treatment may perform prick tests.

TABLE 80
Prick Test Results Given
Semiquantitatively as –, +,
++, +++, ++++ Reactions

Result	Urtica	Erythema
–	–	<3 mm
+	2–3 mm	3–5 mm
++	3 mm	6–10 mm
+++	4–6 mm	11–20 mm
++++	>6 mm	>20 mm

Since performance of the test is inexpensive, it can be done quickly with many different allergens, and there is no need of sterile allergen solutions. The prick test is the most widely used skin test for the diagnosis of a type I *sensitization* (see *Coombs and Gell classification*). Prick test solutions in standardized quality and concentration are available from many commercial sources. A negative (0.9% saline) and a positive control (0.1% *histamine*) must always be performed. As used in *patch tests*, several standardized rows of allergens (e.g., aeroallergens, food allergens, drugs — see *drug allergy*) have been built up for daily routine use. A patient's own substances (e.g., specific food) may be tested, but 10 controls must be performed.

To avoid false negative results, the discontinuation times for certain drugs must be observed (see Table 81).

In patients with *urticaria* factitia, false-positive results are obtained, but this is easily detected by the positive saline prick test reaction. In contrast, false-negative results may not always be detected by a negative histamine prick test reaction.

TABLE 81
Recommended Discontinuation Times
before Prick Testing

Drug	Time Period
Corticosteroid ointments at test site	1 week
Corticosteroid ointments elsewhere	None
High-dose systemic steroids (long-term use)	3 weeks
Astemizole	3 weeks
Other oral *antihistamines*	5 days
Topical antihistamines	1 day
Tricyclic antidepressants	2 weeks
Psychopharmacons with antihistaminic effects	5 days

PRIMARY IMMUNE RESPONSE

Any response of the *immune system* against a new *antigen*, i.e., an antigen that the immune system has never seen and never reacted against before, is called a primary immune response. *Dendritic cells* are by now the only *antigen-presenting cells* (APC) that have been demonstrated to induce a primary immune response. In contrast, many cell types are able to induce *secondary immune responses* (see also *allergen-induced immune responses*).

PRIMARY STRUCTURE

The primary structure is the linear *amino acid* sequence of a protein molecule.

PRIMATE T CELLS

Nonhuman primate species possess *T cell* subpopulations similar to those of humans, which express T lineage-specific markers such as *CD3*, *CD4*, or *CD8* (see *CD antigens*). Additionally, they possess *CD16⁺ NK cells*. *IL-4* is produced by *Th2 cells* and has been shown to promote *lymphocyte* and NK cell trafficking by the induced expression of *adhesion molecules*, such as *VCAM-1,* on vascular *endothelial cells*. Attraction of lymphocytes and *eosinophils* expressing the VCAM-1 ligand *VLA-4* and the production of *T cell cytokines* (e.g., *IL-5*) have been shown to promote selective *eosinophilia* characteristic of chronic *allergic inflammation*.

PRIMER

A primer is a short *oligonucleotide*, usually between 20 and 30 bases in length. It is supposed to bind to a *complementary* sequence of *DNA* during the *polymerase chain reaction* (PCR), but also in other molecular biology techniques in order to initiate DNA synthesis.

PRIMING

(See *granulocyte priming*.)

PROFILIN

Profilin is an allergenic molecule present in plants. Anti-profilin *IgE antibodies* can explain various cross-reactivities (see *cross-reacting allergens*) between *pollen* and food *allergens* (e.g., hazel-*tree pollen* with hazelnut, *birch pollen* with *apple allergen* and stoned fruits, *mugwort pollen* with *celery*, carrot, and spice).

PROGRAMMED CELL DEATH (PCD)

PCD is the physiologic form of cell death. In contrast, *necrosis* is always pathologic. PCD is an active, genetically programmed and evolutionarily conserved process by which cells self-destruct without causing an inflammatory response (see *inflammation*).

> *Apoptosis* is the most common form of PCD and refers to characteristic biochemical and morphological changes of the dying cell.

PROGRESSIVE PIGMENTED PURPURA

Progressive pigmented purpura, or Schamberg's disease, is a chronic, recurrent, progressive, purpuric dermatosis caused by punctate hemorrhages in yellowish–orange–brownish foci on the lower legs, rarely spreading to the thighs, abdomen, and lower arms. A chronic capillaritis in the papillary and subpapillary dermis causes the extravasation of *lymphocytes* and erythrocytes. An allergic *type IV reaction* (see *Coombs and Gell classification*) or an *intolerance* reaction to hypnotics, sedatives (see *adverse drug reactions*), food, or food additives (see *adverse food reactions*) are assumed to be of pathogenetic relevance. Recognition and avoidance of the causative provoking factors are important.

PROMOTER

This is a *DNA* sequence element located 5′ to *genes*, which fixes the site of initiation of *transcription*. The start region for the DNA-dependent *RNA polymerase* II encompasses about +20 bp up to −100 bp upstream around the initiation site of transcription. This region comprises DNA motifs for cis-regulatory *transcription factors*, which direct *RNA* synthesis to one strand as well as control *mRNA* quantity and sometimes tissue specificity. Differences in the promoter sequence of genes (see *genetic predisposition*) may have an influence on gene transcription. Therefore, many research groups currently investigate promoter sequences of *cytokine* genes in patients and control individuals to understand the mechanisms of increased *Th2* cytokine expression in *IgE*-mediated *allergic diseases*. Evidence has been obtained in families with *asthma* that a polymorphism in the *IL-4* promoter is associated with elevated total serum *IgE levels*.

PROPELLANTS

(See *CFC propellants* and *HFA propellants*.)

PROSTAGLANDINS (PGs)

Arachidonic acid metabolites generated via the *cyclooxygenase* pathway. Significant amounts of PGD_2 are generated by *mast cells* and seem to contribute to the immediate asthmatic reaction (see *immediate hypersensitivity*). *Aerosol* administration of PGD_2 causes *airway obstruction* in human subjects and potentiates *airway hyperresponsiveness* to *methacholine* and *histamine* in patients with *asthma*. In addition, PGD_2 is a *chemotactic factor* for human *neutrophils*, augments *leukotriene* B_4-induced neutrophilia, and is a powerful inhibitor of *platelet* aggregation.

> Although a beneficial role could be expected, *nonsteroidal antiinflammatory drugs* (NSAID), which block cyclooxygenases, do not have any role in the management of *allergic diseases*.

PROSTAGLANDIN H SYNTHASE

(See *cyclooxygenase*.)

PROSTANOID

"Prostanoids" is a term used for the products of *cyclooxygenase*, which include *prostaglandins* (PGs) and *thromboxane*.

PROTEASE

Proteases are proteolytic enzymes that hydrolyze the *peptide* bond. They are often named for a feature of their active site; for example, the cysteine or thiol proteases such as papain or actinidin have a conserved cysteine *amino acid* involved in the catalytic mechanism.

> Many proteases are involved in the pathogenesis of *allergic diseases*.

For instance, several *major allergens* are proteases, e.g., the group 1 mite *allergens* are cysteine proteases, and the *cockroach allergen* Bla g 2 is an aspartic protease. Moreover, *mast cells* generate *neutral proteases*, which are important for the initiation and maintenance of *allergic inflammation*. *Metalloproteases* are enzymes that degrade *extracellular matrix* proteins. In addition, many proteins of the *complement system* are proteases. Furthermore, *angiotensin-converting enzyme* (ACE) is a protease that cleaves *angiotensin* I, but also *bradykinin*. For the resolution of *inflammation*, intracellular *caspases* play an essential role in the execution of inflammatory cells (see *apoptosis*).

PROTEASE I AND II

These two chymotrypsin-like *neutral proteases* help to distinguish *rat mast cells*. *Protease* I (rat *chymase* I) is found exclusively in the *connective tissue mast cells* (CTMC), whereas protease II (rat chymase II) is only expressed in *mucosal mast cells* (MMC). Although protease I and II are derived from different *genes*, they appear to belong to a gene family composed of 10 to 15 members. A sensitive *immunoassay* for protease II was developed and used to assess the presence of this enzyme in complex biologic fluids as an indicator of MMC activation (see *mast cell activation*). Concentrations of more than 120 µg/ml were found in blood after intravenous injection of N. brasiliensis into rats.

PROTEIN CONTACT DERMATITIS

This skin disease is an urticarial reaction (see *urticaria*) following the direct contact of foods or other agents to the skin. Repeated contact may result in eczematous lesions (see *eczema*). It is due to either an *IgE*-mediated reaction (*food allergy, latex allergy, animal dander, drug allergy*) or a direct *histamine* release (cinnamaldehyde, nicotinic acids, dimethylsulfoxide). Chefs, sandwich makers, and veterinarians are commonly affected.

PROTEIN KINASE C (PKC)

PKC is a calcium-dependent enzyme (see *calcium mobilization*) associated with the inner surface of the plasma membrane. Its activity is greatly influenced by the action of membrane-associated *diacylglycerol* (DAG), a product generated by *phospholipase C* (PLC) or *phospholipase D* (PLD). PKC phosphorylates intracellular target proteins on serine and threonine residues, and thereby participates in many different *signal transduction* pathways. *Phorbol ester* (e.g., TPA or PMA) can substitute for DAG in the activation of PKC. Interestingly, PKC executes inhibitory *phosphorylation* reactions on *phospholipase C* (PLC). PKC exists in many *isoforms* that are derived both from several *genes* and from *alternative splicing*.

PROTEIN NITROGEN UNIT (PNU)

The PNU is an alternative to the *Noon unit* to quantify the *allergen* content of a test solution. The amount of allergen that contains 0.01 µg of protein nitrogen is defined as 1 PNU.

PROTEIN TYROSINE KINASES

(See *tyrosine kinases.*)

PROTEIN TYROSINE PHOSPHATASES

(See *tyrosine phosphatases.*)

PROTEOGLYCANS

Proteoglycans comprise the major structural unit of the *mast cell granule*. They are large molecules that contain a long protein core of repeating serine and glycine units, to which highly sulfated glycosaminoglycan (GAG) side chains are attached by xylose–galactose–galactose–glucuronic acid links. These links are unique to proteoglycans. It is the nature and degree of sulfation of the GAG side chains which determine the molecular species of proteoglycans, i.e., *heparin* or chondroitin. The length of the protein core determines the molecular weight. Heparin and *chondroitin sulfate E* have been associated with purified human mast cells, whereas *chondroitin sulfate A* is the predominant proteoglycan found in human *basophils*. Heparin is selectively concentrated only in mast cells. However, chondroitin sulfate E has also been found in human *monocytes*.

The presumed biologic functions of proteoglycans are somewhat speculative. These proteoglycans bind to *histamine, neutral proteases*, and *acid hydrolases* at the acidic pH inside of mast cell secretory granules, and may facilitate uptake and packaging of preformed *mediators* into secretory granules. Under these conditions, mast cell proteoglycans may regulate the stability and activities of many of the enzymes present. During mast cell *degranulation*, cationic mediators dissociate from heparin by ionic exchange, initially with Ca^{2+} (*calcium mobilization* as a consequence of *high-affinity IgE receptor* activation), later with Na^+. Mediators with isoelectric points close to neutrality, e.g., histamine and acid hydrolases, dissociate rapidly. In contrast, the process is slower in the case of the highly charged neutral *proteases*.

After release from the mast cell, proteoglycans may continue to affect those substances that remain associated, particularly the neutral proteases. The stabilizing effect of heparin on *tryptase* activity may be crucial for the proteolytic activity of this enzyme.

PROTOONCOGENE

This is a normal cellular *gene* homologous to an *oncogene*.

PROVOCATION TEST

Provocation tests are used to identify a relevant *allergen* or *occupational agent* responsible for the initiation or maintenance of *allergic inflammation* (see *allergen challenge, exposition test, food challenge*, and *bronchial provocation test*). They may also be used to study pathogenic mechanisms (see *local allergen challenge*). In *hymenoptera allergy*, these tests are used to evaluate the success of *immunotherapy*.

PRURIGO

The name "prurigo" is applied to various secondary, firm, and severely itchy skin eruptions. The diagnosis of the three subtypes — acute prurigo of childhood, subacute prurigo, or chronic prurigo — is made on clinical grounds. The primary lesions of this reaction may be itchy urticarial seropapules, urticarial papules (see *urticaria*), or papulonodules, which subsequently become excoriated by scratching. Acute prurigo (synonymous with stropholus infantum) is believed to be secondary to *food allergy* or insect sting reactions. It starts with seropapules and is seen mostly in young children. Subacute prurigo is believed to start with an urticarial *type I reaction*, followed by a *delayed hypersensitivity* reaction (see *Coombs and Gell classification*, type IV) with cellular infiltration of the urticarial lesion. The clinical findings consist of a dimorphic picture, namely excessively scratched primary lesions, and atrophic, pigmented scars. Chronic prurigo resembles the subacute form, but there are no atrophic scars, and the lesions are mostly located on the extremities.

PRURIGO BESNIER

This is a historic synonym of *atopic dermatitis*.

PRURITUS

Pruritus, or itching, is regarded as a nociceptive stimulus, which is linked to the motor response of scratching. Pruritus is one of the most common sensations of the skin. It is not just disturbing, but may cause sleep loss, nervousness, and impaired performance at work or school.

> Pruritus is not a diagnosis, but a symptom which should lead to proper investigation and identification of the underlying pathology.

Atopic dermatitis, allergic *contact dermatitis*, lichen planus, *urticaria*, and epizoonoses (e.g., scabies) are the most common causes of this type of pruritus. However, pruritus may occur without any skin lesion or parasite (see *parasitic diseases*) present. This pruritus sine materia can be produced by systemic diseases. For instance, bile stasis, diabetes mellitus, kidney diseases, Hodgkin's disease, and many other hematopoietic diseases may cause pruritus. If there is no skin disease present, symptomatic therapy may be started with *corticosteroids* or *antihistamines*.

PSEUDOALLERGENS

> Pseudoallergens are agents that do not induce a *primary* or *secondary immune response*, but cause the same clinical manifestations as observed in *allergic diseases*.

Adverse food reactions can be caused by nonspecific *histamine* release (strawberries, tomato, wine), high contents of biogenic amines like histamine, *serotonin*, tyramine (wine, bananas, cheese, chocolate), or intolerance reaction to *food additives* (tartrazine, salicylate, glutamate). Similar mechanisms are responsible for *adverse drug reactions*. Pseudoallergic reactions in patients sensitive to acetylsalicylic acid (see *aspirin*) or *nonsteroidal antiinflammatory drugs* manifest in *urticaria, anaphylactoid reactions, rhinosinusitis, asthma,* or *hypersensitivity pneumonitis*.

PSEUDOALLERGY

Pseusoallergic reactions share the same clinical manifestation as *IgE*-mediated allergic reactions (see *Coombs and Gell classification*, type I).

> The underlying mechanisms of pseudoallergic reactions lack specific *immune responses*.

The term "pseudoallergy" is used by some authors as a synonym for *idiosyncrasy* (see *pseudoallergens*).

PSEUDOGENE

A pseudogene is an inactive or nonfunctional *gene* in the *genome*. The *DNA* sequences have the structures of expressed genes and were presumably once functional, but have acquired *mutations* during evolution that prevent the generation of a functional gene product.

PULMONARY FIBROSIS

(See *cryptogenic fibrosing alveolitis.*)

PULPITE SÉCHE

Pulpite séche is a chronic, nonallergic, probably *irritant*, squamous or fissured, inflammatory skin reaction (see *dermatitis*) of the fingertips or forefeet. The majority of the frequently adolescent patients have severe asteatosis and a personal or familial history of *atopy*. Lubrication of the skin with greasy ointments may lead to substantial improvement.

PULSUS PARADOXUS

Pulsus paradoxus is an exaggeration of the normal variability in pulse pressure that occurs during respiration. Patients with acute *asthma* have a very high negative intraplural pressure during inspiration and a raised intraplural pressure during expiration. This increased variability in intrathoracic pressure affects venous filling of the heart, and hence affects the stroke volume and output pressure of the left heart. Pulsus paradoxus can be detected by sphygmomanometry at the bedside.

PURPURA

A basic dermatologic lesion, defined as a discoloration of the skin or mucosa due to extravasation of blood.

PURPURA CHRONICA PROGRESSIVA

(See *progressive pigmented purpura.*)

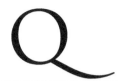

QUALITY OF LIFE IN ASTHMA

Since *asthma* is rarely fatal, the majority of its impact is on quality of life. A variety of *questionnaires* have been developed to quantify the effect of asthma on quality of life. In general, questionnaires, such as the SF-36, that cover all aspects of health are less sensitive to the impact of asthma than questionnaires that are specifically targeted to respiratory problems. Beneficial effects on quality of life are increasingly cited as justification for the introduction of new and expensive *anti-allergic/anti-asthmatic drugs* (see *asthma treatment strategies*). This approach is justified in that a small improvement in *peak expiratory flow rate* (PEF) is not inherently worthwhile, whereas decreases in *asthma exacerbation* rates or improved general quality of life may be worth paying for.

QUESTIONNAIRE

To identify an *asthma*-inducing agent, the following strategy might be helpful (these are sample questions only; their validity and reliability have not been assessed):

☐ Does the patient have symptoms the whole year?

If yes:

☐ Does the patient keep indoor pets and, if so, of what type (see *animal dander, cat allergen*, and *dog allergen*)?
☐ Is moisture or dampness present in any room of the patient's home? (suggests *house-dust mite* or *fungal allergens*)
☐ Is *mold* visible anywhere in the patient's home?
☐ Are there house plants or decaying organic materials in the patient's home?
☐ Has the patient seen *cockroaches* (see *cockroach allergens*) in the home in the past month?

If the patient does not experience symptoms year round:

☐ Do symptoms worsen at particular times? (This may suggest exposure to particular *allergens*: early spring (*tree pollen*), late spring (*grass pollen*), late summer to autumn (*weed pollen*), summer and fall (Alternaria, Cladosporium).

QUINCKE EDEMA

(See *angioedema*.)

R

RADIO ALLERGO SORBENT TEST (RAST)

> The RAST is an in vitro test to measure specific *IgE antibody* levels.

The basis of the test is that the *allergen* of interest is attached to a solid phase (a paper disk is commonly used). The disk is incubated with the patient's serum, and any antibodies that recognize the allergen will bind. The disk is then washed and a radiolabeled detection antibody is used to identify IgE antibodies that have bound to the allergen. The detection antibody will commonly be a mouse anti-human-IgE antibody. The disk is then washed, and the bound radioactivity is proportional to the amount of specific IgE antibodies in the patient's serum (see Figure 39). A similar technique can be used to identify other antibody classes, e.g., IgG_4, IgG_1, etc.

> The original RAST has largely been replaced by alternative methods (see *CAP-system* and *Phadiatop*), but the term "RAST" remains in general use as a description for any measurement of allergen-specific IgE.

The performance of all these tests depends on using a high-quality and consistent *allergen extract* on the solid phase. Therefore, *recombinant allergens* are increasingly used to measure specific IgE antibodies. Such *immunoassays* can be used as an alternative to skin testing (see *prick tests*) for *allergy* diagnosis.

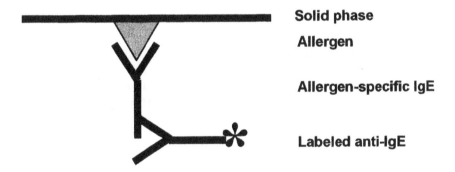

Solid phase

Allergen

Allergen-specific IgE

Labeled anti-IgE

FIGURE 39   Basic principle of the RAST.

RADIOCONTRAST MEDIA

Immediate hypersensitivity reactions to radiocontrast media are quite rare (1% of patients). Table 82 summarizes the suggested pathogenic mechanisms of such reactions, which usually occur within 15 minutes after injection.

Atopy is a predisposing factor for adverse reactions to radiocontrast media. Patients with a previous reaction have a 17 to 35% chance of recurrence on re-exposure. Third-generation radiocontrast media with low osmolarity cause significantly fewer life-threatening reactions. A premedication with *corticosteroids* together with *antihistamines* may decrease the risk of adverse reactions.

TABLE 82
Possible Pathogenic Mechanisms
of Radiocontrast Media-Mediated
Immediate Hypersensitivity Reactions

1. *Complement system*-mediated *mast cell/basophil* activation.
2. Direct *mediator* release from mast cells/basophils.
3. *IgE*-mediated mast cell/basophil activation.

Raf

Raf is a serine/threonine *kinase* and activates *mitogen-activated protein kinase* (MAPK). Raf is activated by *Ras*.

RAGWEED ALLERGENS

Ragweed (Ambrosia) *pollen* contains important *allergens* causing *allergic rhinoconjunctivitis* in North America. Flowers bloom between July and November in most areas, but in some regions, pollen can be counted year round. Some ragweed species can be found in southern Europe, with a main pollen season from August to September.

RAJKA–LANGELAND

This is the most commonly used grading system for the severity of *atopic dermatitis*. Scores from 1 to 3 are given for the criteria extent (<9%, 9 to 36%, >36%), course (>3 months remission/year, <3 months remission/year, continuous course), and intensity (night sleep disturbance by itch: exceptional, intermediate, usual). Scores from 3 to 4 are classified as mild, from 5 to 7 as moderate, and from 8 to 9 as severe atopic dermatitis.

RANTES

RANTES (regulated upon activation, normal T cell expressed and secreted) was initially cloned from *T cells*. It is a *CC chemokine* produced by activated T cells and shown to exert chemotactic activity for memory *CD4⁺* T cells, *eosinophils*, and *basophils*, but not *neutrophils*. Besides T cells, *platelets* also contain large amounts of RANTES, which can be released upon activation (e.g., *platelet-activating factor* activation).

RANTES, *eotaxin*, and *MCP-3* are considered to be the most important specific *chemotactic factors* for eosinophils in *allergic diseases*.

Injection of RANTES into the skin causes eosinophil recruitment, especially in allergic subjects, due to an in vivo *priming* effect. Moreover, along with other chemokines, RANTES is a potent inducer of *histamine* and *mediator* release from basophils (see *histamine-releasing factors*). In addition, RANTES and MIP-1α selectively enhance *IgE* and *IgG₄* production by human *B cells*.

Ras

Ras is a 21-kDa membrane-anchored GTP-binding protein (see *G protein*). It was originally identified as an oncogene in human bladder, lung, and colon carcinomas. Currently, there are more than 50 Ras-related low-molecular-weight GTP-binding proteins. It is now clear that they play an important role in *signal transduction* via many cell surface *receptors* in all mammalian cells. The major pathway leading to Ras activation results from tyrosine *phosphorylation* of a number of intracellular proteins. The *Src* homology 2/a-collagen related

(Shc) is tyrosine phosphorylated by *tyrosine kinases*, and this event leads to an interaction with the small adapter protein, Grb2. Grb2 then interacts with the 150-kDa guanylnucleotide exchange factor for Ras, SOS. SOS is targeted to the plasma membrane, which allows the rapid conversion of Ras from the inactive GDP-bound to the active GTP-bound state (see Figure 40). Ras activation begins its downstream signaling through association with the serine/threonine kinase, *Raf*. Activated Raf phosphorylates and activates *mitogen-activated protein kinases* (MAPKs).

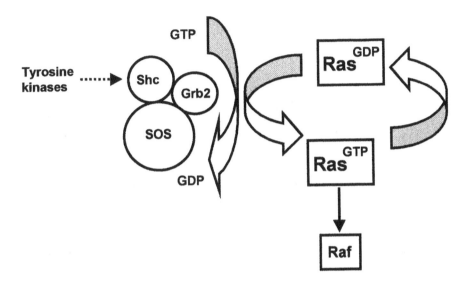

FIGURE 40   Upstream and downstream signaling events related to Ras activation.

RAST

(See *radio allergo sorbent test*.)

RAT BASOPHILIC LEUKEMIA (RBL-2H3)

The RBL-2H3 cell line is a factor-independent tumor analog of *mucosal mast cells* (MMC) that has been used extensively to study the structure and function of the *high-affinity IgE receptor*. In contrast, RBL-2H3 cells are refractory to the actions of many nonimmunological stimuli, including *compound 48/80* and *substance P*.

RAT MAST CELLS

Two distinct populations of rat *mast cells* can be distinguished according to their fixation properties: (1) formalin-sensitive mast cells, which are called atypical or *mucosal mast cells* (MMC), and (2) formalin-resistant mast cells, which are called typical or *connective tissue mast cells* (CTMC). The different staining characteristics of MMC and CTMC reflect differences in their *proteoglycan* content (see Table 83).

> CTMC (skin and peritoneal mast cells) contain mostly *heparin*, and MMC (intestinal and *bone marrow-derived mast cells*) mostly *chondroitin sulfate E*.

CTMC can also be distinguished from MMC by their *neutral protease* content. *Chymase* I (rat mast cell *protease I* found in small intestine, skin, tongue, intestinal serosa, and lung parenchyma) and *carboxypeptidase* are found in CTMC, but chymase II (rat mast cell *protease II* found in intestine and bronchial epithelium) is dominant in MMC. Both types of cells store *histamine,* albeit in different amounts: MMC about 2 pg/cell and CTMC about 35 pg/cell. Stimulation via the *high-affinity IgE receptor* of CTMC leads to the preferential production of *prostaglandin* D_2 (PGD_2), while activated MMCs synthesize *leukotrienes* (LTC_4 and LTB_4) as well as PGD_2. Moreover, MMC and CTMC vary functionally in their sensitivity to different stimuli.

> While both CTMC and MMC can be activated by *IgE*-dependent mechanisms, only CTMC have been shown to be responsive to nonimmunological activation.

Furthermore, disodium *cromoglycate* and *theophylline* inhibit *allergen*-induced histamine release from serosal CTMC (see *immediate hypersensitivity*), but not from MMC isolated from intestine (see also *mast cell heterogeneity*).

TABLE 83
Characteristics of Rat Mast Cells

Characteristics	CTMC	MMC
Size	10–20 mm	5–10 mm
Formaldehyde fixation	Resistant	Sensitive
Staining	Safranin	Alcian blue
T cell dependence	No	Yes
Protease content	Protease I	Protease II
Proteoglycans	Heparin	Chondroitin
Histamine	35 pg/cell	2 pg/cell
PGD_2	+	+
LTC_4	–	++
Activation by		
IgE *cross-linking*	Yes	Yes
Compound 48/80	Yes	No
Substance P	Yes	No
Inhibition by cromoglycate	Yes	No

REACTIVE AIRWAYS DYSFUNCTION SYNDROME (RADS)

RADS was first described in patients who developed *airway hyperresponsiveness* and *asthma*-like symptoms after a single exposure to high concentrations of *irritant* or toxic fumes. Subsequently, it has become clear that a similar process can occur after multiple exposures to irritants, and the term "irritant-induced asthma" is now preferred by many authorities. A wide variety of causative agents have been implicated including acids, alkalis, ammonia, smoke (see *smoking*), *sulfur dioxide* (SO_2), chlorine, aldehydes, *isocyanates*, etc.

> In contrast to *allergic asthma*, with RADS the patient need not have a latent interval (a period of exposure without symptoms).

The patient does not show specific *sensitization* and does not necessarily show a positive *bronchial provocation test*. Airway hyperresponsiveness or peak flow variability is a required element in the diagnosis. The histology of irritant-induced asthma is somewhat different from that found in ordinary allergic asthma or ordinary *occupational asthma*. Typically the basement membrane thickening (see *subepithelial fibrosis*) is much more exuberant, and there may be prominent *edema* with relatively less cellular *inflammation*. *Eosinophils* are sometimes apparent on conventional microscopy, but they and their *granule* products (see *eosinophil granule proteins*) will usually be demonstrable by *immunohistochemistry*. The natural history of irritant-induced asthma is for gradual improvement, although not all patients make a full recovery. Compensation arrangements for this disease vary between countries and, in some cases, irritant-induced asthma is regarded as an industrial injury and is handled under regulations different from those applied to cases of occupational asthma (see also *isocyanate-induced asthma*).

REACTIVE OXYGEN SPECIES

(See *oxygen metabolites*.)

READING FRAME

The reading frame is one possible way of reading a *nucleotide* sequence as a series of triplets. An open reading frame (ORF) contains no termination *codons* (see *stop codon*) and provides a continuous series of sequence information for the *translation* into protein.

RECEPTOR

A receptor is a molecule that can bind other molecules (= ligands). Many receptors are located on cell surfaces and can initiate, as a consequence of *cross-linking*, a variety of cellular responses that require *signal transduction* (see *high-affinity IgE receptor*, *cytokine receptors*, *death receptors*, *CD40*, *G protein-coupled receptors*, *T cell antigen receptor*, and *B cell antigen receptor*). Other receptors are intracellularly located (e.g., *corticosteroid receptor*).

RECEPTOR CROSS-LINKING

(See *cross-linking*.)

RECESSIVE

This means that the manifestation of a trait is only expressed in *homozygotes* (see *dominant*).

RECOMBINANT ALLERGEN

Traditional methods of diagnosis and treatment of *allergic diseases* have relied on the use of heterogeneous *allergen extracts*. The problems with these extracts are that the absolute potency is difficult to define, and some patients have adverse reactions when the extracts are injected (during *immunotherapy*) that can be life-threatening (see *anaphylactic reaction*).

> Following *cloning of allergens*, the generation of purified recombinant *allergens* expressed in bacteria, yeast, or insect cells offers the prospect of using defined proteins for both diagnosis and treatment.

An increasing number of recombinant allergens have been produced, and it is possible to investigate whether cocktails of three to four allergens would be suitable for clinical purposes. Typical *vectors* in which allergens have been expressed include pGEX and pET (in E. coli); pSAY-1 (in the yeast Saccharomyces) and pPIC 9 (in the yeast *Pichia pastoris*), and the baculovirus system, yielding 1 to 10 mg/l. The allergens can be obtained with a high degree of purity (see Figure 41), and in many cases have excellent immunoreactivity when used in *prick tests* or *immunoassays* to detect *IgE antibodies* in serum (see *RAST*, *Phadiatop*, *CAP-system*). Recombinant allergens from *house-dust mite* (Der p 2, Blo t 5, Der p 5), *aspergillus* (Asp f 1, Asp f 4, Asp f 6), *cockroach* (Bla g 4, Bla g 5), and *grass pollen* (Phl p 1, Phl p 5) have good biologic activity on skin testing and elicit positive wheal and flare reactions using picogram doses of protein.

> Recombinant allergens are essential for providing sufficient quantities of highly purified protein for structural studies.

It is possible to manipulate allergen sequences and to produce partial constructs for investigation of functional or immunologic activity. Using site-directed mutagenesis, site-specific variants of Der p 2 have been produced that have reduced binding for IgE antibodies. These experiments allow *B cell epitopes* to be localized and can also be applied to investigate functional domains of the allergen, for example, the active sites of enzyme activity or the ligand binding regions. Moreover, the *sequence homology* between allergens and other protein families can be used to generate molecular models of the *tertiary structure* of allergens. Two examples involve mite allergen Der p 1, whose structure has been modeled on the cysteine *protease, papain*, and *cockroach allergen*, Bla g 4, which has been modeled on other calycin structures for which X-ray crystal (see *X-ray crystallography*) coordinates were known (see Figure 15 in *cloning of allergens*). The X-ray crystal structures of several allergens have been determined, including mouse and rat urinary proteins (Mus m 1 and Rat n 1), *ragweed* Amb a 5, and chironomid hemoglobin, and *birch pollen* allergen Bet v 1. The tertiary structure of the Group 2 mite allergens has been determined by *nuclear magnetic resonance (NMR) spectroscopy.*

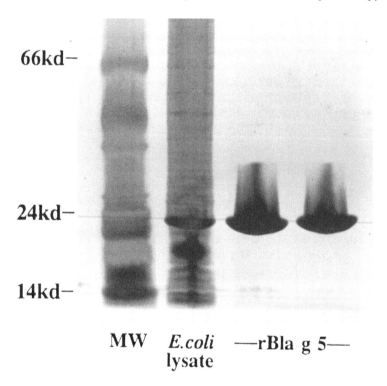

FIGURE 41   The cockroach allergen Bla g 5 was produced as a recombinant protein. Gel electrophoresis and protein staining show that the allergen is obtained with a high degree of purity. (From Arruda, L.K., Vailes, L.D., Platts-Mills, T.A.E., Hayden, M.L., and Chapman, M.D., Induction of IgE antibody responses by glutathione *S*-transferase from the German cockroach (*Blattella germanica*), *J. Biol. Chem.*, 272, 33, 1997. With permission.)

RECOMBINANT PEPTIDE VACCINES

Besides synthetic *peptides*, several strategies exist for the production of recombinant peptide vaccines. These include *recombinant allergens* and *epitopes*, recombinant chimeric proteins associated with the *major histocompatibility complex* (MHC), *immunoglobulin* variable regions or surface *antigen receptors* of *T* and *B cells*, as well as genetic immunization with *DNA* fragments encoding *antigens* (see *DNA immunotherapy*). The treatment of *allergic diseases* would be directed at inducing *anergy* (see *immunotherapy*) or *apoptosis* of allergen-reactive *T cell clones*, whereas a target for prophylactic "vaccine" treatment would be more difficult to rationalize. These technologies are relatively new and will require development.

RECOMBINATION

A recombination is the formation of new combinations of linked *genes* by *crossing-over* (breakage and rejoining) between their loci (see *gene rearrangement*).

RECOMBINATION HOTSPOT

A *recombination* hotspot is any *DNA* sequence that is associated with an abnormally high frequency of recombination.

RECRUITMENT OF INFLAMMATORY CELLS

Inflammatory cells are recruited from the blood into the tissue. In *allergic inflammation*, *eosinophils* preferentially migrate into allergic inflammatory sites. Several mechanisms contribute to the development of tissue *eosinophilia*, such as expression of specific *adhesion molecules* on *endothelial cells*, *chemotactic factors*, or delayed *eosinophil apoptosis* (see also *homing*).

REDUNDANCY

Redundancy describes the property of overlapping functions that almost all *cytokines* bear.

> One single cytokine can often be replaced by another.

This view has been confirmed by observation in *knockout mice* that lack particular cytokine *genes* and demonstrate no abnormalities in their *immune responses*. Redundancy can also be observed between *mediators* that do not represent cytokines. For instance, both *histamine* and *cysteinyl-leukotrienes* alter vasopermeability and induce *mucus* secretion.

RELATIVE RISK (RR)

The RR can be determined by the odds ratio if the disease or event is rare. The odds (incidence of a disease) of exposed people developing the disease compared to the odds of nonexposed people developing the disease serve to determine whether the disease of interest is associated with a certain exposure in a population. An RR larger than 1 in exposed people provides evidence for a possible *association* between the factor and the disease. If the RR is smaller than 1, the factor might have protective effects in terms of the disease. In genetic studies, the term RR indicates how many times more frequent the disease is in individuals positive for a specific *allele* compared to individuals negative for the allele (see *risk*).

REMODELING

(See *airway remodeling*.)

REPRESSOR

A repressor is a *DNA*-binding factor that can downregulate or block transcriptional activity (see *transcription*). Synonymous with "silencer."

REPROTEROL

This is a *β2-agonist*.

RESIDUAL VOLUME

The amount of air left in the lungs after a *forced expiratory maneuver.*

RESOLUTION OF INFLAMMATION

An *inflammation* caused by bacteria, viruses, or *allergens* is resolved as a consequence of *antigen* removal. This might be due to successful *primary* and *secondary immune responses,* by antigen elimination (e.g., treatment with *antibiotics* or antiviral drugs) or, in the case of *allergic diseases,* by avoidance of the antigen (see *allergen avoidance*). If the antigen is unknown or if it cannot be removed for other reasons (e.g., in cases such as *autoallergy, autoimmunity,* or when an allergen cannot completely be avoided), the resolution of inflammation can be induced, at least partially, by antiinflammatory drugs (e.g., *anti-allergic/anti-asthmatic drugs*). Like antigen removal, these drugs reduce either directly (*corticosteroids*) or indirectly (*antihistamines, leukotriene antagonists, cromones*) the expression of *cytokines* at inflammatory sites. This results in the induction of *apoptosis* in antigen-activated and expanded *T* and *B cells,* as well as in *granulocytes* (see *eosinophil apoptosis*), since the *survival factors* are less present or completely removed (see Figure 42). The induction of *T cell apoptosis* occurs via *Fas ligand* (FasL)/*Fas receptor* (FasR) molecular interactions, which is prevented by *IL-2* and *IL-4* during an inflammatory response. In granulocytes, the expression of *Bcl-2* family members changes due to survival factor withdrawal, leading to the induction of apoptosis.

With the specific induction of apoptosis in those cells which had been expanded due to the inflammatory response, the cellular homeostasis is reestablished.

Moreover, with the reduction of cytokine *gene* expression, both the generation of inflammatory cells in the *bone marrow* and the *recruitment of inflammatory cells* are reduced.

RESPIRATORY BURST

All *phagocytes,* including *eosinophils* and *neutrophils,* can generate toxic *oxygen metabolites,* which are essential for the phagocytic oxidative killing mechanism. This generation of oxygen radicals is called "respiratory burst." At least in *granulocytes,* the induction of the respiratory burst requires both *priming* (e.g., *GM-CSF*) and triggering agents (e.g., *PAF, C5a*). Thus, it appears that the cell requires both tyrosine *phosphorylation* of certain target proteins and *calcium mobilization* for the generation of oxygen radicals.

RESPIRATORY FAILURE

This is a failure to maintain normal arterial *blood gas* tension. Two distinct forms are recognized: Type 1 respiratory failure in which there is *hypoxia* with normal or low p_aCO_2, and Type 2 respiratory failure in which there is hypoxia with an elevated p_aCO_2. Type 1 respiratory failure is mainly due to *ventilation–perfusion mismatch* and is characteristic of patients with *emphysema,* acute *asthma,* pulmonary *fibrosis* (see *cryptogenic fibrosing alveolitis*), etc. Patients with Type 1 respiratory failure remain sensitive to CO_2 and can be given high concentrations of oxygen to breathe. Type 2 respiratory failure always involves alveolar hypoventilation, but other causes of hypoxia present as well. Patients with Type 2 respiratory failure have usually lost their responsiveness to CO_2 and rely on hypoxic drive to maintain their respiration. If given high concentrations of oxygen to breathe, they will often stop breathing. The presence of Type 2 respiratory failure in acute asthma is an indication for elective *ventilation,* but when Type 2 respiratory failure occurs in *COPD,* care must be taken not to ventilate people who will not be able to be weaned off the ventilator. It is therefore

Inflammation

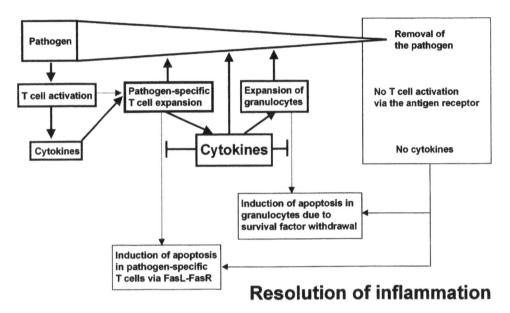

FIGURE 42   Mechanisms of inflammatory responses and the resolution of inflammation as a consequence of apoptosis induction.

important to accurately diagnose asthma versus COPD, based on previous history, knowledge of lung physiology, etc.

RESPIRATORY SYNCYTIAL VIRUS (RSV)

RSV is an *RNA* paramyxo virus that is the single most important agent causing infantile bronchiolitis and pneumonia. RSV infection is an important cause of childhood wheezing (see *wheeze*) and may lead to *asthma*.

RESTRICTION ENZYMES

(See *endonucleases*.)

RESTRICTION FRAGMENT LENGTH POLYMORPHISM (RFLP)

RFLP is a variation in a *DNA* sequence that alters the length of a restriction fragment due to *mutations* in a specific recognition site for a restriction *endonuclease* which either destroy or create a restriction site. RFLPs are usually biallelic and convenient DNA *markers* for *linkage* analyses. Both *genotypes* can thus be distinguished by enzymatic digestion with a specific endonuclease.

REVERSIBILITY

Patients with *asthma* will usually show improved *lung function tests* after inhaling a *β2-agonist*. This reversibility is a characteristic feature of asthma, but is not absolutely essential to the diagnosis. Patients with good lung function may not be capable of further improvement, but will show *peak flow variability* when serial *peak expiratory flow rate* (PEFR) measurements are made. Alternatively, they may show marked *airway hyperresponsiveness*. Patients with *COPD* may show some reversibility or may have irreversible *airway obstruction*.

RFLP

(See *restriction fragment length polymorphism.*)

RHEUMATOID ARTHRITIS (RA)

RA is an autoimmune disease (see *autoimmunity*) that is, in contrast to *IgE*-mediated *allergic inflammation*, characterized by an aberrant *Th1 cell* function. Moreover, overproduction of *TNF-α* and consequent *inflammation* of the synovia of joints appear to be central in the pathogenesis of the disease. Treatment with anti-TNF-α *monoclonal antibodies* (mAbs) has been successful in clinical trials (see *anticytokine therapy*).

RHINITIS

Rhinitis can be classified into allergic (perennial and seasonal *allergic rhinitis*) and nonallergic (see *vasomotoric rhinitis*). The traditional symptoms of rhinitis are nasal blockage, itching, sweating bouts, and increased nasal surface fluid. Rhinitis is most common in patients aged 15 to 25 and is rare in patients over 45. As with other *allergic diseases* (see *asthma epidemiology*), the prevalence of rhinitis is steadily increasing. Allergic rhinitis involves an early phase (see *immediate hypersensitivity*), largely mediated through *mast cells*, and a late phase (see *delayed hypersensitivity*) that involves cellular infiltration and *mediator* release. Studies of the nasal mucosa have shown that the total number of mast cells is increased in allergic rhinitis. Moreover, the numbers of both mast cells and *eosinophils* increase in the mucosa during the *pollen* season.

RHINITIS MEDICAMENTOSA

This form of *rhinitis* is caused by the prolonged use of *decongestant* nose drops or sprays, or other medications.

RHINOCONJUNCTIVITIS

Coexistent *rhinitis* and *conjunctivitis*, often associated with *allergy* to seasonal *allergens* such as *pollens* (see *allergic rhinoconjunctivitis*).

RHINOMANOMETRY

Rhinomanometry is a method to measure airway resistance in the nose by analyzing the nasal air flow. It is performed with a face mask and a pneumotachograph. The resulting pressure change is measured with a manometer via a tube either to one nostril or through the mouth to the back of the nose. The method is frequently used in *exposition tests* and in clinical studies.

RHINOSINUSITIS

Rhinosinusitis is a coexistent *inflammation* of the nasal mucosa (see *rhinitis*) and paranasal sinuses. Chronic inflammation may cause *nasal polyps*.

RHINOVIRUS

Rhinovirus particularly affects nasal *epithelial cells* and causes common cold. It contains a single strand of *RNA*. Rhinovirus infection is associated with the majority of *asthma exacerbations* in children (see *childhood asthma*) by upregulating *inflammation* in the lung. It could be demonstrated that rhinovirus infection followed by *allergen challenge* leads to an increased infiltration of *eosinophils*.

RHONCHI

Old-fashioned term for *wheezes*.

RIBONUCLEIC ACID (RNA)

RNA almost always exists as a single-stranded polymer of four different *nucleotides*. In RNA, the sugar is ribose. The base *thymine*, which occurs in *DNA*, is replaced by uracil (U). RNA is synthesized *complementary* to a DNA template by *RNA polymerases*. RNA molecules serve different functions in the eukaryotic cells (see also *gene*). They are either translated into proteins (see *messenger RNA* and *translation*) or have structural functions (ribosomal RNA) or are part of enzyme complexes (e.g., spliceosome).

RISK

The absolute risk is defined as the incidence of a disease in a population (see *relative risk*).

RISK FACTORS

There has been an increase in *asthma* (see *asthma epidemiology*) and other atopic diseases (see *atopy*) throughout the world. Table 84 lists apparent factors associated with a higher risk for *IgE*-mediated *allergic diseases*. Moreover, it appears that *smoking* and *allergen* exposure during pregnancy represent additional risk factors for *childhood asthma* (see *gene environmental interactions*).

TABLE 84
Risk Factors for Atopic Diseases

1. Positive family history
2. Male sex
3. Low birth weight
4. Maternal smoking
5. Higher parental socioeconomic status
6. Smaller family size
7. Good hygienic conditions
8. Low frequency of infections during early childhood

RNA

(See *ribonucleic acid.*)

RNA POLYMERASE

This enzyme transcribes *DNA* into *RNA* (see *transcription*). RNA polymerase I produces ribosomal RNA. In contrast, most of the cellular *genes* are individually transcribed by RNA polymerase II.

RODENT ALLERGY

This form of *allergy* has to be considered in workers at laboratory animal facilities. *Allergic rhinoconjunctivitis* and *asthma* (see *occupational asthma*) are frequently the consequences of mouse, rat, and guinea pig exposure. Most of the relevant *allergens* occur primarily in urine. Hair, dander, and dust act as carriers of urine allergens.

RODENT T CELLS

Rodent *T cell* systems have been used extensively in characterization of *primary* and *secondary immune responses*. The major T cell surface markers (see *CD antigens*) and functional phenotypes were first identified in mice, and subsequently confirmed in human systems. As in humans, *Th1*, *Th2*, and *Th0* functional phenotypes orchestrate immune responses by the production of *cytokines* and by cognate interactions (see *cognate/noncognate interactions*) with other immune cells.

ROTADISK

This is a multidose *dry powder inhaler* that is breath-activated and delivers the micronized drug together with a carrier powder of lactose or glucose (see also *turbohaler*).

RSV

(See *respiratory syncytial virus.*)

RUSH IMMUNOTHERAPY

In this form of *immunotherapy* with bee or wasp venom (see *hymenoptera allergy*), the initial course is condensed into a short period of one or a few days, during which the top dose is reached. Patients then continue on maintenance therapy.

S

SALBUTAMOL

Salbutamol is a *β2-agonist*.

SALMETEROL

Salmeterol is a *β2-agonist*.

SANDBOX DERMATITIS

Sandbox *dermatitis* (dermatitis papulosa juvenilis) consists of small, white or pale papules, and is frequently seen in children with an atopic constitution (see *atopy*). Individual lesions may coalesce to a plaque with a rough or raspy feel. A spontaneous remission is common.

s_aO_2

The saturation of oxygen in arterial blood. Due to the sigmoid nature of the hemoglobin oxygen dissociation curve, 90% saturation is achieved when the p_aO_2 is approximately 7.6 kPa. When the p_aO_2 falls below this, there is a sharp fall in s_aO_2. The three principal determinants of oxygen delivery to the tissues are s_aO_2, the hemoglobin concentration, and the cardiac output.

SAR

(See *scaffold-associated region*.)

SARCOIDOSIS

Sarcoidosis is a relatively common multisystem disorder that often affects the lungs. In its most benign form, it causes bilateral hilar lymphadenopathy sometimes associated with iritis, arthritis, skin rashes (*erythema nodosum*) and infiltration of old scars. Sarcoidosis can affect the central *nervous system*, causing a wide variety of clinical disorders. In the lungs, sarcoidosis can cause a diffuse granulomatous process seen radiographically as widespread nodular shadowing.

> Immunophenotyping of the *bronchoalveolar lavage* (BAL) *lymphocytes* is often useful, since the disease is associated with an accumulation of *CD4+ T cells* in the lungs.

Typically the patient will have relatively normal lung function at presentation, although there may be some reduction in carbon monoxide *transfer tests*. If the disease is widespread and progresses, it can cause pulmonary *fibrosis*, which will lead to worsening lung function (characteristically a restrictive pattern), poor gas transfer, and a degree of *respiratory failure*.

> The etiology of sarcoidosis is unknown, but there are environmental and genetic predispositions.

For example, the disease is more common in Ireland and in the Caribbean and appears to behave differently in people of African origin living in the U.S. Acute sarcoidosis does not require specific treatment, unless the eyes are affected or the plasma calcium is elevated.

Chronic sarcoidosis will usually respond to oral *corticosteroids*, and the duration of the course is judged by serial *lung function tests*.

SARCOMA (Src) TYROSINE KINASES

This is a family of *tyrosine kinases*. Table 85 lists some *receptors* important in *allergic inflammation* that are known to be associated with Src family tyrosine *kinases*. Another member, Src, is activated by *arrestin*, which links *G protein* and tyrosine kinase pathways.

TABLE 85
Associations of Src Family Kinases with *Antigen Receptors, Cytokine Receptors*, and Other Receptors

Receptor	Involved Src Kinase
T cell antigen receptor	Lck, Fyn
B cell antigen receptor	Lyn, Btk, Fyn
High-affinity IgE receptor	Lyn
Fc receptors	Lyn, Fgr
IL-5 receptor	Lyn
Fas receptor	Lyn
CD4	Lck
CD8	Lck
CD19	Lyn

SCAFFOLD-ASSOCIATED REGION (SAR)

SARs are *DNA* sequences that are bound to the *nuclear matrix* in the nucleus in vivo. They define transcriptionally active *chromatin* loops. Proteins binding DNA take part in the unfolding process of chromatin in a cis-acting manner. SAR-containing *transgenic mice* show an integration site-independent, copy number-dependent level of *transcription* (see also *DNase hypersensitivity*).

SCALE

A basic dermatologic lesion, defined as a falt plate or flake of stratum corneum. The subtypes of collarette scale, furfuraceous scale, ichthyosiform scale, and psoriasiform scale are distinguished on clinical grounds and are characteristic for the underlying skin disease.

SCF

(See *stem cell factor*.)

SCHAMBERG'S DISEASE

(See *progressive pigmented purpura*.)

SCHISTOSOMIASIS

Raised *IgE* levels and *eosinophilia* are characteristic immunological findings in subjects infected with Schistosoma spp. Various stages in the life cycle of the parasite are able to elicit immunological responses, including juvenile and adult worms and soluble egg *antigens*. Schistosome egg antigens sequestered in inflammatory granuloma are presented to *CD4+* *T cells*, which respond with the production of *Th2 cytokines*. This response can be reduced by *IL-12* or anti-*IL-4* treatment (see *cytokine therapy* and *anticytokine therapy*). It is thought that antilarval IgE may be protective and that IgG_4 production antagonizes this activity. Factors other than T-cell-mediated immunological mechanisms are important in resistance to, and infectivity of, schistosomes (see also *parasitic diseases*).

SCHNITZLER SYNDROME

This rare syndrome is a combination of *urticaria vasculitis*, IgM-paraproteinemia, hyperfibrinogenemia, and painful bone involvement.

SCHÖNLEIN–HENOCH PURPURA

(See *allergic vasculitis*.)

SCLERODERMA

Scleroderma is a chronic disease of unknown cause that may affect the skin or may occur as a systemic disease (systemic sclerosis).

In both its forms, there is a diffuse involvement of connective tissue characterized by *fibrosis* of the skin, and in systemic sclerosis, also of various internal organs. Skin biopsies of scleroderma patients exhibit elevated levels of *collagen* type I *gene* expression in *fibroblasts*. *Mast cells* have been demonstrated in increased numbers in the skin lesions of "early" inflammatory stages of scleroderma, but not in clinically uninvolved skin of the same patients nor in the skin of patients with "late" quiescent scleroderma.

SCORAD

This is a scoring system for the severity of *atopic dermatitis*, established by the European task force on atopic dermatitis in 1993. *Erythema*, *edema*/papulation, oozing/*crusts*, *excoriation*, and *lichenification* are scored on a 0 to 3 scale; the affected areas are estimated on a 0 to 100 scale using the rule of nine; subjective symptoms are scored separately; and a final, total score is calculated from these data.

SCRATCH TEST

The scratch test is a *skin test* based on scratching the *epidermis* with a blood lancet; otherwise quite similar to the *prick test*.

SEASONAL ALLERGENS

Seasonal *allergic rhinoconjunctivitis* is caused by *grass pollen, tree pollen, weed pollen allergens*, or fungal spores (see *fungal allergens*). In Europe, tree pollination occurs from March to May, whereas pollination of grasses is at its peak in June or early July. Weed pollination takes place in July and August. *Mold* spores can be counted in August and September. *Pollen* grains may be disseminated by airstream for many miles (see *aeroallergens*). *Pollen counts* are usually very high on warm, dry, and sunny days. Rainfall washes pollen from the air. The highest pollen counts occur in the morning and in the late afternoon. Patients suffering from *hay fever* should avoid outdoor activities during these periods (see *allergen avoidance*). During the spring and summer, pollen counts are reported in the weather forecast in many locales.

SEBOSTASIS

(See *dry skin*.)

SECONDARY IMMUNE RESPONSE

Any response of the *immune system* against a known *antigen*, i.e., an antigen the immune system has seen before and reacted against before, is called a secondary immune response. *Antigen-presenting cells* (APC) such as *dendritic cells, monocytes, macrophages*, and *B cells* have been demonstrated to induce secondary immune responses.

SEGMENTAL ALLERGEN CHALLENGE

(See *local allergen challenge*.)

SEGREGATION

This term is used in genetics and describes the separation of allelic *genes* during *meiosis*.

SELECTINS

Selectins are single chain glycoproteins which currently includes three members: L-selectin (found on *leukocytes*, ligands include mannose-6-P), E-selectin (found on *endothelial cells*, ligands include sialylated Lewis X) and P-selectin (found on *endothelial cells*, ligands include Lewis X and CD15).

> Selectins are important *adhesion molecules* that bind to polysaccharides, and are important in the first step of leukocyte/endothelial cell interactions required for the *recruitment of inflammatory cells*.

P-selectin is carried inside of endothelial cells in *granules* known as *Weibel–Palade bodies* and is redistributed to the cell surface within minutes following exposure to *leukotrienes* (e.g., LTB_4), *complement factors* (e.g., *C5a*), or *histamine*.

SELECTION

The action of environmental factors on a particular *phenotype*, and hence its *genotype* is based on differences in biological fitness. Survival of the fittest is called selection.

SENSITIZATION

Patients who have *IgE antibodies* against *allergens* are said to be sensitized.

> Sensitization can be demonstrated by skin *prick tests* or *immunoassays* (see *RAST, Phadiatop, CAP-system*), but this does not necessarily mean that the patient has an *allergic disease* as a result of that IgE antibody.

In most settings, there is an initial, symptom-free period of exposure leading to *T cell sensitization*, in which an *allergen-induced immune response* occurs. In a further period of allergen exposure, the patient may proceed to develop clinical symptoms as a consequence of *immediate* and *delayed hypersensitivity* reactions.

SEQUENCE HOMOLOGY

Sequence homology describes the extent to which two or more sequences (either *DNA* or protein, see *DNA sequencing*) are the same. Using computerized databases, the relationship between sequences can be determined. This information is useful for placing new sequences within previously identified families of *genes* or proteins, for identifying common motifs and functional domains. DNA databases include GenBank (Los Alamos National Laboratory) and the EMBL Data Library (European Molecular Biology Laboratory, Heidelberg). The Brookhaven National Laboratory Protein Database is a repository for protein structures.

SEROTONIN

5-Hydroxytryptamine (serotonin), derived from tryptophan, can be found in certain *rat mast cells*, but is not in human *mast cells*. The rat mast cell cannot synthesize serotonin, but takes it up from extracellular sources by an active uptake process in the cell membrane, which is similar to that found in *platelets*.

SERUM SICKNESS

Serum sickness arises after systemic injection of a foreign *antigen*, causing type III *hypersensitivity* reaction (see *Coombs and Gell classification*). It is characterized by fever, urticarial rushes (see *urticaria*), arthritis, and nephritis. It develops 7 to 10 days after antigen application, and may persist for 2 to 3 weeks.

SEX-LINKED DISEASE

This is a disease caused by a defective *gene* carried on a sex *chromosome*.

SHIP

This is a *tyrosine phosphatase* that blocks *phosphatidylinositol-3-kinase* (PI3-kinase).

SHP-1

This is a *tyrosine phosphatase* involved in negative *signaling* (see *immunosuppressive mechanisms*).

SHP-2

This is a *tyrosine phosphatase* that can act as an adapter molecule or as a negative regulator of *signaling* pathways.

SHOCK

(See *anaphylaxis*.)

SIB PAIR ANALYSIS

The presence of a disease in affected siblings is compared with the frequency with which each sib has none, one, or two *alleles* in common at the test *locus*, as each sib has a 1 in 2 chance of receiving each allele at a locus from each parent (see *twin studies*).

SIGNALING

(See *signal transduction*.)

SIGNAL TRANSDUCER AND ACTIVATOR OF TRANSCRIPTION (STAT)

Similar to *signal transduction* pathways, the same *transcription factors* are often activated by many different cell surface *receptors*.

It is not completely clear at the moment how selective *gene* activation is mediated.

One possibility is that, besides transcription factors (see *guanine–adenine and thymine–adenine repeats*), additional changes in the chromatin structure are needed for gene activation (see *DNase hypersensitivity*). However, there are also some specific transcription factors that are specifically activated following stimulation of a single *cytokine receptor*. At least part of such a mechanism involves STAT proteins. There are currently six known members of the

STAT family with masses from 84 to 113 kDa. STATs transduce a signal from a cytokine receptor to a *transcription* regulatory element of *DNA*.

STAT proteins are cytoplasmic proteins that are activated by *Janus kinases* (Jaks).

Phosphorylated STATs dimerize and move to the nucleus, where they bind to specific DNA elements, activating transcription (see Figure 43).

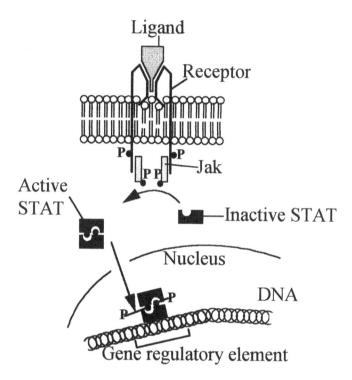

FIGURE 43   Diagram showing simplified Jak/STAT interaction. Receptor dimerization and molecular complexing with Jaks catalyzes *phosphorylation* and activation of cytosolic inactive STAT molecules to the active state. The active STAT translocates to the nucleus, where it binds to a gene regulatory element on the DNA and initiates transcription.

Each cytokine receptor is specific for a certain STAT or STATs, and each activated STAT activates transcription of only certain genes (see Table 86).

Th1 differentiation is driven by *IL-12* and requires the IL-12-responsive transcription factor STAT4, while *Th2* differentiation is elicited by *IL-4* and requires the IL-4-responsive transcription factor STAT6.

This view has clearly been demonstrated using STAT4- and STAT6-*knockout mice*.

SIGNAL TRANSDUCTION

Ligands such as *antigens*, *cytokines*, inflammatory *mediators*, *neuropeptides*, or hormones bind to specific *receptors*, which are usually expressed on cell surfaces.

A common element in signal initiation is the *cross-linking* of receptors or receptor subunits, which juxtaposes their cytoplasmic domains and allows the receptor to engage the intracellular signaling machinery.

TABLE 86
Activation of STAT Proteins by Cytokines

STAT	Mass (kDa)	Cytokine
1α, 1β	91, 84	*IFN-α, IFN-β, IFN-γ*
2	113	IFN α/β (with STAT1)
3	92	*IL-2, IL-6*, IL-7, *IL-9, IL-10*, IL-11, *IL-15*, EGF, *G-CSF*
4	89	IL-12
5A, 5B	77, 80	IL-2, *IL-3, IL-5*, IL-7, IL-15, *GM-CSF*
6	94	IL-3, IL-4, *IL-13*

This machinery consists of a network of proteins that transform multiple external stimuli into appropriate cellular responses. Molecules from this network can be placed into ordered biochemical pathways in which signal propagation occurs through the sequential establishment of protein–protein and small-molecule–protein interactions. Some of the best-studied intracellular cascades are the *tyrosine kinase* and *G protein-coupled receptor* pathways. In the cases of receptor tyrosine *kinases* (e.g., growth factors such as EGF or PDGF) and *cytokine receptors,* recruitment of specific adapter proteins (Grb2 and Shc) creates a tyrosine phosphoprotein scaffold that is anchored at the plasma membrane and serves as an organizing center for components of the *mitogen-activated protein kinase* (MAPK) pathways. G protein-coupled receptors and *antigen receptors* activate *phospholipase C*, which results in intracellular *calcium mobilization*. However, these receptors may also activate MAPK (see Figure 44). This example illustrates the dilemma in current signal transduction research. At present, it is mostly unclear how specificity arises in connecting a given input signal with the appropriate cellular response (see also *adrenergic receptors, B cell antigen receptor, CD40, chemokine receptors, cytokine receptor signal transduction, death receptors, high-affinity IgE receptor, interleukin-4 receptor, interleukin-5 receptor, T cell activation*, and *T cell antigen receptor*).

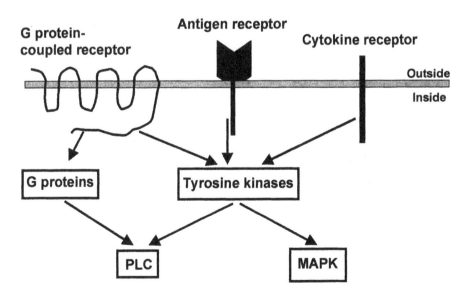

FIGURE 44 Multiple receptors activate PLC and MAPK pathways.

SILENCER

(See *repressor.*)

SILENT CHEST

In acute *asthma exacerbations*, the chest is normally wheezy (see *wheeze*), but if the disease becomes really severe, the amount of air moving through the chest may drop and the chest becomes silent. This is a very bad sign and should prompt consideration of elective *ventilation*.

SILENT MUTATION

This is a *mutation* within a triplet that does not alter the *codon*, usually in the third position.

SINGLE-GENE DISORDER

This is a disease caused by a single mutant *gene*.

SINUS

Air cavities within facial bones are called sinuses. They are lined with mucosa similar to those in other parts of the airways.

SINUSITIS

Sinusitis is an *inflammation* of the mucous membrane of the *sinuses*, often caused by bacterial or viral infection. However, it is also commonly associated with *allergic disease*. Moreover, sinusitis can be due to structural problems of the ostio-meatal complex. Patients with sinus disease often have post-nasal drip, and this can cause *cough* and, in some cases, *asthma exacerbations*. Treatment of the sinus disease may therefore lead to improvement in the lower respiratory symptoms.

SKIN-ASSOCIATED LYMPHOID TISSUE (SALT)

The concept of SALT was proposed by Wayne Streilein in 1978, extending the concept of already established *gut-associated lymphoid tissue* (GALT). In its original meaning, the term summarizes all immunologically active cell systems of the skin such as *keratinocytes, Langerhans cells*, skin *homing T cells, endothelial cells*, and the skin-draining *lymph nodes*. In 1990, Streilein extended his concept by subdivision into endoSALT and exoSALT. However, the dendritic epidermal *gamma/delta (γ/δ) T cells*, which play a crucial role in this extended concept, have been demonstrated in mice but not in humans.

SKIN IMMUNE SYSTEM (SIS)

The concept of the skin *immune system* (SIS) was proposed by Jan Bos in 1986, and proposed that *keratinocytes, Langerhans cells, T cells*, vascular and lymphatic *endothelial cells*, tissue *macrophages, monocytes*, tissue *dendritic cells*, and *mast cells* have to be regarded as *immune-response* associated. In contrast, melanocytes, merkel cells, *fibroblasts*, eccrine and apocrine glandular cells, sebocytes, pericytes, Schwann cells, and *smooth muscle* cells may not be involved in immune reactions. A few years later, constituents of the humoral immune system such as *immunoglobulins* (Igs), *cytokines, neuropeptides, complement factors, prostaglandins, leukotrienes*, fibrinolysins, and free *oxygen metabolites* were included in the concept as well. Besides simply listing the cellular and humoral constituents of SIS, a resident part (keratinocytes, endothelial cells, mast cells, and macrophages), a recruited part (monocytes, *granulocytes*, mast cells, epitheloid cells), and a recirculating part (*NK cells*, dendritic cells) of SIS were outlined.

SKIN-MIXED LYMPHOCYTE REACTION (SMLR)

The SMLR, a standard laboratory procedure, is defined as a co-culture of epidermal cells (see *epidermis*) and *peripheral blood mononuclear cells* (PBMC) or subsets thereof. The epidermal *Langerhans cells*, which may be enriched or purified for this purpose, act as an *antigen-presenting cell* (APC), whereas the *T cells*, which may also be purified, act as responder cells. Tritium-labeled thymidine incorporation assays are the standard method used as a readout system (see *lymphocyte transformation test*).

SKIN TEST

A skin test is used to determine *immediate* or *delayed hypersensitivity* or immunity to an *allergen* or *antigen*.

Multiple skin test methods have been established to assess the reaction state of an individual toward *allergens*. Type I *allergies* (see *Coombs and Gell classification*) are diagnosed by *prick tests*, *scratch tests*, and *intradermal tests* (see *immediate hypersensitivity skin tests*). In contrast, *type IV reactions* are detected by *patch tests*. In addition, photoallergic reactions (see *photoallergy*) may be detected by the *photopatch test*. The *tuberculin test* is an example of delayed hypersensitivity skin testing.

SLOW-REACTING SUBSTANCES OF ANAPHYLAXIS (SRS-A)

SRS-A is a mixture of *mediators* derived from *arachidonic acid* (AA) that are now called *leukotrienes* (LTs).

SMOG

This term describes an extensive increase in *air pollution*. Two types of smog are differentiated: an acid and a photochemical type. The acid type may occur in industrial areas during the winter. High concentrations of *sulfur dioxide* (SO_2), nitric oxides (NO_x), and particulate matter are characteristic. In contrast, photochemical smog arises during the summer when *ozone* is formed by the action of sunlight on *nitrogen dioxide* (NO_2) in the presence of hydrocarbons. These *pollutants* come primarily from car exhaust, fuel combustion, and industrial processes.

SMOKING

Tobacco smoking may be considered as an important *indoor air pollutant*. Several epidemiological studies (see *asthma epidemiology*) show that exposure to tobacco smoking during pregnancy or in infancy is associated with an increased incidence of airway infections, and a higher rate as well as early onset of *asthma* in children (see *childhood asthma*). Subjects exposed to cigarette smoke through active or passive routes may demonstrate *airway hyperresponsiveness*. Smoking affects both the upper and lower airways by inducing *mucus* secretion and nasal mucosal blood flow. In children exposed to tobacco smoke, as well as in smokers, elevated total *IgE* levels and *eosinophil* numbers can be measured.

SMOOTH MUSCLE

The airways are surrounded by smooth muscle from the trachea down to the small *bronchioli*. In the trachea and larger *bronchi*, the muscle is largely posterior and is attached to the semicircular cartilages. Upon contraction, the muscle brings the free ends of the cartilage together, narrowing the bronchus, but the bronchus remains open due to the structural support provided by the cartilages. Further down the bronchial tree (see *airway anatomy*), the smooth muscle is distributed more evenly around the bronchi, so contraction of the smooth muscle leads to a concentric narrowing of the lumen. In the peripheral airways, the fibers run spirally, and so contraction will shorten the bronchi as well as narrowing the lumen (see *airway obstruction*).

The tone in airways smooth muscle is maintained by cholinergic constrictor signals (see *acetylcholine*) carried in branches of the vagus nerve, and adrenergic *bronchodilator* tone is driven by the sympathetic *nervous system*. The sympathetic influence is thought to act predominately at the parasympathetic ganglion level rather than directly at the smooth muscle fibers. This is thought to underlie the ability of the sympathetic neurotransmitter *noradrenaline* to reduce *bronchodilation* when released from sympathetic fibers, and its lack of effect when administered by inhalation. However, airway smooth muscle cells have β2-*adrenergic receptors* and can be relaxed directly by *β2-agonists*. Bronchial tone is also affected by local *hypoxia* and physical reflexes mediated through stretch *receptors*.

SMOOTH MUSCLE HYPERTROPHY

In *asthma*, the *smooth muscle* is hypertrophied (see *airway remodeling*), and shows increased sensitivity to constrictor substances compared to muscle from normal subjects (see *airway hyperresponsiveness*).

SODIUM CROMOGLYCATE

(See *cromoglycate*.)

SOMATIC CELL

Any cell of an organism not belonging to the germ line.

SOMATIC MUTATION

This is a *mutation* that occurs in a *somatic cell* sometime in the life of an individual. Therefore, somatic mutations are not inherited. Cancer is caused by somatic mutations.

SOUTHERN BLOT

This is a technique in molecular genetics first described by Edward Southern to transfer *DNA* fragments separated by agarose gel electrophoresis onto a membrane. These transferred membrane-bound DNA fragments can be further analyzed for the presence of specific DNA sequences by *hybridization* with labeled *oligonucleotides* or fragments.

SOYBEAN ALLERGY

Immediate hypersensitivity reactions, including *anaphylaxis*, due to the ingestion of soybean have shown increasing incidence in the last years. Because of their nutritional and functional benefits, soybean proteins are incorporated into a variety of food products at levels high enough to cause *food allergy*. Soybeans are a member of the legume family of plants that also includes peanuts (see *peanut allergy*).

SPACER DEVICES

Many conventional *metered dose inhalers* deliver their *aerosol* at high speed, and much of the material deposits in the oropharynx. To reduce the oropharyngeal deposition and the need for precise coordination of the activation of the inhaler with inspiration, a number of spacer devices have been developed. These allow the aerosol to be generated in the chamber of the spacer, and patients then breathe in at their own convenience. Spacer devices have been shown to be as effective as *nebulizers* in the treatment of acute severe *asthma*. Spacer devices are also useful for giving inhaled medication to children, provided that appropriate valves are fitted that allow the child to draw in the drug without undue resistance.

SPECIFIC AIRWAYS CONDUCTANCE

This is an alternative method to measure lung function (see *bronchial provocation test*).

SPECIFIC IgE DETECTION

Allergen-specific *IgE* is detected by *immediate hypersensitivity skin tests* and *immunoassays* (see *RAST, Phadiatop, CAP-system*).

SPECIFIC IgE INDUCTION

(See *allergen-induced immune responses, sensitization, allergic inflammation, immunoglobulin class switching*.)

SPHINGOMYELIN

Sphingomyelin (N-acetylsphingosin-1-phosphocholine) is a phospholipid that is cleaved by *sphingomelinase*. The result of this enzymatic reaction is the generation of *ceramide*.

SPHINGOMYELINASE

Sphingomelinase is a *sphingomyelin*-specific *phospholipase C* (PLC). Besides other possible *receptors*, this enzyme is activated by *death receptors* and contributes to the induction of *apoptosis*.

SPIROMETER

A variety of spirometers have been developed for performing *lung function tests*. Historically most of these measured volume against time using a wedge bellows, but most newer spirometers rely on a pneumotach (a small turbine that measures flow rate). The flow rate is then integrated to obtain the volume of air exhaled. The pneumotach-based spirometers make it easy to display the expiratory part of the *flow volume loop* as well as the *forced expiratory maneuver*. Predicted values vary according to height, age, and gender. Most modern spirometers include a program that calculates the predicted values, but tables are available for use with older spirometers. Individual devices are usually consistent, but there is some variation between devices. Therefore, studies that depend on measurement of small differences should always be done with the same spirometer.

SPIROMETRY

Measurement of the bellows function of the lung, either by *forced expiratory maneuvers* using a *spirometer* or with a body plethysmograph (see *body plethsmography*).

SPLICING

Splicing is the process of excision of intronic sequences by a specialized enzyme complex recognizing the *exon/intron* boundaries (GU-AG) in the transcribed *RNA* and subsequent joining of the exon sequences to obtain mature *mRNA*.

SPONGIOSIS

Spongiosis is the secondary loss of cohesion between epidermal cells as a consequence of tissue fluid influx into the *epidermis*. It is the histopathological hallmark of an acute *dermatitis*.

SPUTUM

Material coughed up from the lower respiratory tract, usually consisting of *mucus* and inflammatory cells. In *asthma*, *epithelial cells* may be shed (creola bodies), and the mucus may form spirals (Curshmann's spirals). By microscopy, intact or apoptotic (see *apoptosis*) *eosinophils* may be seen as well as crystals derived from the *major basic protein* (*Charcot–Leyden crystals*).

SPUTUM CYTOLOGY

This is the microscopic examination of cells in *sputum*. The technique is in routine use for diagnosis of lung cancer and has research applications for studying the cellular composition of sputum in *asthma* both in resting state and after *asthma exacerbations* or *allergen challenge*. Following *corticosteroid* therapy, apoptotic (see *apoptosis*) *eosinophils* can be observed in the sputum of asthmatics.

Src

(See *sarcoma tyrosine kinases*.)

ST2

(See *T1*.)

STAPHYLOCOCCUS AUREUS (S. aureus)

S. aureus is a bacterium believed to contribute to *atopic dermatitis* exacerbation. S. aureus could be isolated from the skin of more than 80% of patients with atopic dermatitis, whereas the normal skin is resistant to bacterial colonization. The mechanisms of how S. aureus may intensify skin *inflammation* in these patients may include their ability to secrete bacterial *superantigens*.

STAT

(See *signal transducer and activator of transcription*.)

STATUS ASTHMATICUS

An old term for acute severe *asthma*. Strictly speaking, status asthmaticus was an *asthma exacerbation* that had lasted for at least 24 hours and was unresponsive to standard antiasthma therapy (see *asthma treatment strategies*). However, recognizing that some patients with acute severe asthma deteriorated very rapidly and could even die within the first 24 hours of an exacerbation, the term status asthmaticus was replaced by "acute severe asthma."

STEM CELL FACTOR (SCF)

SCF, also called c-kit ligand or *mast cell* growth factor, is a glycoprotein that is the *gene* product of the Steel (Sl) locus and a ligand for the protooncogene c-kit tyrosine *kinase receptor* (CD117, see *cytokine receptors*). A variety of cells can produce SCF, including *bone marrow* stromal cells and *fibroblasts*. SCF exists in a membrane-bound or proteolytically released soluble form. Together with other *cytokines* such as *IL-3*, *IL-4*, *IL-9*, and *IL-10*, SCF critically regulates the *migration* and survival of *mast cell precursors*, and promotes the differentiation and proliferation of both immature and mature mast cells. Moreover, SCF enhances *IgE*-mediated *histamine* secretion from human lung, heart, uterine, and skin mast cells. Sl mutations result in *mast-cell-deficient mice*.

STEROIDS

(See *corticosteroids*.)

STEROID-DEPENDENT ASTHMA

(See *corticosteroid-dependent asthma.*)

STEROID-RESISTANT ASTHMA

(See *corticosteroid-resistant asthma.*)

STEVENS–JOHNSON SYNDROME

Target-shaped skin lesions with *erosions* and blister formation in limited areas in combination with extensive erosions of the oral mucosa and systemic malaise are the main characteristics of Stevens–Johnson Syndrome. The prognosis of this subtype of drug *intolerance* is good (<1% lethality) (see *adverse drug reactions*).

STOP CODON

Three *codons* cause translational termination (see *translation*) in the synthesis of polypeptides: UAG, UAA, and UGA.

STORAGE MITES

The nonpyroglyphid storage mites belong to two families: Acaridae (genera Acarus and Tyrophagus) and the Glycyphagidae (genera Glycyphagus and Lepidoglyphus). Storage mites feed on decaying vegetation and are most prominent in agricultural environments, where they infest hay and grain. *Allergens* from storage mites are a source of occupational exposure (see *occupational agents*), best documented among Scandinavian farmers who suffer from *asthma* and *rhinoconjunctivitis. Allergy* to storage mites has also been documented in Scotland and the Netherlands. Although these farmers are exposed to many allergens including *pollens, molds* (see *fungal allergens*), *animal dander*, and *house-dust mites*, the prevalence of positive *RAST* was highest to L. destructor in a study examining *sensitization* among Swedish farmers.

STRIDOR

A musical noise caused by partial obstruction of the trachea or larynx. Characteristically, stridor is heard during inspiration, whereas *wheezes* are mainly heard during expiration. The inspiratory timing of stridor is attributed to the greater flow rate of air during inspiration compared to expiration.

SUBEPITHELIAL FIBROSIS

> Increased amounts of *collagen* type III and type V are deposited beneath the basement membrane of the asthmatic airway.

This is observed in all grades of *asthma* and is present to a minor degree in patients with *allergic rhinitis* but no clinical evidence of asthma. The precise significance of subepithelial *fibrosis* is debated, but it seems likely that it has some effects on airways mechanics, and may contribute to nonspecific *airway hyperresponsiveness*. The collagen is deposited by *fibroblasts*. Fibroblast growth and collagen production is regulated by growth factors (e.g., *TGF-β* and *IL-4*) released by *eosinophils* and *mast cells*. On the other hand, fibroblasts produce *GM-CSF*, which contributes to the survival of *eosinophils* in the airways (see *eosinophil apoptosis*), indicating close cellular interactions between these two cell types within chronic inflammatory responses. Subepithelial fibrosis is therefore a marker of ongoing *allergic inflammation* in the airways (see also *airway remodeling*).

SUBMUCOSAL GLANDS

As well as *mucus*-secreting *goblet cells* in the bronchial epithelium (see *epithelial cells*), there are specialized glandular structures in the airways beneath the *smooth muscle* layer. These submucosal glands contribute to the production of airways mucus as well as antibacterial substances such as lysozyme, lactoferin, and a low-molecular-weight anti-*protease*. Submucus gland numbers are normal in *asthma*, but reduced in *COPD*.

SUBSTANCE P

Substance P is a *neuropeptide* that belongs to the family of *tachykinins*. Specific substance P *receptors* are present on airway *smooth muscle* cells, *submucosal glands*, blood vessels, and inflammatory cells. Substance P stimulates *airway obstruction* and *mucus* production, indicating a role of the *nervous system* in the pathogenesis of *asthma*. In addition, it is a potent vasoconstrictor and can also cause microvascular leakage. Moreover, and similar to *compound 40/80*, it activates *mast cells* to release *histamine* in a *G protein*-dependent manner, however independently from *calcium mobilization* and *phospholipase C* activation. *Degranulation* of *eosinophils* by substance P has also been reported (see *neurogenic inflammation*). The amount of substance P in the airways is increased following *ozone* exposure. Substance P is metabolized by *proteases* such as *angiotensin-converting enzyme* (ACE).

SULFITES

This is a group (sodium and potassium sulfites, bisulfites, and metabisulfites) of *food additives* involved in idiosyncratic (see *idiosyncrasy*) food and drug reaction (see *sulfite sensitivity*). These preservatives are added to salads, wine, dehydrated fruits, potatoes, seafood, baked goods, and tea mixtures, to name a few.

SULFITE SENSITIVITY

Ingestion of *sulfites* may produce *asthma* and *anaphylaxis* in some individuals due to *intolerance* reactions. Sulfites are added to foods and drugs as preservatives (see *food additives*). In the acid environment of the stomach, sulfites are converted into *sulfur dioxide* (SO_2) and sulfurous acid (H_2SO_3), which, after inhalation, may cause *airway obstruction*. *Bronchial provocation tests* confirm the diagnosis. Other possible symptoms include flushing, itching, *urticaria*, *angioedema*, and nausea.

SULFUR DIOXIDE (SO_2)

SO_2 is an *outdoor air pollutant* produced by combustion of coal and other fuels containing sulfur. It may also be generated from *sulfites* in the stomach (see *sulfite sensitivity*). This gas, even when encountered at concentrations as high as 0.6 ppm, has little effect on normal individuals. However, persons with *asthma* have been shown to experience remarkable *bronchospasm* after experimental exposure to SO_2. This is thought to be mediated by airway neurons (see *nervous system*). Environmental disasters experienced decades ago, including the killer *smogs* of Donora, PA, in the 1950s and those experienced in London in the last century, were thought to be due in large part to very high levels of SO_2 encountered over a short period of time (see also *irritants*).

SUPERANTIGEN

Superantigens are high-molecular-weight molecules with unique features in terms of *T cell antigen receptor* (TCR) stimulation. In contrast to normal *antigens*, superantigens do not require classical *antigen processing* by *antigen-presenting cells* (APCs). Superantigens bind directly to the β-chain of *MHC class II molecules* (see Figure 45).

Whereas normal antigens can only activate *T cells* carrying the antigen-specific TCR (see *antigen recognition*), superantigens can directly activate all TCRs that belong to a certain TCR family.

For *Staphylococcus aureus* (S. aureus)-derived superantigens, this means that up to 25% of the T cells can be activated. Therefore, the activation of the TCR by superantigens does not occur in a *major histocompatibility complex* (MHC)-restricted fashion (see *MHC restriction*), and may result in *T cell proliferation*, *cytokine* production, or *T cell apoptosis*. In addition to T cell activation, binding of the superantigen to MHC class II molecules also results in the stimulation of the APCs, leading to *TNF-α* and *IL-1* secretion and consequent upregulation of *adhesion molecules* on *endothelial cells*. Although it remains to be shown that superantigens can be the direct cause of a disease, it is clear that they play a central role in the maintenance and exacerbation of inflammatory processes (see *inflammation*). Superantigens from S. aureus have been implicated in the pathogenesis of *atopic dermatitis*. Note that a superantigen may also specifically stimulate T cells as *allergen*, resulting in an anti-superantigen *IgE* response.

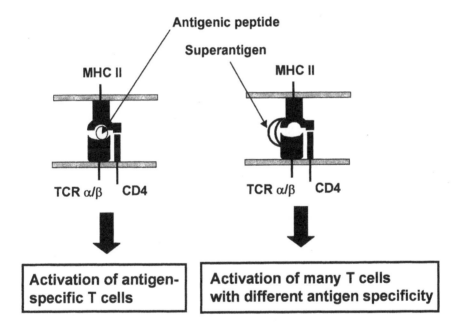

FIGURE 45   Activation of T cells by antigens and superantigens.

SUPEROXIDE ANION (O_2^-)

O_2^- is a highly reactive and destructive oxygen radical (see *oxygen metabolite*) that is generated from oxygen by *NADPH oxidase*.

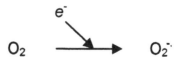

SUPEROXIDE DISMUTASE

This enzyme scavenges *superoxide anion* (O_2^-) to *hydrogen peroxide* (H_2O_2) (see *oxygen metabolites*). It is found in all cells.

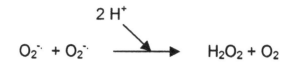

$$2 \, H^+$$
$$O_2^{-} + O_2^{-} \longrightarrow H_2O_2 + O_2$$

SURFACE MOLECULES

Surface molecules are expressed at cell membranes. Many of them are listed within the *CD antigen* classification. Surface molecules usually contain extracellular, transmembrane, and intracellular parts. *Cross-linking* of these molecules by ligand binding often initiates a signal that, following *signal transduction*, is then associated with a functional response(s) of the cell. Some molecules are specific for cell populations. Such *lineage-specific markers* (see *T cell surface markers* and *B cell surface markers*) can be detected by *monoclonal antibodies* (mAbs) and *flow cytometry*. For instance, *lymphocyte* subpopulations are routinely analyzed for diagnostic reasons as well as for immune monitoring (e.g., *extrinsic allergic alveolitis*, *sarcoidosis*, *T cell lymphoma*, *acquired immunodeficiency syndrome*).

SURFACTANT

Surfactant is a compound that reduces the surface tension of a liquid. This way, another lipid can be mixed with it. In the lungs, surfactant is secreted by type II alveolar cells. Surfactant decreases the surface tension of the alveolar wall during expiration, which stabilizes the alveolar spaces as they expand and contract during respiration. Absence of surfactant in premature infants results in respiratory distress syndrome. Surfactant principally consists of dipalmitoyl phosphatidylcholine. Surfactant also contains variable amounts of phosphatidyl glycerol, cholesterol, and surfactant apoproteins.

SURVIVAL FACTORS

Survival factors are *mediators* that prolong the survival of cells. Most of the survival factors represent *cytokines*. Many cells die due to *apoptosis* in the absence of survival factors. In contrast, in the presence of survival factors, they can have a long residence time in tissues. For instance, *eosinophil apoptosis* is delayed in *allergic inflammation* by overexpression of *IL-5*, a mechanism that contributes to the development of *eosinophilia*. In addition, *mast cells* depend on *SCF*. Moreover, *allergen*-activated *T cells* may not die as a consequence of *Fas ligand/Fas receptor* interactions as long as they are exposed to *IL-2* and *IL-4*.

SUSCEPTIBILITY

Susceptibility is the disposition for a certain disease that is caused by inherited factors (see *genetic predisposition*).

SYSTEMIC REACTION

(See *anaphylaxis*.)

T

T1

This is a cell *surface molecule* with >25% sequence *homology* to the type I *IL-1 receptor*. However, it does not bind *IL-1α*, IL-1β, or *IL-1-receptor antagonist*. In the mouse, T1 is exclusively expressed on the surface of *Th2*, but not *Th1 cells* (see *Th1/Th2 markers*). Some functional data suggest that T1 is a co-stimulatory molecule (see *co-stimulation*). The physiological ligand of T1 is currently unknown.

TACHYKININS

Tachykinins are a family of *neuropeptides* characterized by a common C-terminal sequence (Phe-x-Gly-Leu-Met-NH$_2$). Three principal tachykinins have been described in mammals: *substance P*, as well as the *neurokinins* A and B. Tachykinins are almost exclusively localized to neurones, both in the central and peripheral *nervous system*. Substance P and neurokinin A are found in the airways, and the levels of these tachykinins are affected by age, cigarette *smoking*, and various pathological processes. Tachykinin *receptors* are present on *smooth muscle*, *submucosal glands*, and vascular *endothelial cells* in the airways, and mediate nonadrenergic noncholinergic (see *nonadrenergic noncholinergic nerves*) *airway obstruction*.

TACROLIMUS

Tacrolimus (FK506) is an immunosuppressant macrolide (see *immunosuppressive drugs*) produced by the fungus Streptomyces tsukubaensis.

> Similar to *cyclosporin A* (CsA), tacrolimus inhibits *T cell antigen receptor* (TCR)-mediated *calcineurin* activation and consequent *cytokine gene* expression.

Due to its physicochemical properties, tacrolimus penetrates the stratum corneum of inflammatory skin, and is therefore suitable for topical treatment of *atopic dermatitis* and some other inflammatory skin diseases. The clinical effectiveness of oral tacrolimus has been confirmed in psoriasis and atopic dermatitis in controlled clinical trials. Topical administration of tacrolimus has also been effective in atopic dermatitis.

TANDEM REPEAT

Arrays of multiple copies of a specific *DNA* sequence. Due to their length variations in the population and their detection by *polymerase chain reaction* (PCR), they present useful markers for *linkage* analyses and in forensic medicine. Tandem repeats are distinguished based on the size of the repeat array into *microsatellite* (small repeat block of often less than 0.1 kb), minisatellite with an intermediate size array of less than 20 kb, and macrosatellite with stretches larger than 20 kb of tandemly repeated DNA. Macrosatellite DNA constitutes the *centromere* of *chromosomes*.

TATA BOX

This is a common *adenine* and *thymine*-rich *DNA* motif, which is located about 21 to 27 bp upstream of the initiation site of *transcription* of many *genes*. Some authors call it the Hogness box. It can interact with *RNA polymerase* II to initiate transcription. Another *promoter* element found frequently is the G/C-rich element of the *transcription factor* SP-1. Besides the function of correct local initiation of transcription by *RNA* polymerase II, TATA-binding proteins and Sp-1 can cooperate with each other (see *general transcription factors*) and furthermore with inducible transcription factors to increase *mRNA* synthesis rates.

Tc1

> Tc1 cells are *CD8⁺ T cells* able to secrete *cytokines* with a profile similar to *Th1* cytokines. They may participate in the *delayed hypersensitivity* reactions of allergic *contact dermatitis* and in some cases of *autoimmunity.*

These cells have been classified as Tc1 (T cytotoxic type 1 or sometimes Ts1 suppressor type 1) cells. *IFN-γ, IL-12*, and *IL-18* induce Tc1 cell differentiation from CD8 precursors. Tc1 cells have been isolated from patients with tuberculoid leprosy. Cytotoxicity mediated by CD8⁺ T cells does not appear to be greatly affected by the cytokine-secreting profile of the T cell (Tc1 or *Tc2*). Cross-regulation between Tc1/Th1 and Tc2/*Th2* has been demonstrated.

Tc2

> Tc2 cells are a functional phenotype of *CD8⁺ T cells* expressing a *cytokine* pattern similar to *CD4⁺ Th2 cells*; they may participate in the *delayed hypersensitivity* reactions of *allergic diseases.*

They represent a minority of CD8⁺ T cells and require high levels of *IL-4* for their induction from CD8 precursors. Tc2 cells do not provide cognate help to *B cells* (see *cognate/noncognate interactions*) due to their cytolytic activity and the inability of CD8⁺ T cells to interact with *MHC class II molecules* on B cells. However, noncognate help effected by secretion of *immunoglobulin* potentiation cytokines (e.g., *IL-4, IL-6*, and *IL-13*) is possible. Moreover, Tc2 may produce large amounts of *IL-5* generating *eosinophilia.*

> Tc2 cells have disease associations with *allergic asthma*, *atopic dermatitis*, *acquired immunodeficiency syndrome* (AIDS), *hyper-IgE syndrome* (HIES), lepromatous leprosy, and lymphocytic choriomeningitis virus infection.

T CELL

> T cells are *lymphocytes* and belong to the white blood cell (*leukocyte*) compartment of the blood.

In common with most *B cells* (from which they are microscopically indistinguishable) and *monocytes*, they are mononucleated (see *peripheral blood mononuclear cells*, PBMC) and, in the blood, usually spherical. They have a mean diameter of approximately 18 μm, but can range in size from about 10 to 25 μm in diameter. When resident in tissues such as the spleen or *thymus*, they can deform to accommodate available space, which allows for intimate contact of T cells with each other and with other cell types. T cells and other PBMC can be separated from whole blood by density gradient centrifugation (they have a density below 1.077g/l). T cells can be further distinguished by their functional activity, but are more generally categorized by the expression of specific *surface molecules*. These *T cell surface markers* can be individually identified by their binding characteristics to specific fluorescence-labeled *antibodies* (see *flow cytometry*).

> T cells are distinguished by the presence of the *T cell antigen receptor* (TCR), which binds *antigen* presented by *major histocompatibility complex* (MHC) molecules of *antigen-presenting cells* (APCs).

Nearly all T cells also express a co-receptor associated with the TCR in the form of either a *CD4* or *CD8* molecule. T cells play a central role in the pathogenesis of *allergic inflammation*.

T CELL ACTIVATION

The molecular events associated with *T cell* activation involve complex cascades of enzymes. At least three protein *tyrosine kinases* have been associated with T cell activation: p59fyn and ZAP70 associated with the cytoplasmic domain of the ζ-chain, and p56lck associated with *CD4* and *CD8* molecules following *antigen recognition* due to interactions between *T cell antigen receptor* (TCR) and *major histocompatibility complex* (MHC). These protein tyrosine *kinases* then phosphorylate p21*Ras* leading to activation of the *mitogen-activated protein kinase* (MAPK) pathway, phosphatidylinositol-specific *phospholipase C* leading to *calcium mobilization*, and activation of the *protein kinase C* (PKC) pathway. Therefore, at least three distinct *signal tranduction* pathways stem from the TCR (see Figure 46), leading to the activation of *transcription factors* with consequent *cytokine* production and *T cell proliferation*. Many transcription factors bind to the *IL-2 promoter* to induce *cytokine gene activation*; one of the most important is *nuclear factor of activated T cells* (NF-AT). However, several other transcription factors including *nuclear factor-κB* (NF-κB) and *activator protein 1* (AP-1) also need to bind to the IL-2 promoter for T cell activation.

T CELL ANERGY

(See *anergy* and *immunotherapy*.)

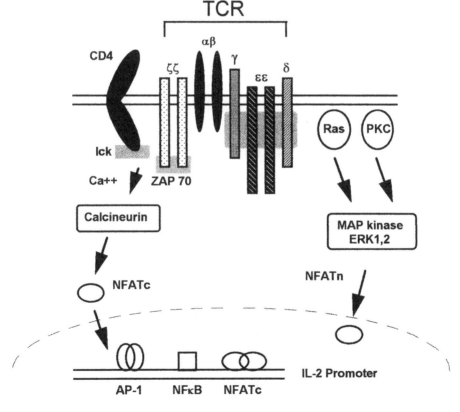

FIGURE 46 Signal transduction pathways activated by the T cell antigen receptor leading to the induction of cytokine genes.

T CELL ANTIGEN PRESENTATION

There is evidence that under certain conditions *T cells* can present *antigen* to other T cells. The mechanism of this process is uncertain, as T cells do not express high levels of *MHC class II molecules*, and therefore they are poor *antigen-presenting cells* (APCs). Little *co-stimulation* by *CD4* or *CD8* is possible and co-stimulatory molecule expression is unlikely to be complementary. However, it is possible that the requirement for CD4 or CD8 ligation can be overcome (as in *superantigen* presentation), possibly by high antigen concentrations, and that high levels of *cytokine receptor* occupancy may substitute for co-stimulatory input. Occupancy of the *T cell antigen receptor* (TCR) by antigen or *antigenic peptides* in conditions of antigen excess is also a possible mechanism for induced *anergy* (see *immunotherapy*), or may provide signals for *apoptosis*.

T CELL ANTIGEN RECEPTOR (TCR)

> The TCR is responsible for *antigen recognition* and initiates *antigen*-specific *T cell activation*.

It is composed of two transmembrane polypeptide chains (α/β or less frequently *gamma/delta* *(γ/δ) T cells*) which are associated with several other polypeptides including ζ, γ, ε, and δ chains that together form the TCR-*CD3* complex. Molecular models predict that the α and β chains are members of the *immunoglobulin superfamily*. The extracellular portion has a structure similar to an *antibody Fab* fragment, containing one variable and one constant domain. Interestingly, the *signal transduction* pathways initiated via the TCR (Figure 47) are very similar to those stimulated through the *B cell antigen receptor* (Figure 10). Several accessory molecules such as *CD2*, CD5, and *CD28* can also synergize with the TCR (see *co-stimulation*) to initiate T cell activation.

> The result of proper T cell activation is upregulation of cell *surface molecules* and production of *T cell cytokines* (see *cytokine gene activation*) with consequent antigen-specific *T cell proliferation*.

Of particular importance is the expression of *IL-2 receptors* (see *CD25*) and production of IL-2, leading to an autocrine loop and T cell expansion.

T CELL ANTIGEN RECEPTOR (TCR) GENE REARRANGEMENT

(See *gene rearrangement*.)

T CELL–APC INTERACTIONS

T cells interact with *antigen-presenting cells* (APCs). The most important interactions for the shaping of the T cell repertoire are thymic epithelial, cortex and medullary cells, *dendritic cells*, *macrophages*, *monocytes*, *fibroblasts*, and *B cells*. Specialized APCs such as *Langerhans cells* and *M cells* (specialized sampling, processing, and presenting cells of the gut epithelium) are important in the process of *T cell sensitization*.

T CELL APOPTOSIS

T cells undergo activation-induced *apoptosis* after an *immune response*.

> T cell apoptosis is needed to keep cell homeostasis of *antigen*-specific T cells.

Therefore, T cells produce not only molecules needed for proliferation (e.g., *IL-2*, *CD25*), but also molecules required for their own death (*Fas ligand*, *Fas receptor*). In the presence

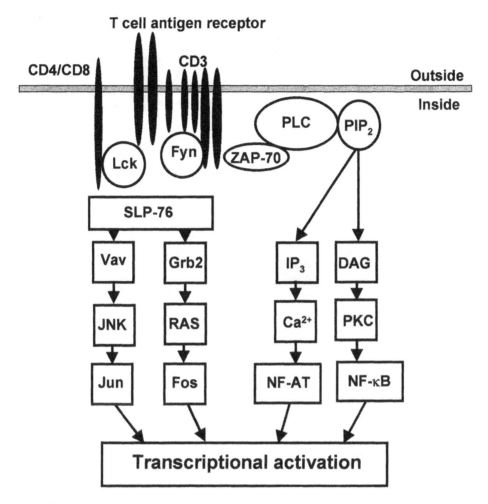

FIGURE 47 Signal transduction pathways initiated via the TCR and co-receptors.

of IL-2, *IL-4*, or *IL-15*, activated T cells fail to die following Fas ligand/Fas receptor inter-actions (Figure 48). Failure to die via apoptosis may result in chronic *inflammation* and/or lymphoproliferative diseases (see *hypereosinophilic syndrome*). Therefore, apoptosis is a natural homeostatic mechanism controlling proliferative responses in T cells following acti-vation by antigens.

T CELL CLONE

A T cell clone is a population of *T cells* that originates from one T cell.

In vitro, peripheral T cells are stimulated with *antigen*, and the resulting blasts are separated by gradient centrifugation and cultured under limiting dilution conditions. The result is a single cell per culture. Upon antigen stimulation, the cells that grow out of this culture will be clones of the seed T cell.

The study of T cell clones has served to illustrate T cell heterogeneity, and also to define functional and phenotypic parameters.

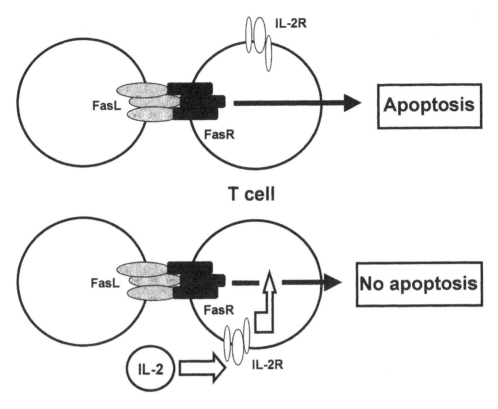

FIGURE 48 Activated T cells undergo Fas receptor (FasR)-mediated apoptosis when Fas ligand (FasL) activation occurs, a mechanism needed to downregulate numbers of antigen-specific T cells after an immune response. If inflammation is maintained, T cells do not undergo apoptosis, although they express all molecules needed for activation-induced apoptosis.

For instance, it was first recognized that mouse T cell *CD4+* T cell clones can be divided into functional phenotypes, which either augment cell-mediated immune reactions or *humoral immune responses*. Furthermore, analysis of the *cytokine* secreting profile of those clones revealed a mechanistic basis for the functional divergence and the *Th1/Th2* paradigm.

> Th1 T cell clones were found to produce *TNF-β, IFN-γ*, and *IL-2,* whereas Th2 cells produced *IL-4, IL-5*, and *IL-13.*

This fundamental observation has been developed and refined to include T cell clones with mixed or apparently unrestricted cytokine profiles *(Th0)* and has been established and accepted in human T cell clone systems. It is also now recognized that T cell clones of different phenotypes (CD4+ and *CD8+*) have compartmentalized cytokine secretion patterns and that a wide range of functional heterogeneity exists. Several functional phenotypic subsets have been described including CD4+ Th1, Th2, *Th3 (TGF-β*-producing), Th0, Th(c)1, and Th(c)2 (the latter two are CD4+ T cells with cytotoxic activity), and CD8+ *Tc1, Tc2*, Ts1, and Ts2 (cytotoxic and suppressor). *Tr1* (T regulatory) cells are CD4+ T cells that generate large amounts of *IL-10*. T cell clones have been created with a wide range of divergent antigens and *allergens* and remain a powerful tool for elucidating immunological mechanisms of disease.

T CELL CYTOKINES

The *cytokines* produced by *CD4+* and *CD8+ T cells* can be conveniently split into three categories using the *T helper (Th) cell* functional subset convention (which could also be applied to CD8+ cells). These are the *Th1*, *Th2*, and *Th0*. Expression and major functional subgroups are shown in Table 87.

TABLE 87
Cytokine Expression and Function of Major Th Cell Subsets

	Th1	Th2	Th0
Function			
B cell help	+	++	++
Support for *eosinophils* and *mast cells*	–	++	?
Macrophage activation	++	–	+
Delayed hypersensitivity	++	–	+
Cytokine			
IL-2	+	–	+
IFN-γ	++	–	++
TNF-β	++	–	?
TNF-α	++	+	?
GM-CSF	++	+	+
IL-3	++	+	++
IL-4	–	++	++
IL-5	–	++	++
IL-6	–	++	?
IL-10	–	++	++
IL-13	–	++	+
IL-15	+	–	+

In addition to cytokines produced by T cells, there are a number of important cytokines produced by other cells that have profound regulatory functions on T cell activity. For instance, *IL-12* and *IL-18*, which are produced by *monocytes/macrophages*, are potent inducers of IFN-γ production by Th1 cells and indirect inhibitors of Th2 cell differentiation. Moreover, certain *chemokines*, such as *RANTES*, which can also be produced by T cells, are able to specifically recruit *memory T cells* to sites of *inflammation*.

T CELL CYTOKINE KINETICS

The levels of *cytokines* generated in vivo or in vitro that are subsequently detectable depend on rates of synthesis, rates of accumulation, rates of removal or breakdown, and homeostatic control mechanisms of *gene* activation and deactivation. Binding of certain cytokines to their specific *receptors* (see *cytokine receptors*) can have direct control over other cytokines, either enhancing or inhibiting their synthesis. Acute-phase cytokines (*TNF-α, IL-1,* and *IL-6*) can be produced within minutes upon immune cell stimulation, rapidly reach peak production, and then decline. These early cytokines are generally produced by cells of the myeloid lineage, and can include cytokines such as preformed *IL-4* released from *basophils* or *mast cells*. Production of *T cell cytokines* is generally a slower process that depends on the nature of the stimulus and number of responding cells. T cell cytokine production in vitro can be compressed into a 24- to 48-hour window when using T cell lines or *T cell clones*, or be spread out over several days when using low densities of *peripheral blood mononuclear cells* (PBMCs). The characteristic profile of a lag phase after stimulation (during which *cytokine gene activation* occurs) followed by a period of rapid production and accumulation before a peak or plateau is reached (where production is equal to consumption), and then a period of decline is common to most cytokines (see Figure 49).

> The first T cell cytokines generally expressed are *IL-2* and IL-4, which are primarily responsible for *T cell activation*, proliferation, and functional phenotype selection (*Th1* or *Th2*).

Next appear the cytokines responsible for continued recruitment and activation of inflammatory effector cells such as *IL-3* and *GM-CSF* (*mast cells, basophils,* and *macrophages*), *IL-5* (*eosinophils*), and *IL-8* (*neutrophils*). These are followed by cytokines with major homeostatic regulatory roles such as *IL-12* and *IFN-γ* (induce Th1 differentiation) and *IL-10* (limits *inflammation*). Finally, continuous *TNF-α* production would maintain inflammation. The order in which the cytokines appear following stimulation indicates the predominant functional phenotype of the responding T cells. Where IL-2, IFN-γ, and TNF-α predominate in *antigen*-specific responses but IL-4, IL-5, IL-6, and *IL-13* are absent, the response is primarily Th1 in nature. This is exemplified by the profiles seen for bacterial recall *antigens* that induce *delayed hypersensitivity*. In contrast, allergenic stimulation of PBMC from sensitive subjects results in Th2 cytokine production, but includes low levels of IL-2.

T CELL DIFFERENTIATION

(See *T helper cell differentiation*.)

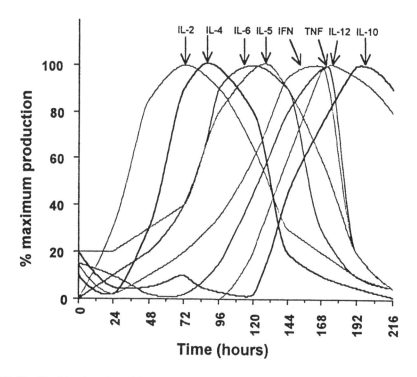

FIGURE 49   The kinetics of cytokine production of PBMC upon stimulation with antigen.

T CELL EPITOPES

Unlike *antibodies*, which recognize soluble protein *antigens*, *T cells* see antigen in the form of short *peptides* (see *linear epitopes*) on the surface of another cell.

> The T cell *epitope* is a peptide fragment of an antigen recognized specifically by the *T cell antigen receptor* (TCR).

The TCR binds to peptide antigens that are held within the groove of *MHC class I* and *II molecules*. Precise identification of T cell *epitopes* has been aided by developments in peptide synthetic chemistry as well as the ability to clone T cells (see *T cell clone*). Once the primary *amino acid* sequence of an antigen has been determined (usually by protein sequencing or *DNA cloning*), synthetic peptides that span the entire sequence can be generated. These peptides can be used to specifically stimulate *T cell proliferation*, to identify the portion of the antigen, or epitope, recognized by the TCR (see *lymphocyte transformation test*). This approach is possible, because crystallographic data (see *X-ray crystallography*) suggest that only peptides of a certain length (13 to 17 amino acids) can be presented by MHC class II molecules and recognized by T cells (see *antigen recognition*), and even shorter peptides (8 to 12 amino acids) by MHC class I molecules.

> Many environmental *allergens* are comprised of multiple reactive antigens.

For example there are at least eight *antigenic peptides* of the *house-dust mite* (Der p 1 through Der p 8). Identification of T cell epitopes is a prerequisite in the emerging field of *peptide immunotherapy*, where it is possible that more specific, more potent, and safer forms of *immunotherapy* may be developed. Administration of high doses of peptides in the absence of *antigen-presenting cells* (APCs) or appropriate *co-stimulation* by, for example, *CD28/B7* results in specific T cell unresponsiveness (*anergy*), which can downregulate *Th2 cell* help, which drives *allergic inflammation*. Many allergens have been T cell epitope mapped and the most potent allergenic peptides identified by limiting dilution and proliferation assays.

T-CELL-MEDIATED APOPTOSIS

CD8⁺ *T cells* can kill target cells by inducing *apoptosis*. This process is important in the defense against viruses and cancer, and involves *Fas ligand/Fas receptor* molecular interactions.

T CELL PROLIFERATION

> *T cell* proliferation is important for the expansion of *antigen*-specific T cells during host defense mechanisms.

In the context of *allergic diseases*, in vitro stimulation of T cells (either as part of the *peripheral blood mononuclear cell* compartment, purified T cells, T cell lines, or *T cell clones*) with specific *allergen* can result in proliferative responses (see *lymphocyte transformation test*). This response is usually restricted to *CD4⁺* T cells, and allergenic stimulation results in production of *Th2 cytokines* in association with the proliferative response (see *cytokine gene activation*). *IL-2* and *IL-4* synergize to sustain proliferative responses. At a cellular level, CD4⁺ T cell proliferation is induced by signals derived from ligation of the *T cell antigen receptor* (TCR), the co-receptor CD4 molecule, and various co-stimulatory interactions such as *CD28*. A complex series of *signaling* pathways (see *T cell activation*) leads to the induction of *nuclear factor κB* (NF-κB), one of many *transcription factors* able to activate various *genes* in the nucleus of the cell. NF-κB translocates from the cytoplasm to the nucleus and activates, among others, cyclin genes, *DNA polymerase-α*, and thymidine kinase (hence tritiated thymidine incorporation assays to measure proliferation) as the cell progresses from the G1 to S phase of the cell cycle. The proliferative responses can effectively be inhibited by *corticosteroids*, *cyclosporin* A (CsA), or other *immunosuppressive drugs*. Proliferative responses have been used to define important *T cell epitopes* of allergens.

T CELL SENSITIZATION

Thymocytes undergo repertoire selection and maturation in the *thymus*, and those that survive emerge as predominantly CD4+/CD8− or CD8+/CD4− *T cells* or more rarely as CD4−/CD8− *gamma/delta (γ/δ) T cells*.

> T cell sensitization is the process whereby a naive T cell (see *naive lymphocytes*), which leaves the thymus, is activated on exposure to a specific *antigen* presented to the *T cell antigen receptor* (TCR) in the groove of a *major histocompatibility complex* (MHC) molecule.

In order to sensitize a T cell, there are three major requirements that have to be met. First, the appropriate antigen (usually an *antigenic peptide*) presented in the groove of the MHC of *antigen-presenting cells* (APCs) (*MHC class I molecules* for *CD8* and *MHC class II molecules* for *CD4*) must be complementary and recognized by the TCR. Second, there must be engagement of either CD4 or CD8 with the appropriate MHC molecule ligand. Third, there is an obligatory requirement for *co-stimulation* of the T cell, either by interaction with cell *surface molecules* of the APC or by soluble *mediators*, such as *cytokines* acting on surface *receptors* of the T cell. The result of sensitization is to activate the T cell such that subsequent exposure to the same antigen can lead to rapid clonal expansion (see *T cell proliferation*), expression and secretion of cytokines, and active cognate interactions (see *cognate/noncognate interactions*) with *B cells* to provide help for *antibody* production.

> Sensitization of T cells is an initiating step in allergic *sensitization* that is subsequently manifested by *immediate* and *delayed hypersensitivity* reactions in *allergic inflammation*.

T cell sensitization usually occurs across mucosal surfaces, but can occur via the skin or systemically. The activation, differentiation, and development of sensitized T cells depend to a large extent on the environment in which they mature (see the three requirements above). For instance, if a naive T cell is stimulated by an *allergen*, it is likely that this cell will develop into a *Th2 cell* when large amounts of *IL-4*, but only little *IFN-γ*, is present in its microenvironment (see *T helper cell differentiation*).

T CELLS IN ALLERGIC ASTHMA

T cells are one of the best studied cells in *allergic diseases* and are recognized as having an extremely important role in the regulation of *immune responses*, which are responsible for initiating, enhancing, perpetuating, modifying, and resolving pathological mechanisms (see *allergic inflammation* and *resolution of inflammation*) in *asthma*. Asthma has been categorized as intrinsic (see *intrinsic asthma*) or extrinsic (see *allergic asthma*).

> A role for the T cell as an inducer and coordinator of the inflammatory response is suspected in both allergic and intrinsic asthma.

CD4+ and *CD8+* T cells can produce numerous *cytokines*, which are relevant to the development of asthma, although it is clear that cytokines elaborated by other cells are also important. Major problems in addressing the importance of *T cell cytokines* in asthma are (1) accurately determining the source of the cytokines produced (see *cytokine detection methods*), (2) determining the target of those cytokines (see *cytokine receptors*), and (3) determining the mechanisms that control such cytokine production (see *cytokine gene activation*).

> In asthma, the focus has naturally fallen on the *Th2* cytokines, among which *IL-4*, *IL-5*, and *IL-13* are thought to have significant functions.

Infiltration of asthmatic airways by T cells that exhibit increased levels of mRNA for IL-4 and IL-5 has been illustrated by *in situ hybridization*. In addition, a high proportion of T cells recovered from *bronchoalveolar lavage* (BAL) fluids of asthmatic lungs also expressed IL-4, IL-5, and IL-13. Functional assays clearly suggest that IL-4 and IL-13 are responsible for *IgE isotype* selection (see *immunoglobulin class switching*) and upregulation of *adhesion molecules* on vascular *endothelial cells*. IL-5 is known to be an important growth, differentiation, *priming*, and *survival factor* for *eosinophils*. This is evidently of considerable functional and clinical significance and helps to explain the observation of pulmonary *eosinophilia* associated with asthma. In severe asthma (see *asthma exacerbation*), IL-5 can often be detected in the serum. The role of *IL-10* in asthma remains enigmatic, since, besides acting as a general immunosuppressant by downregulating both Th1 and Th2 cytokines, it synergizes with IL-4 and IL-13 in the upregulation of *mast cell* responsiveness.

> The control of T cell cytokine production in asthma is a poorly understood subject.

As in *atopic dermatitis*, there appears to be a lack of Th1 cells in *asthma*, perhaps due to a genetically determined (see *genetic predisposition*) reduced capacity to generate *IL-12* and/or *IFN-γ*. Since Th1 and Th2 cells are known to be cross-regulatory, this might explain the overexpression of Th2 cytokines in these diseases. However, cytokines from other cells such as *monocytes/macrophages*, *mast cells*/basophils, eosinophils/*neutrophils*, *NK cells*, and *platelets* may also play an important role in regulating Th2 cytokine production of T cells.

T CELLS IN ALLERGIC INFLAMMATION

(See *allergic inflammation*.)

T CELLS IN ALLERGIC RHINOCONJUNCTIVITIS

(See *allergic inflammation*.)

T CELLS IN ATOPIC DERMATITIS

As with the *T cells in allergic asthma*, *T cell* responses in *atopic dermatitis* are largely of the *Th2* type.

> *Immunohistochemistry* studies have shown that the majority of the infiltrating T cells in skin lesions carry the homing *receptor cutaneous lymphocyte antigen* (CLA), and express large amounts of *IL-5* and *IL-13*.

In contrast, *IL-4* and *IFN-γ* are expressed in relatively small amounts. The help for *B cells* to generate large amounts of *IgE* is therefore largely the consequence of IL-13 overexpression. Overexpression of IL-5 is associated with *eosinophilia*. Some authors describe a shift from Th2 to *Th1* responses in chronic lesions; however, this is not a generally accepted concept at the moment. It is more likely that the T cells from atopic dermatitis patients have a genetic defect that precludes production of sufficient amounts of IFN-γ (see *genetic predisposition*), and therefore patients develop a chronic Th2-driven *allergic inflammation*.

T CELLS IN AUTOIMMUNITY

(See *autoimmunity.*)

T CELLS IN DELAYED HYPERSENSITIVITY

Delayed hypersensitivity reactions are characterized by an inflammatory cell infiltrate, which includes *CD4+ T cells*, particularly *memory T cells* (CD45RA$^-$/RB$^+$) (see *Coombs and Gell classification*, type IV).

> The role of T cells in the development of delayed hypersensitivity without the need for *immediate hypersensitivity* reactions was demonstrated using *antigenic peptides*, which represented *T cell epitopes* of *allergens*.

T cells are specifically attracted by the *chemokine RANTES*, and perhaps also by *eotaxin*. Activated T cells play an important role at sites of *allergic inflammation* by the secretion of *cytokines* and by cognate interactions (see *cognate/noncognate interactions*) with resident or recruited *antigen-presenting cells* (APCs). *Th2* cytokines are particularly important in allergic inflammatory response, where *IL-4* and *IL-5* synergize in the development of *eosinophilia*. Although T cells occupy principally a regulatory role, there is also evidence for direct cytopathic effects, particularly by subsets of cytotoxic *CD8+* T cells. Moreover, *TNF-α*, a product of *Th1 cells* as well as *monocytes/macrophages*, can directly affect the pathology of *asthma*.

T CELLS IN IMMEDIATE HYPERSENSITIVITY

Immediate hypersensitivity reactions are characterized by cell-bound *IgE* interactions with *allergen*, resulting in *degranulation* of *mast cells* and/or *basophils*. The *T cell* component to this reaction is restricted to the potentiating role of *T cell cytokines* on (1) *IgE isotype* selection (see *immunoglobulin class switching*), and (2) *priming* of mast cells for *mediator* release. For instance, the growth factors *IL-3* and *GM-CSF* serve to enhance mast cell reactivity, priming these cells for the release of *histamine* and other proinflammatory mediators.

T CELLS IN IMMUNOGLOBULIN ISOTYPE SELECTION

> *Immunoglobulin* (Ig) *isotype* production and the magnitude of the *B cell* response in vivo depends largely on the influence of *cytokines* produced by *CD4+ T cells*.

IL-4 and *IL-13* select exclusively for *IgE* production (see *immunoglobulin class switching*), whereas IL-4 and *IFN-γ* together select *IgG*. During *immunotherapy*, IgG1 and IgG4 are upregulated, which has been shown to correlate with a reduction of *allergen*-specific *Th2* responses (see *anergy*). The process of Ig class switching might also be influenced by cytokines from sources other than T cells.

Besides cytokines, co-stimulatory activity between B and T cells during cognate interactions (see *cognate/noncognate interactions*) also influence isotype selection. Moreover, the type of *antigen-presenting* cell (APC) is important. For instance, when *antigen* is presented by APCs with high constitutive *MHC class II molecule* expression, such as *dendritic cells* or B cells, T cell responses generally favor *Th1* development. This is associated with IgG production. In contrast, presentation by *macrophages* can induce not only IgG, but also IgE production.

T CELLS IN IMMUNOTHERAPY

(See *immunotherapy.*)

T CELLS IN INTRINSIC ASTHMA

In patients with *intrinsic asthma*, there is no obvious cause related to *allergen* exposure or *atopy* in general. The underlying pathophysiological mechanisms are the same as in *allergic asthma*, but the initial or sensitizing triggers are unknown. Intrinsic *asthma* is not associated with *immediate hypersensitivity* reactions, but is etiologically similar to the *late-phase response* in allergic asthma (see *delayed hypersensitivity*).

> *T cells* in intrinsic asthma express *Th2 cytokines*, especially *IL-5*, explaining the chronic *eosinophilic infiltration* of the airways.

Moreover, the clinical efficacy of *corticosteroids* and *cyclosporin A* (CsA) suggests that *T cell activation* is also central to the mechanisms of this form or asthma.

T CELLS IN INTRINSIC ATOPIC DERMATITIS

As in the extrinsic form of *atopic dermatitis*, *T cells* also appear to play a major role in the pathogenesis of the intrinsic form of atopic dermatitis (see *intrinsic atopic dermatitis*).

> *Immunohistochemistry* studies have shown that the majority of the infiltrating T cells in skin lesions carry the *homing receptor cutaneous lymphocyte antigen* (CLA) and generate significant amounts of *IL-5* and *IL-13*.

In contrast, *IL-4* and *IFN-γ* are expressed in relatively small amounts. Although skin T cells express IL-13, the amount may not reach the *threshold* needed for *immunoglobulin class switching* and consequent *IgE* production by *B cells*. Interestingly, as observed in the extrinsic form of atopic dermatitis, the T cells appear to express a genetically determined low capacity to generate IFN-γ (see *genetic predisposition*). Low IFN-γ expression may contribute to the development and maintenance of a chronic *Th2* response.

T CELLS IN PARASITIC DISEASES

(See *parasitic diseases*.)

T CELL SUBSETS

> There are several distinct functional subsets of *T cells*, some of which can be distinguished by the expression of *surface molecules*, while others are categorized by their *cytokine* secreting profiles.

CD4+ and CD8+ T cells

The earliest recognized functional categories were helper–inducer T cells (see *T helper cells*), and suppressor–cytotoxic T cells, subsequently shown to express the *CD4* and *CD8* surface molecules, respectively, and mutually exclusively. A small subset of T cells that expresses neither CD4 nor CD8 is categorized by having only the gamma and delta (γ/δ) chains (see *gamma/delta T cells*) expressed in the *T cell antigen receptor* (TCR). The differentiation of the following functional subtypes depends on the cytokine environment, *antigen* dose (see *antigen dose responses*), the nature of the *antigen-presenting cell* (APC), and *co-stimulation* mechanisms (see *T helper cell differentiation*).

Th0, Th1, Th2, and Th3 cells

It has been shown that CD4+ cells can be further divided by their cytokine secreting profiles into cells with distinct functional characteristics. Studies have demonstrated the existence of compartmentalization in CD4 cells in both mice and humans into the now-recognized *Th1*, *Th2*, and *Th0* functional phenotypes (see *T cell cytokines* and *Th1/Th2 markers*). Recently,

T cells were called *Th3* cells when they express *TGF-β* (see *immunosuppressive mechanisms*). Th2 responses are important in the development of *allergic diseases*. *IL-4* production induces *IgE isotype* selection and can lead to *immediate hypersensitivity* reactions mediated by *mast cell*/IgE/*allergen* interactions, resulting in *degranulation* and release of inflammatory *mediators* from those cells. *IL-5* is important in recruiting, activating, and expanding *eosinophil* populations in *delayed hypersensitivity* responses.

Tc1 and Tc2 cells

CD8⁺ T cells can be subdivided regarding their cytokine profile into *Tc1* and *Tc2* cells. In contrast to CD4⁺ T cells, CD8⁺ T cells are activated by antigens on *MHC class I molecules*. Tc2 cells have been shown to induce delayed hypersensitivity reactions in *asthma*. Tc1 may be involved in *contact dermatitis* and *autoimmunity*.

Tr1 cells

This is a recently described subgroup of immunosuppressive T cells that generate large amounts of *IL-10*. Such cells appear to be generated during allergen-specific *immunotherapy*. Besides Tr1 cells, other cells such as *monocytes* and *B cells* were reported to be able to generate IL-10.

T CELL SURFACE MARKERS

T cells express a number of different *surface molecules* that can be used to identify them. These markers are defined by their ability to bind *antibodies* raised against surface-expressed *antigens*. The antibodies are coded according to cluster differentiation patterns (*CD antigens*) in a widely accepted system. Surface marker expression varies, depending on the maturation and differentiation stage of the T cell. Thus markers expressed early during ontogeny may be lost during later development, although, once expressed, certain markers such as *CD3*, *CD4*, and *CD8* remain for the lifetime of the T cell and may be used as functional markers (see T cell subsets). Table 88 shows a number of important markers associated with T cells (although not necessarily exclusive to them).

T cells also express numerous activation-associated markers (see *T cell activation*) such as *CD25*, *CD30*, CD71, or *HLA*-DR, as well as inducible molecules mediating adhesion such as CD11/CD18 (see *LFA-1*). In addition, many *cytokine receptors* are transiently expressed depending on the activation state of the T cell. The *T cell antigen receptor* (TCR) is expressed on all T cells (α/β or *gamma/delta* (γ/δ) *T cells*), and antibodies have been raised that recognize these structures.

T CELL TRAFFICKING

> *Homing* and *migration* are the two main mechanisms by which *T cell subsets* move to appropriate sites at appropriate times.

Homing involves the interactions between *adhesion molecules* such as *ICAM-1* (ligand CD11/CD18), *VCAM-1* (ligand CD49/CD29 complex), and *selectins* on *endothelial cell* surfaces with *integrins* on *leukocytes*. The result is attachment of leukocytes and transendothelial migration into tissue spaces. *CD44* (also called *extracellular matrix receptor* III), and some *CC chemokines* such as *RANTES* and *MIP-1* play an important role in T cell migration. RANTES is particularly important in T cell trafficking, with the apparent ability to selectively attract *memory T cells* (CD4⁺/CD45RO⁺), but not *B cells* or other T cells. Activated memory T cells are central in chronic *allergic inflammation*, such as bronchial *asthma*, and in *autoimmunity*.

TABLE 88
Selected T Cell Surface Molecules

Marker	Mol. wt. (kDa)	Expression	Ligand (if known)	Associated function
CD1a	49	Cortical thymocytes, dendritic cell subset, Langerhans cells, B cell subset		Restricted presentation to B cells, associated with β2-microglobulin
CD1b	45			
CD1c	43			
CD2 (LFA-2)	50	T cells, most NK cells	CD58 (LFA-3)	Sheep RBC receptor
CD2R	50	Activated T cells, NK cells	CD2	Thymic and peripheral T cell activation
CD3	20–50	T cells		Complex formation with TCR, signal transduction
CD4	59	Helper/inducer T cells, monocyte subset, cortical thymocyte subset	(MHC class II)	Co-recognition of MHC class II with the TCR, HIVgp120 receptor
CD5	67	Mature T cells, thymocytes, B cell subset	CD72	T cell proliferation
CD6	100	Mature T cells, thymocytes, B cell subset		T cell proliferation
CD7	40	T cells, NK cells, immature myeloid subset	Fc receptor for IgM	T cell and NK cell activation
CD8	32	Cytotoxic/suppressor T cells, NK cell subset, cortical thymocyte subset	(MHC class I)	Co-recognition of MHC class I with the TCR
CD27	55	Mature T cells, B cell subset	CD70	TNF receptor–like protein, T cell activation and proliferation
CD28	44	T cell subset	CD80, CD86	T cell co-stimulation
CD38	45	Plasma cells, thymocytes, activated T and B cells, monocytes, precursor cells		Leukocyte activation
CD39	78	Mature B cells, endothelial cells, subset of activated T cells and NK cells		Signal transduction
CD45 (LCA)	180–240	Leukocytes		Tyrosine phosphatase, involved in signal transduction
CD45RA	205–220	T cell subset, B cells, monocytes, macrophages, granulocytes		Naive T cells
CD45RB	205–220			
CD45RO	180	Thymocytes, activated T cells		Memory T cells
CD95	45	T cell subset, activated T cells, many other cells	CD95L	T cell apoptosis
CD98	80/40	Broad		T cell signaling, activation, proliferation
CD99	32			
CD100	150			
CD152 (CTLA-4)	44	Activated T cells	CD80, CD86	Downregulation of T cell activation
CD153	40	T cells	CD30	TNF family, co-stimulatory molecule, apoptosis
CD154 (CD40L)	32–39	Activated T cells	CD40	Major co-stimulatory molecule for B cell help

TCR

(See *T cell antigen receptor.*)

TELOMERE

The tips of the *chromosomes* have a specific sequence that ensures the stability of a chromosome (see *centromere*).

TERBUTALINE

(See *β-agonists.*)

TERFENADINE

(See *antihistamines.*)

TERMINATION CODON

(See *stop codon.*)

TERTIARY STRUCTURE

This is the *three-dimensional structure* of a protein formed from the spatial arrangement of primary and secondary structural elements and disulfide bonds.

TGF-β

(See *transforming growth factor-β.*)

Th CELL

(See *T helper cell.*)

Th0 CELL

(See *T helper 0 cell.*)

Th1 CELL

(See *T helper 1 cell.*)

Th2 CELL

(See *T helper 2 cell.*)

Th3 CELL

(See *T helper 3 cell.*)

Th1/Th2 MARKERS

(See *T helper 1/T helper 2 markers.*)

T HELPER (Th) CELL

Th cells are defined as *T cells* expressing *CD4* on their surface. CD4⁺ T cells are further divided into functional phenotypes, *Th1* and *Th2 cells*, according to the pattern of secreted *cytokines*.

> Generally, Th cells are important in providing optimal support for humoral (Th2) and cell-mediated (Th1) immune responses.

Th cells provide help to *B cells* for the production of *antibodies*. T cell help is achieved either by direct contact with B cells, resulting in *surface molecule* and respective complementary ligand *signaling*, or by paracrine interactions involving signaling mediated by the engagement of T-cell-elaborated cytokines with the relevant *cytokine receptor* on the B cell (see *cognate/noncognate interactions*).

T HELPER (Th) 0 CELL

Th0 cells represent either a distinct intermediate functional phenotype of *Th cells* between the *Th1* and *Th2* extremes, capable of secreting both Th1 and Th2 *cytokines*, or a mid-point on a continuum of response between these extremes. Often referred to as a precursor or differentiation stage of Th functional phenotype, this remains to be unequivocally determined.

T HELPER (Th) 1 CELL

> Th1 cells are a functional phenotype of *CD4⁺ Th cells*, which produce and secrete so-called Th1 *cytokines* such as *IFN-γ, IL-2, IL-15,* and *TNF-β.*

Th1 cells are induced in the presence of IFN-γ, *IL-12*, and *IL-18*, and their cytokine secretion enhances cell-mediated *immune responses*, particularly *macrophage* activity, but can also cause *delayed hypersensitivity* reactions (type IV, see *Coombs and Gell classification*). Th1 cells provide *B cell* help for opsonizing *IgG* production.

> Overactivity of Th1 cells or overexpression of Th1 cytokines is often associated with autoimmune diseases (see *autoimmunity*) such as *rheumatoid arthritis* and *multiple sclerosis.*

Th1 cytokines antagonize the effects of, and are cross-regulated by, *Th2* cytokines. They are derived from a common *T helper precursor (Thp) cell* under the influence of cytokines, antigen dose (see *antigen dose responses*), type of *antigen-presenting cell* (APC), and *genetic predisposition*. There has recently been some progress in the identification of *surface molecules* specific for Th1 cells (see *Th1/Th2 markers*).

T HELPER (Th) 2 CELL

> Th2 cells are a functional phenotype of *CD4⁺ Th cells* that produce and secrete so-called Th2 cytokines such as *IL-4, IL-5, IL-6, (IL-9),* and *IL-13.*

IL-10 was originally described as a Th2 cytokine. However, it is also produced by *Th1 cells*, *B cells*, and *monocytes*. Moreover, unlike other Th2 cytokines, IL-10 downregulates not only Th1 but also Th2 cytokine production. Th2 cytokines generally augment humoral *immune responses*, providing B cell help, and synergistically upregulate *IL-2*-dependent *T cell proliferation*.

> When Th2 cells are overactivated, as observed in *allergic diseases*, IL-4 and IL-13 induce *immunoglobulin class switching* with consequent high *IgE* production. The action of IL-5 contributes to *eosinophil* production in the *bone marrow*, *eosinophil infiltration*, eosinophil *priming*, and *delayed eosinophil apoptosis.*

Th2 cells appear to be heterogenous in their capacity to synthesize Th2 cytokines. Therefore, they may be further subdivided. For instance, it is clear that some patients have high expression of IL-4, but little IL-5, and one can find patients with the opposite constellation. Moreover, *T cell clones* were identified that produced either IL-4 or IL-5.

> Th2 cells do not necessarily synthesize all Th2 cytokines in large amounts, and may therefore be heterogenous in their specific function.

Th2 cells are derived from a common *T helper precursor (Thp) cell* under the influence of cytokines, antigen dose (see *antigen dose responses*), type of *antigen-presenting cell* (APC), and *genetic predisposition*. There has recently been some progress in the identification of *surface molecules* specific for Th2 cells (see *Th1/Th2 markers*).

T HELPER (Th) 3 CELL

Th3 cells should not be called *Th cells*, since they have potent inhibitory or immunosuppressive properties by secreting high levels of *TGF-β*. They might be involved in the limitation and/or resolution of *inflammation* (see *immunosuppressive mechanisms*).

T HELPER (Th) CELL DIFFERENTIATION

There are several factors that influence the developing *Th cell* response following *T cell activation*. These include the *antigen* dose (see *antigen dose responses*), the type of *antigen-presenting cell* (APC) and *major histocompatibility complex* (MHC) class II haplotype, but probably most important is the effect of *cytokines*.

> *Th1* and *Th2* subsets exhibit mutually exclusive cytokine production (see *T cell cytokines*), and these cytokines generally have antagonistic or inhibitory activity on cytokine-mediated responses of the opposing phenotype.

This has been extensively demonstrated in vitro where Th2 cells expand in the presence of homologous cytokines (e.g., *IL-4*), but are inhibited by Th1 cytokines. Likewise, Th1 cells are selected and expand in a Th1 cytokine environment (*IL-12, IFN-γ*), but are downregulated by Th2 cytokines. Moreover, it is now clear that Th1 and Th2 cytokines serve as their own autocrine growth factors and promote differentiation of naive T cells (see *naive lymphocytes*) to their respective phenotypes. This positive feedback mechanism, and the cross-inhibition between the functional phenotypes, tends to polarize responses to particular antigens.

> Strong polarized Th1 and Th2 cytokine responses are often associated with disease.

For instance, autoimmune diseases (see *autoimmunity*) are often associated with a pathologic Th1 cell response, whereas *allergic diseases* are often the consequence of abnormal Th2 activation. In most cases, however, T cell responses to antigen probably encompass a wide range across the polarized spectrum, and it has been recognized that modulation of the specific functional subset response could have important therapeutic potential (see *anticytokine therapy* and *cytokine therapy*).

T HELPER (Th) 2 CYTOKINE GENE CLUSTER

The first evidence of *linkage* of *genetic markers* near the *IL-4 locus* at *chromosome* 5q31.1 encoding a large number of *cytokines* (*IL-3*, IL-4, *IL-5*, *IL-9*, *IL-13*, *GM-CSF*) was reported in 1994. This region was associated with total *IgE levels* in Pennsylvania Amish people representing an isolated group with large family size and a high degree of intermarriage. Further studies carried out in other populations, including families with *asthma* patients, partly supported the *association* of high IgE levels and markers in the chromosomal segment 5q31-q33. However, it should be noted that mapping of a major IgE control locus to this cytokine *gene* cluster does not discriminate so far whether an IL-4/IL-13 *allele* or a variant at the linked loci confers disease susceptibility (see *genetic predisposition*).

T HELPER PRECURSOR (Thp) CELLS

Thp cells are naive T cells (see *naive lymphocytes*) that have not been committed to any particular functional phenotypic development pathway. Several factors influence the development toward either *Th1* or *Th2* (*Tc1* or *Tc2*) cells. These include the *antigen* dose (see *antigen dose responses*), the type of *antigen-presenting cell* (APC) and *major histocompatibility complex* (MHC) class II haplotype, and the *genetic predisposition* of the immunological response. However, probably most important is the effect of *cytokines*, which are present in the microenvironment of the Thp cell (Th2 drives Th2 development, Th1 drives Th1). *T helper (Th) cell differentiation* can be induced to "switch" by altering the local cytokine environment and by other interrelated factors such as induction of *anergy* by increasing antigen dose (see *immunotherapy*). Thp cells can express either *CD4* or *CD8* co-*receptor* molecules.

T HELPER 1/T HELPER 2 MARKERS

Since the *Th1/Th2* paradigm has greatly helped to improve our understanding of pathologic responses of the *immune system* as they occur in *allergic diseases*, there is a great need to identify these different *T helper (Th) cells* in diseases using simple methods. Therefore, besides the measurement of characteristic *cytokines*, researchers and clinicians would like to have other specific markers for Th1 and Th2 cells. A suitable marker could be a *surface molecule*, since labeled *antibodies* could then be used for protein expression studies (see *flow cytometry* and *immunohistochemistry*). There is some progress in the field of identifying mutually exclusive surface structures on Th1 and Th2 cells (see Table 89). However, suitable antibodies are not frequently available against these surface molecules at the moment.

TABLE 89
Differentially Expressed Surface Molecules on Th1 and Th2 Cells

	Th1	Th2
IL-1 receptor	–	+
IFN-γ receptor β-chain	–	+
IL-12 receptor β-chain	+	–
IL-18 receptor α-chain	+	–
CD30	–	+
P-selectin ligand	+	–
CCR3 (see *chemokine receptors*)	–	+*
CCR4	–	+
CCR5	+	–
T1/ST2	–	+

* There are controversial findings regarding the expression of CCR3 on Th2 cells.

THEOPHYLLINE

Theophylline is a nonspecific *phosphodiesterase* (*PDE*) *inhibitor*, thereby increasing intracellular *cAMP* levels. This results in relaxation of bronchial *smooth muscle* cells in patients with *airway obstruction* (see *asthma* and *COPD*). In addition, theophylline may have anti-inflammatory effects. Besides its role as a PDE inhibitor, low doses of theophylline may block *adenosine receptors*. This latter effect may be responsible for theophylline-mediated *eosinophil apoptosis*. Blood theophylline measurements are useful to ensure that the patient falls into the therapeutic range (10 to 20 μg/ml).

THORACIC DEFORMITY

Children with severe *asthma* may develop marked chest deformity, such as pectus excavatum, pectus carinatum, or kyphosis. This is due to the highly compliant thoracic cage in childhood (see *childhood asthma*).

THREE-DIMENSIONAL STRUCTURE

The three-dimensional structure of proteins can be determined by *X-ray crystallography* or NMR. In general, this knowledge is important to understanding how a certain protein can perform its function. For instance, the three-dimensional structures of *allergens* explain the formation of *conformational* and *B cell epitopes*.

THRESHOLD

Dose required for a measurable or expected effect. *Co-stimulation* may modulate the threshold. For instance, *CD28* reduces the threshold of *T cell antigen receptor* stimulation needed for *T cell proliferation* and *cytokine* production.

THROMBOCYTOPENIC PURPURA

An acquired thrombocytopenic bleeding in the skin and mucous membranes due to anti-*platelet antibodies* is the pathophysiological basis of thrombocytopenic purpura (see *Coombs and Gell classification*, type II), also known as idiopathic thrombocytopenic purpura (ITP) or Werlhof's disease. Purpura on the limbs and upper thorax, sometimes with mucosal bleeding but without lymphadenopathy, a positive Rumpel–Leede test, a low platelet count, and a prolonged bleeding time are the diagnostic hallmarks of ITP. Two subtypes of ITP are distinguished:

Acute ITP occurs most frequently in children between 2 and 6 years old, and is preceded in most of the children by a viral infection (e.g., measles, influenza, chickenpox) a few weeks prior. The prognosis of acute ITP is excellent, since recurrence is rare (<10%) and the mortality is low.

Chronic ITP is diagnosed if the bleeding persists for longer than 6 months. In those patients, spontaneous remission is rare (<10%) and fine petechial skin hemorrhages are scattered around the lower legs. Minor skin injuries induce extensive blood extravasation.

Therapy of acute ITP is not needed in the majority of cases, whereas in chronic ITP, *corticosteroids*, *azathioprine*, cyclophosphamide, *cyclosporin* A (CsA), high-dose *intravenous immunoglobulin* (*IVIG*) *preparations*, or even splenectomy should be considered.

THROMBOXANE A$_2$ (TXA$_2$)

TXA$_2$ is an intermediate of the *arachidonic acid* metabolism. It is produced by *platelets* and *macrophages*, and has a very short life (30 seconds) in vivo. TXA$_2$ is a very potent bronchoconstrictor, but is produced only in very small amounts. However, some *prostaglandins* (PGD$_2$ and PGF$_2$) may bind to and stimulate thromboxane *receptors* to cause *airway obstruction* in *asthma*.

THYMINE

A pyrimidine base that is an essential component of *DNA*.

THYMUS

The thymus is a central lymphoid organ in which *T cell* progenitors derived from pluripotent *bone marrow* stem cells differentiate and mature to emerge into the circulation as *naive T cells* bearing specific *T cell antigen receptor* (TCR) reactivity.

One of the earliest events in the life of a developing thymocyte is a process known as somatic *DNA* recombination, in which *genes* responsible for the production of the TCR complex are activated. This process of *receptor gene rearrangement* permits the combination of the constant domains of the TCR with the variable (future *antigen* binding) domains, represented principally by the α and β variable chains, but in a minority of cases with γ and δ chains. About 90 to 99% of T cells that exit the thymus are α/β T cells; the remainder are *gamma/delta (γ/δ) T cells*.

The importance of the thymus in T cell development was first discovered through observations in immunodeficient children. In the DiGeorge syndrome, the thymus fails to form, and the affected individual produces *B cells*, but only a few T cells.

TIDAL VOLUME

The volume of air inspired and expired during normal resting breathing.

TIFFENEAU TEST

(See *forced expiratory maneuver.*)

TISSUE INHIBITORS OF METALLOPROTEASES (TIMPs)

TIMPs are naturally occurring inhibitors of *metalloproteases*, and may therefore limit tissue damage and inflammatory responses (see *inflammation*).

T LYMPHOCYTES

(See *T cells.*)

TNF-α

(See *tumor necrosis factor-α.*)

TNF-β

(See *tumor necrosis factor-β.*)

TNF-RECEPTOR-ASSOCIATED FACTOR (TRAF)

TRAF proteins belong to a family of proteins that bind to the intracellular domain of members of the *TNF receptor superfamily*. There are six known members of the TRAF family, TRAF-1 through TRAF-6. TRAF-2, TRAF-3, TRAF-5, and TRAF-6 bind directly to *CD40*, and therefore they may have important functions in *immunoglobulin class switching*. TRAF proteins share a conserved C-terminal TRAF domain. In addition, TRAF-2 through TRAF-6, but not TRAF-1, contain an N-terminal RING finger and five zinc binding motifs that are found in a number of *DNA*-binding proteins and *transcription factors*. Functional analysis demonstrated that TRAF-2 is a common signal transducer for TNF *receptor* II (see *TNF receptors*), *CD40*, and *CD30* that mediates activation of the transcription factor *nuclear factor-κB* (NF-κB) by these receptors. Moreover, TRAF-2 was shown to bind TRADD, an adapter molecule associated with the TNF receptor I. This way, TNF receptor I-mediated signals can also activate NF-κB. TRAF-5 and TRAF-6 have also been reported to mediate NF-κB activation. The role of TRAF-3, which binds CD40 is not well defined, but has been shown to mediate CD40-induced upregulation of *CD23* in *B cells*.

TNF RECEPTORS

(See *tumor necrosis factor receptors.*)

TNF RECEPTOR SUPERFAMILY

(See *tumor necrosis factor receptor superfamily.*)

TNF SUPERFAMILY

(See *tumor necrosis factor superfamily.*)

TOBACCO SMOKE

(See *smoking.*)

TOLERANCE

Self-reactive *T cells* are deleted in the *thymus*, resulting in tolerance toward self-*antigens*. Tolerance toward self-antigens is most important for a functional *immune system*, and its loss leads to autoimmune diseases (see *autoimmunity*). Specific recognition of exogenous antigens by *lymphocytes* may lead either to an *immune response* or to antigen-specific *anergy*. The decision of the immune system toward either of the two directions is dependent on many microenvironmental factors, such as the protein characteristics and dose of the specific antigen, the presence of adjuvants or immunosuppressive *cytokines* (e.g., *IL-10*), and the expression of co-stimulatory molecules (see *co-stimulation*). *B cell tolerance* is often achieved by lack of T cell help.

TOTAL ALLERGY SYNDROME

(See *multiple chemical sensitivity.*)

TOTAL LUNG CAPACITY

Total amount of gas that the lungs can hold.

TOTAL SERUM-IgE

Allergen-specific *IgE* is a key factor for *immediate hypersensitivity* reactions (see *Coombs and Gell classification*, type I). Determination of the total serum *IgE levels* has been used to determine the reaction state of an individual toward IgE-mediated responses. Normal ranges are assumed at less than 100 kU/l, with 1 Unit corresponding to 2.14 ng of IgE. In atopic patients (see *atopy*), the total serum IgE is increased, with *atopic dermatitis* patients showing the highest values.

TOXIC EPIDERMAL NECROLYSIS

Extensive formation of large, subepidermal blisters in areas of disseminated exanthema are the characteristics of toxic epidermal necrosis. This type of drug *intolerance* (see *adverse drug reactions*) frequently shows mucosal involvement, as well as general malaise. The prognosis is questionable (30% lethality). Excessive *apoptosis* of the epidermal cells (see *epidermis*) is the consequence of *Fas ligand/Fas receptor* molecular interactions that can be disrupted by blocking anti-Fas receptor *antibodies*, which are present in *intravenous immunoglobulin* (*IVIG*) preparations (see *dermatitis exfoliativa*).

Tr1 CELL

(See *T regulatory 1 cell.*)

TRAF

(See *TNF-receptor-associated factor.*)

TRAIT

This is any detectable phenotypic characteristic (see *phenotype*).

TRANS-ACTING

This term is used for regulatory influences not acting on the same *DNA* molecule (*chromosome*), i.e., proteins encoded by other chromosomes or viral proteins that regulate *transcription*.

TRANSCRIPTION

Transcription is the process by which the genetic information in genes is copied into *RNA*. Synthesis of RNA on a *DNA* template is accomplished by *RNA polymerase* as well as ATP, CTP, GTP, and UTP as RNA precursors. The action of proteins in cells is predominantly controlled at the level of *gene* transcription. The transcriptional start point is dictated by a *promoter* sequence, typically located a few hundred base pairs upstream of the gene and requires *general transcription factors*. Transcription normally terminates shortly after the RNA polymerase and encounters a special sequence, usually a variant of the consensus sequence AATAAA (= *polyadenylation site*). The mechanisms of increased gene expression, especially of *cytokine* genes (see *cytokine gene activation*), are of great interest for our understanding of pathogenic principles of *inflammation*. It is now recognized that there are so-called *transcription factors* that bind to specific recognition motifs in the promoter regions of genes. However, the same transcription factors are often activated by many different cell surface *receptors*. Therefore, it is not clear at the moment how a specific cellular response is achieved upon activation of a cell. For example, many transcription factors are involved in the activation of both *Th1* and *Th2* cytokine gene expression. There is evidence that cell activation results not only in activation of transcription factors, but also in changes of the *chromatin* structure, allowing the molecular interaction between transcription factors and promoter sequences of genes (see *DNase hypersensitivity* and *scaffold-associated regions*).

TRANSCRIPTION FACTORS

Transcription factors are proteins that bind to *promoter* sequences and regulate *gene* transcription. The interaction between protein and *DNA* can result in either induction or repression of the gene.

Cytokines and *antigen receptors* usually activate, in a cascade of intracellular *signal transduction* events, transcription factors to upregulate gene expression in *inflammation* (Figure 50). This includes the possibility that they are able to upregulate their own gene expression, at least in some cases. Transcription factors are usually located in the cytosol. However, upon cell stimulation, they translocate to the nucleus in order to be able to influence transcription. Transcription factors important in the pathogenesis of *allergic diseases* are *activating protein*-1 (AP-1), *nuclear factor-κB* (NF-κB), *nuclear factor of activated T cells* (NF-AT), *signal transducers and activators of transcription* (STATs), *guanine–adenine and thymine–adenine repeats* (GATA), and the *corticosteroid receptor/corticosteroid* complex. Combinatorial responses are often required and specific requirements for any particular gene activation remain to be elucidated (see *general transcription factors*).

TRANSCRIPTION START SITE

(See *initiation site of transcription*.)

TRANSFECTION

This is a method that allows the transfer of *genes* or a gene segment into bacteria or eukaryotic cells.

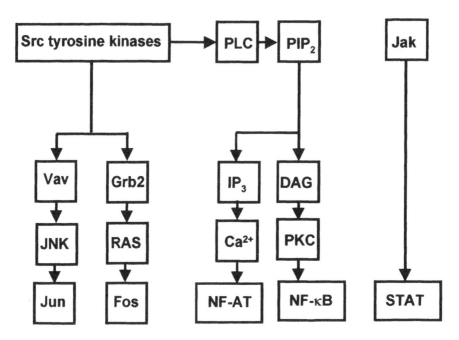

FIGURE 50   A simplified view of some signaling pathways leading to the activation of transcription factors.

TRANSFER FACTOR

The ability of the lungs to transfer oxygen from the alveolar space into the bloodstream is assessed by using the surrogate gas carbon monoxide. A known concentration of carbon monoxide and helium is breathed in, and the breath is held for a fixed period (usually about 10 seconds). The exhaled gas is analyzed for helium and CO content, and the amount of carbon monoxide absorbed per unit alveolar volume per unit time is calculated. Transfer factor is usually normal or slightly increased in *asthma*, but is characteristically low in *emphysema* and fibrotic lung disease (see *cryptogenic fibrosing alveolitis*). Transfer factor is also reduced by anemia, low cardiac output, and pulmonary *edema*.

TRANSFORMING GROWTH FACTOR (TGF)-β

TGF-β is produced by a variety of cells including *eosinophils*. It stimulates the differentiation of bronchial *epithelial cells* as well as the growth and differentiation of *myofibroblasts*. Therefore, TGF-β contributes to the process of *airway remodeling* in *asthma*. However, TGF-β is also an immunoregulatory *cytokine* produced by *Th3 cells* with immunosuppressive properties (see *immunosuppressive mechanisms*). For instance, TGF-β has been shown to suppress *T cell proliferation* and to block *IL-5-receptor*-mediated *signal transduction* in eosinophils. TGF-β *knockout mice* die of overwhelming inflammatory disease.

TRANSGENIC

This is an organism in which a foreign *DNA* sequence has been introduced into the *genome*, usually by genetic manipulation of the zygote to alter the *genotype* (see *transgenic mice*).

TRANSGENIC MICE

Important advances in our understanding of the role of *cytokines* in *allergic inflammation* were accomplished using *knockout mice* (mice deficient in a particular protein) and transgenic mice

(mice overexpressing a particular protein). For instance, the *IL-4* and *IL-5* transgenic mice clearly demonstrated the important role of these cytokines for elevated *IgE* and *eosinophil* levels. Results obtained with several cytokine-overexpressing mice are summarized in Table 90.

TABLE 90
Abnormalities Found in Cytokine Transgenic Mice

Cytokine	Abnormalities
IL-4	High total and specific IgE level
	Inflammatory lesions of the external eye with eosinophils, *lymphocytes*, and *mast cells*
IL-5	Increased eosinophil generation in the *bone marrow*
	Peripheral blood and tissue *eosinophilia*
IL-9	Airway inflammation including *T cell* and eosinophil infiltration
	Mast cell hyperplasia
	Airway hyperresponsiveness
GM-CSF	Accumulation of activated *macrophages*
	Mild eosinophilia

TRANSLATION

The process of protein synthesis is called translation. The four-letter alphabet of *mRNA* (see *base pair*) is translated into the entirely different alphabet of proteins, which consist of *amino acids*. Translation is a much more complex process compared to *transcription*. More than a hundred macromolecules are involved. Translation occurs on ribosomes, which consist of large and small subunits. Proteins are synthesized in the amino-to-carboxyl direction, and mRNA is translated in the 5′ to 3′ direction. The initiation amino acid is in most cases methionine. Cycloheximide can be used to block protein synthesis in experimental systems (e.g., inhibition of *cytokine* production in *T cells*).

TRANSPLANTATION ANTIGENS

Major histocompatibility complex (MHC) *antigens* that in an allogeneic situation lead to transplant rejection.

TREE POLLEN

Besides *grass pollen*, wind-pollinating trees are an important source of *allergens* in the outdoor environment (see *aeroallergens*). Tree *pollens* of various genera are morphologically distinct, and pollen identification is based on visible characteristics under light microscopy. Pollen grains range between 15 and 50 μm in size and tend to be spherical or ellipsoid in shape. Allergenically important genera of the Betulaceae family include birch (Betula, see *birch pollen*), hazel (Corylus), and alder (Alnus, see *alder pollen*). Other important tree pollens include Japanese cedar, oak, and maple.

T REGULATORY 1 (TR1) CELL

Tr1 cells are *CD4+ T cells* that generate large amounts of *IL-10*, but little or no *IL-4*.

Tr1 cells were first described as cells that prevent colitis in animal experiments. They appear to play a general role in the limitation and resolution of inflammatory response (see *immunosuppressive mechanisms*). This is also true for *allergic inflammation*. For instance, *allergen*-specific *immunotherapy* is associated with the occurrence of IL-10-producing T cells.

TRIAMCINOLONE

This is a potent *corticosteroid* for systemic, inhaled, and topical use.

TROLEANDOMYCIN

Troleandomycin is a macrolide *antibiotic* that has been used as a *corticosteroid*-sparing agent. However, this is not the consequence of an antiinflammatory effect of troleandomycin. Instead, it slows down the metabolism of corticosteroids. This way, the therapeutic and adverse effects of steroids are both achieved by a smaller dose. Thus, although a smaller steroid dose can be used to achieve a given effect, there is no real therapeutic gain in terms of reducing side effects.

TRYPTASE

Expression

Tryptase (MW 140 kDa as a tetramer) is the principal *protease* with trypsin-like activity of *mast cells*, first detected by histochemical techniques (see *neutral proteases*). It is the major protein constituent of human mast cells, regardless of the mast cell subtype (see *heterogeneity of mast cells*). Substantial amounts of tryptase are present in mast cells (10 to 35 pg/cell). These quantities appear to account for 20 to 50% of the entire protein in a mast cell.

> Since other cell types have no detectable tryptase, the enzyme is a discriminating marker of human mast cells.

Antibodies against tryptase are useful for identifying mast cells in tissue biopsies by *immunocytochemistry*. Two tryptase *genes* (α and β) are expressed by human mast cells at the level of *mRNA* and protein. Both mast cell tryptase genes are encoded on human *chromosome* 16. The *amino acid* sequence of α-tryptase is 90% identical with that of β-tryptase. α-tryptase is not stored in secretory *granules*, but instead is constitutively secreted by mast cells and is the predominant form of tryptase found in the blood of both healthy subjects and those with systemic *mastocytosis* under nonacute conditions (normal tryptase level is <1 ng/ml).

> Blood tryptase levels are elevated during *anaphylactic reactions* (1 to 10 ng/ml).

Measuring tryptase levels is particularly useful in *anaphylaxis* associated with anesthesia (see *anesthetic allergy*) to differentiate it from other causes of intraoperative hypotension.

Enzymatic activity

Conversion of the inactive monomeric form of β-tryptase to the active homotetramer requires an acid pH and *heparin*.

> Tryptase is uniquely stabilized in its active tetrameric form by heparin, to which it is ionically bound under physiologic conditions.

When free in solution, tryptase subunits rapidly dissociate into inactive monomers, without any evidence for autodegradation. Dissociation of tryptase from heparin may represent the primary means of regulatory tryptase activity in vitro. Tryptase is stored within the secretory granules as a fully active tetramer. It hydrolyzes *peptides* and proteins on the carboxyl side of basic *amino acids* (Lys, Arg).

Biological functions

Various activities have been described for tryptase (see Table 91). Therefore, tryptase appears to play an important role in several disease etiologies, and therefore constitutes a unique target of intervention. Its pathophysiologic role in *allergic inflammation* such as *asthma* has been confirmed from studies using selective tryptase inhibitors.

TABLE 91
Biological Processes Influenced
by the Proteolytic Activity of Tryptase

- *Bradykinin* generation
- Cleavage of fibrinogen
- Degradation of *VIP* and *CGRP*, but not *substance P*
- *Epithelial cell* and *fibroblast* proliferation
- Expression of *ICAM-1*
- *IL-8* release
- *Leukocyte migration* and activation
- Mast cell *degranulation*
- *Mucus* secretion
- Tissue degradation
- Vascular exudation (see *edema*)

T SUPPRESSOR/CYTOTOXIC CELLS

T suppressor/cytotoxic cells are defined as *T cells* expressing *CD8* on their surface. CD8$^+$ T cells have a major function in mediating direct cytotoxicity by mechanisms that include *Fas receptor/Fas ligand*-mediated as well as perforin-mediated *apoptosis*. During defense immune reactions, they preferentially recognize short *antigen-presenting cell* (APC)-processed bacterial or viral *peptides*.

CD8-expressing T cells can also be induced to secrete *cytokines* with subset distinctions similar to *CD4$^+$* T cells (*Tc1* and *Tc2 cells*, as opposed to *Th1* and *Th2 cells*).

The predominance of *IFN-γ* production (Tc1) by CD8$^+$ cells may explain the suppressive effects often noted on humoral *immune responses*. Tc1 and Tc2 cells may play a role in *delayed hypersensitivity* reactions in several *allergic diseases*.

TUBERCULIN TEST

T-cell-mediated immunity can be studied using this *skin test*. Small amounts of tuberculin are injected into the skin. After two days, the skin responds with a red and hard papule due to a local reaction of preexisting *memory T cells* (see *Coombs and Gell classification*, type IV). Cellular immunodeficiency is often associated with a decreased tuberculin reaction.

TUMOR NECROSIS FACTOR (TNF)-α

TNF-α can be generated by LPS-stimulated *macrophages* and *monocytes*, but also by activated *Th1* or *Tc1 cells*, *NK cells*, *mast cells*, and *eosinophils*. Several other *cytokines* are structurally related (see *TNF superfamily*). TNF-α causes, at low concentrations, *endothelial cells* to express *adhesion molecules*, contributing to recruitment of *eosinophils* and other *leukocytes* at local sites of *allergic inflammation*. However, since almost all cells express *TNF receptors*, TNF-α can have a variety of different biological effects (see Table 92).

TUMOR NECROSIS FACTOR (TNF)-β

TNF-β, also known as *lymphotoxin* (LT), is exclusively produced by activated *Th1* or *Tc1 cells*.

In contrast to *TNF-α*, TNF-β is synthesized as a primary secretory protein without a transmembrane region. Both TNF molecules compete for binding to the same *receptors* (see *TNF*

TABLE 92
Biological Effects of TNF-α

TNF-α production	Biological Effects
Low (local actions only)	• Increased expression of adhesion molecules on endothelial cells
	• Activation of *phagocytes* to kill microbes and to generate *IL-1*, *IL-6*, TNF-α itself, and *chemokines*
	• Increased expression of *MHC class I molecules* on virus-infected cells
	• *Apoptosis* in sensitive (neoplastic) cells
	• Activation of *myofibroblasts* to produce *collagen* (see *subepithelial fibrosis*)
Medium (release in circulation)	• Increased synthesis of *prostaglandins* (PGs) in hypothalamic cells and consequent development of fever
	• Stimulation of endothelial cells to release IL-1 and IL-6 into the circulation
	• Activation of hepatocytes to synthesize acute phase response proteins
	• Suppression of *bone marrow* stem cell division and consequent development of *lymphopenia*
	• Activation of coagulation
	• Appetite suppression and cachexia
High	• Increased expression of *NO synthase* and consequent decreased myocardial contractility
	• Relaxation of vascular *smooth muscle* tone and consequent decreased blood pressure
	• Disseminated intravascular coagulation
	• Overutilization of glucose by muscle cells

receptors). Therefore, TNF-α and TNF-β have the same biological effects (see Table 92). However, and in contrast to TNF-α, its production never reaches levels that are high enough to generate systemic effects, and therefore TNF-β acts as a paracrine factor only.

TUMOR NECROSIS FACTOR (TNF) RECEPTORS

TNF-α and *TNF-β* are able to engage two TNF *receptors* (the 55-kD and 75-kD TNF receptors). Both receptors are expressed on many cells, explaining the many biological functions mediated by both TNFs. The TNF receptors belong to the *TNF receptor superfamily*. The 55-kD receptor (TNF receptor I) can mediate *apoptosis*, and belongs therefore to the *death receptors*. Since TNF has many different biological functions, it is likely that TNF receptors initiate many different *signaling* pathways. Several molecules bind to TNF receptors (e.g., *TRAF* proteins and TRADD).

TUMOR NECROSIS FACTOR (TNF) RECEPTOR SUPERFAMILY

All members of the *TNF receptor* superfamily are believed to be transmembrane proteins. The family is defined by a cysteine-rich *amino acid* motif that recurs three to six times in the extracellular domain. The cytoplasmic domains vary more than the extracellular domains. Depending on the structure of the cytoplasmic domains, the TNF receptor superfamily can be subdivided. One subgroup represents the so-called *death receptors*, because it is possible to induce *apoptosis* by activation of these receptors in sensitive cells. They can be distinguished from other members of the family by the presence of a 60-residue cytoplasmic sequence (= death domain), which is essential for activation of *caspases* (Table 93).

TUMOR NECROSIS FACTOR (TNF) SUPERFAMILY

TNF is only one of several known members of a family of structurally related ligands that activate members of the *TNF receptor superfamily*. All members of the TNF family are believed to consist of three polypeptide chains. All except *TNF-β*, which is entirely secreted, and *TNF-α*, which is predominantly secreted, are transmembrane proteins that stimulate their

TABLE 93
Members, Expression, and Function of TNF Receptor Superfamily Members

Member	Distribution	Function
Death Receptors		
TNF receptor I	Many cells	Inflammation
Fas receptor	Many cells	*Lymphocyte* homeostasis
TRAMP receptor (DR3)	Many cells	ND
TRAIL receptor 1 (DR4)	Many cells	ND
TRAIL receptor 2 (DR5)	Many cells	ND
DR6	Many cells	ND
Non-Death Receptors		
NGF receptor	Neurons, other cells	Neuron growth, *mast cell* function
Lymphotoxin-β	Lymphocytes	ND
TNF receptor II	Many cells	inflammation
CD27	*T cells*	ND
CD30	T cells	ND
CD40	*B cells,* T cells	*Ig isotype* selection, *T cell activation*
CD137	T cells, *granulocytes*	T cell activation, limitation of survival
OX-40	T cells	*Th2* differentiation

Note: ND, not determined.

receptors via cell-to-cell contact (see *cognate/noncognate interactions*). Besides the two TNF molecules, *Fas ligand* and CD40 ligand (see *CD154*) are known to be important members of this family in the context of *allergic inflammation*.

TUNEL TECHNIQUE

Terminal deoxynucleotidyl Transferase (TdT) uridine triphosphate (UTP) nick end labeling method to detect apoptotic cells (see *apoptosis*) in purified cells or tissues. Using this technique, free 3′ OH-ends of *DNA* fragments (see *DNA fragmentation*) are labeled with FITC-dUTP (purified cells, analysis by *flow cytometry*) or ^{35}S-dATP (tissues, analysis by light microscopy).

TURBOHALER

This is a multidose *dry powder inhaler* that delivers the micronized drug alone (see also *rotadisk*).

TWIN STUDIES

Twin studies are the epidemiologic survey of incidence and prevalence in twins. Genetic characters should show a higher concordance in monozygotic (genetically identical) than dizygotic twins. Twin studies have shown a greater prevalence of atopic diseases (see *atopy*) in monozygotic twins, supporting the concept of *genetic predisposition*. These studies could demonstrate a 36 to 60% estimated heritability for *asthma*. Monozygotic twins show 71% concordance regarding their *IgE* levels to *common allergens*.

TYPE I REACTION

Any *IgE*-mediated *immediate hypersensitivity* reaction, as classified by Coombs and Gell (see *Coombs and Gell classification*).

TYPE II REACTION

Any cytotoxic reaction, as classified by Coombs and Gell (see *Coombs and Gell classification*).

TYPE III REACTION

Any *immune complex* reaction, as classified by Coombs and Gell (see *Coombs and Gell classification*).

TYPE IV REACTION

Any *delayed hypersensitivity* reaction caused by *allergen-specific T cells*, as classified by Coombs and Gell (see *Coombs and Gell classification*).

TYPE V REACTION

A granulomatous reaction to a given *antigen* (e.g., injection granuloma). This type of reaction has been added later to the *Coombs and Gell classification*.

TYPE VI REACTION

These include all pathogenic effects caused by binding of an *antibody* to a biological structure (e.g., myasthenia gravis). This type of reaction has been added later to the *Coombs and Gell classification*.

TYROSINE KINASE

> Tyrosine *kinases* play a critical role within *signal transduction* pathways initiated via many surface *receptors*.

Their activity is also required for homeostasis of the cell. Tyrosine kinases are enzymes that catalyze the transfer of the γ-phosphoryl group from ATP to tyrosine hydroxyls of proteins (see *phosphorylation*). Many growth factors (e.g., EGF, PDGF) bind to cell-surface receptors that contain intrinsic tyrosine kinase activity. These receptors phosphorylate themselves and other intracellular proteins on tyrosine residues and, through a poorly understood mechanism, initiate cell growth and division.

> Uncontrolled activity of tyrosine kinases leads to various animal and human cancers.

Other receptors, such as *cytokine receptors*, do not have an intrinsic tyrosine kinase activity and need cytoplasmic tyrosine kinases (e.g., *Janus kinases* or *sarcoma tyrosine kinases*) for signal transduction (see *cytokine receptor signal transduction*).

TYROSINE PHOSPHATASE

The tyrosine *phosphatases* are classified as *receptor*-like enzymes and nonreceptor-like phosphatases. The first includes enzymes such as *CD45*. The latter includes *Src* homology domain 2 (SH2)-containing tyrosine phosphatase-1 (SHP-1, previously called HCP, SHPTP1, PTP1C), SHP-2, and SH2-containing inositol-5′-phosphatase (SHIP). In general, tyrosine phosphatases dephosphorylate proteins, which are phosphorylated on tyrosine residues. Receptors with *immunoreceptor tyrosine-based inhibition motifs* are usually able to bind and activate SHP-1, SHP-2, and SHIP following tyrosine *phosphorylation* of the motif by *tyrosine kinases*. These phosphatases therefore play an important role in negative *signaling* of *antigen receptors* (see *immunosuppressive mechanisms*).

U

ULTRAVIOLET (UV) LIGHT

UV light covers a range from 200 to 400 nm of the electromagnetic spectrum and is subdivided according to its wavelength into UV-A, UV-B, and UV-C.

> The most important biological effects of UV-A (320 to 380 nm) are the induction of skin aging (histologically evident as elastosis) and the disease spectrum of photoallergic reactions (see *photoallergy*).

UV-A radiation leads to an immediate darkening of skin pigment due to melanin oxidation, with 40 to 60 J/cm^2 UV-A as the typical minimal tanning dose in clinical dermatology. Due to its long wavelength, UV-A penetrates into the dermis. A wavelength of 335 nm exerts the strongest therapeutic effect in psoriasis, but is associated with the strongest photocarcinogenic effect as well. In clinical dermatology, UV-A is most frequently used in combination with photosensitizers such as topically or systemically applied 8-methoxy-psoralene (8-MOP).

> UV-B (280-320 nm) leads to *dermatitis* solaris (sunburn) and skin pigmentation.

Typical values for the minimal *erythema* dose (MED) of UV-B are 50 to 100 mJ/cm^2, with 311 nm exerting the strongest therapeutic effect in inflammatory skin diseases such as psoriasis and *atopic dermatitis*. Due to its short wavelength, the UV-C (200 to 280 nm) from sunlight is effectively filtered by the atmosphere and does not reach Earth. However, artificial light sources may emit significant amounts of UV-C, leading to severe sunburn and *keratoconjunctivitis*. UV-C is lethal to many microorganisms.

The defense mechanisms of human skin against UV irradiation include thickening of the *epidermis* and stimulation of melanin synthesis (mostly induced by UV-B) as well as oxygenation of preformed melanin, resulting in immediate pigment darkening (mostly induced by UV-A). Defects in the different repair enzymes of human skin cells lead to the different types of xeroderma pigmentosum, a rare skin disease characterized by the development of multiple types of skin cancer in early childhood.

> *Langerhans cells* are extremely sensitive to UV radiation.

UV-B is a potent inducer of Langerhans cell depletion (by *apoptosis*) from the epidermis (see *UV-therapy*). Furthermore, pretreatment of a skin site before *hapten* application may lead to hapten-specific *tolerance* instead of hapten-specific sensitization (see *T cell sensitization*).

ULTRAVIOLET (UV) THERAPY

UV light penetrates the skin in a wavelength-dependent manner, where it induces a dose-dependent immunosuppression as well as wavelength-dependent side effects. UV-A (320 to 380 nm) penetrates the dermis, with 335 nm as a maximum for therapeutic antiinflammatory activity as well as unwanted photocarcinogenic activity. Oxygen-dependent melanin-oxidation leads to an immediate pigment-darkening effect.

Topical or systemic pretreatment of the skin with photosensitizers such as 8-methoxy-psoralene has made the combined psoralene/UV-A (PUVA) treatment a standard therapy of *atopic dermatitis*, psoriasis, and other inflammatory skin diseases.

The wide use of UV-A for tanning purposes in sun studios has made many people aware of the skin-aging side effects of UV-A. UV-B (280 to 315 nm) induces a thickening of the *epidermis* and leads to a depletion of *Langerhans cells* from the epidermis due to induction of *apoptosis*. UV-B has a strong immunosuppressive effect on the epidermis, but penetration into the deeper dermis is minimal.

URTICARIA

Definition
Urticaria is a group of common skin diseases with highly pruritic wheal and flare lesions. A classification based on clinical courses and pictures divides acute (duration less than 6 weeks) and chronic urticaria (duration longer than 6 weeks).

Pathogenesis

Urticaria is the clinical expression of many possible immunological and nonimmunological pathogenic mechanisms, which all lead to the activation of cutaneous *mast cells* and consequent *mediator* release.

For instance, an increased concentration of *histamine* could be demonstrated in the skin of patients with many different forms of chronic urticaria. In contrast, the mechanisms of *mast cell activation* may vary widely among patients.

The pathogenesis of urticaria is heterogenous, and there is no generally accepted classification available.

Table 94 presents a new classification of different urticaria forms, although it should be clear that it does not contain all possible pathogenic mechanisms.

As Table 94 suggests, cutaneous mast cell activation may occur via *high-affinity IgE receptor* (allergic urticaria) or *complement factor* receptor (e.g., *C5a* receptor) activation (complement factors-mediated urticaria). This process might be modulated by *neuropeptides* (physical urticaria). In addition to histamine, the additional release of *cytokines* may amplify and prolong the reaction. For instance, in several forms of chronic urticaria, increased expression of *TNF-α* and *IL-3* has been reported, even in uninvolved skin. This suggests an underlying systemic *inflammation* in these patients.

Diagnostic procedures
Allergic urticaria can be diagnosed using *prick tests* and *immunoassays* (*RAST*, *Phadiatop*, *CAP-system*). Pseudoallergic reactions and physical urticaria are diagnosed by *provocation tests*. Besides exercise, cholinergic urticaria can be diagnosed by the *carbachol* test. The identification of autoantibodies (see *autoimmunity*) can usually be performed in research laboratories only. Please note that in approximately 70% of all cases of chronic urticaria, no cause can be identified (= idiopathic urticaria).

Therapy
It is most important that identified causes should be avoided. Most patients respond to *antihistamines*. Moreover, a number of patients with chronic urticaria who experience flare ups at times of psychological stress benefit from the central anxiolytic action of sedative antihistamines. Drugs known to exacerbate urticaria, such as *NSAIDs* and *ACE* inhibitors,

---

TABLE 94
Classification of Types of Urticaria Based on Pathogenic Mechanisms

Type	Involved Pathogenic Mechanisms
1. Allergic urticaria	
1.1. *Type I reaction*	• *Allergen*-specific *IgE antibodies*
	• Anaphylactic anti-IgE antibodies
1.2. *Type III reaction*	• Immune complexes (see *urticaria vasculitis*)
2. Pseudoallergic urticaria (see *pseudoallergy*)	• Direct histamine release (foods, *food additives*, drugs, insect bites)
	• Generation of *leukotrienes* (*NSAIDs*)
	• Generation of *bradykinin* (blockers of *ACE*)
3. Complement factors-mediated urticaria	• Inherited lack of *C1 inhibitor*
	• Anti-C1 inhibitor antibodies
	• C2 and C4 defects
	• Anti-α-chain *IgERI* antibodies
	• Vaccination
	• Infectious diseases
4. Physical urticaria	
4.1. Mechanical	• ?
4.2. Heat	• *VIP, substance P*
4.3. Cold	• VIP, substance P
	• IgE-like antibody
	• C2 and C4 defects
4.4. Solar	• IgE-like antibody
4.5. Exercise	• Cholinergic nerves (see *nervous system*)
5. Idiopathic urticaria	• ?

---

should be avoided. A diet free of food additives (see *food adverse reactions*) is recommended in all patients sensitive to these substances and those with idiopathic urticaria. In exceptional circumstances, if antihistamines provide inadequate control of symptoms, a short course of *corticosteroids* or *cyclosporin A* (CsA) may be helpful. In chronic urticaria and urticaria vasculitis, treatment with dapsone alone or in combination with pentoxyphylline can be tried. *Antibiotics* should be given in cases of infection with Helicobacter pylori, and also in cold urticaria.

URTICARIA PIGMENTOSA

Although the name implies that this condition is one of the many forms of *urticaria*, it should not be considered as such, because wheals are not a typical feature of this disorder.

URTICARIA PROFUNDA

This term is often used for an *angioedema* of the trunk or extremities.

URTICARIA VASCULITIS

This is a rare subtype of *urticaria* with histologic features of both urticaria and vasculitis. In contrast to normal urticaria, skin lesions tend to persist for longer than a day and show a hemorrhagic infiltrate upon diascopy. A hypocomplementemic and a normocomplementemic subtype are distinguished, with the latter including the more severe cases. An association with IgM-paraproteinemia (Schnitzler's syndrome) has been described.

UV LIGHT

(See *ultraviolet light.*)

UV-THERAPY

(See *ultraviolet therapy.*)

V

VACCINATION

Vaccination is therapeutic induction of an *immune response* by injection of *antigen*. It is usually used to prevent infectious diseases. *Immunotherapy* is also a form of vaccination and is used to treat *IgE*-mediated *allergic diseases*.

VACUUMING

Vacuuming once or twice a week can keep *house-dust mite allergens* from accumulating (see *indoor air pollutants*). Patients who are sensitive to constituents of house dust should avoid recently vacuumed rooms and try not to be around when vacuuming is occurring. If patients must vacuum, they should wear a dust mask and consider using a central vacuum with a collecting bag outside the home or a vacuum cleaner with a high-efficiency particulate arresting (HEPA) filter or a double bag (see *allergen avoidance*).

VARIABLE NUMBER OF TANDEM REPEATS (VNTR)

This is a type of *genetic polymorphism* that, due to differences in the copy number of any *tandem repeat*, is generally used in human genetics to describe highly polymorphic minisatellite *DNA* sequences.

VARIANT

Polymorphic variants of the same *allergen* are called variants or *isoforms*.

VASCULAR CELL ADHESION MOLECULE-1 (VCAM-1)

VCAM-1 is an *adhesion molecule* expressed on the surface of *endothelial cells* by proinflammatory *cytokines* such as *TNF-α* or *IL-1*. It mediates adhesion and *migration* between cells by combining with its specific ligand *very late antigen-4* (VLA-4), a member of the β1 *integrin* family expressed on *eosinophils* and *T cells*, but not *neutrophils*. Interestingly, VCAM-1 is upregulated by *IL-4*.

> It is believed that VLA-4/VCAM-1 interactions may favor the recruitment of eosinophils and T cells into allergic inflammatory sites (see *allergic inflammation*).

VASCULITIS ALLERGICA

(See *allergic vasculitis*.)

VASOACTIVE INTESTINAL PEPTIDE (VIP)

VIP is a *neuropeptide* (see also *nervous system*) that relaxes *smooth muscle* in airways and prevents *airway obstruction* triggered by *histamine, prostaglandin* $F_{2\alpha}$, *kallikrein, leukotriene* D_4, *endothelin*, and *tachykinins*. In addition, VIP is a potent vasodilator. VIP may also have significant antiinflammatory activity, because it increases *cAMP* in cells that carry specific VIP *receptors* (see *immunosuppressive mechanisms*).

> VIP is markedly depleted in asthmatics, and it appears that loss of VIP correlates with *asthma* severity.

Tryptase, which is increased in asthma due to *mast cell activation*, cleaves VIP to inactive forms.

VASOMOTORIC RHINITIS

This term should be replaced by idiopathic *rhinitis*, because the mechanisms involved are not known. Patients demonstrate rhinorrhea or nasal congestion. There is an increased sensitivity of the nasal mucosa to nonspecific triggers, such as perfumes, domestic sprays, and solvents, as well as to changes in environmental temperature and humidity, and to *irritants* such as *dust*, tobacco smoke (see *smoking*), and motor vehicle exhaust (see *outdoor air pollutants*). Patients with vasomotoric rhinitis usually do not have eye or chest symptoms. Intranasal *capsaicin* treatment is clinically effective in vasomotoric rhinitis.

VCAM-1

(See *vascular cell adhesion molecule-1*.)

VECTOR

This is a *phage-* or *plasmid*-derived *DNA* for propagating DNA inserts in bacteria used for clonal replication and thus *amplification* of recombinant DNA (see *DNA cloning*). A cloning vector carries a replication origin and a *gene* conferring resistance to an *antibiotic* for selection in bacteria, and a multiple cloning site containing unique recognition sequences for a number of restriction enzymes for insertion of the foreign DNA fragment.

VEILED CELLS

Veiled cells are defined as dendritically shaped cells mostly resembling epidermal *Langerhans cells* in phenotype and ultrastructure, including the presence of *Birbeck granules*. They are present in or isolated from the lymph vessels. Veiled cells are regarded as epidermal Langerhans cells on their way from the *epidermis* to the regional *lymph node*, progressing from an immature *dendritic cell* stage to the fully matured dendritic cells present inside the lymph node.

VENOMS

Some components of insect venoms are known to be potent *allergens* (see *hymenoptera allergy*). Most research has concentrated on honeybee, bumblebee, yellow jacket (Vespula spp.), yellow hornet, white-faced hornet, and polistes wasp (hymenoptera) venoms. Bee venom contains a number of allergens, including *bee venom phospholipase A_2* (PLA$_2$), *hyaluronidase*, acid *phosphatase*, melittin, apamin, *kinins*, and various other *minor allergens*, any or all of which can be responsible for specific *IgE*-mediated *immediate hypersensitivity* reactions, including potentially fatal *anaphylaxis*. Wasp venom contains additional components such as *antigen* 5. *Major allergens* for bee venom PLA$_2$ (Api m 1), melittin (Api m 3), and hornet antigen 5 (Dol m 5) have been sequenced and *epitope* mapped. *B cell epitopes* have been shown to comprise discontinuous sequences recognized due to the folded *tertiary structure*, whereas the shorter 11 to 14 mer *T cell epitopes* are generally comprised of contiguous *amino acids* of the primary sequence.

VENTILATION

Elective ventilation for *asthma* is rarely necessary, but should be considered if a patient with an acute *asthma exacerbation* begins to tire or shows a rising p_aCO_2. High inflation pressures may be necessary, and it is well recognized that the change from a high-negative to a high-positive intrapleural pressure may lead to circulatory collapse. Great care should be taken to ensure adequate hydration before putting an asthmatic patient on a ventilator. The principal purpose of ventilation is to allow the acute exacerbation to be treated and let the exhausted respiratory muscle recover (see *respiratory failure*). It can sometimes be difficult to differentiate a sick asthmatic patient from a sick *COPD* patient. Ventilation in COPD is justified if the patient has pneumonia or other intercurrent disease that is remediable, and if there is a realistic chance of weaning the patient from the ventilator. If neither of these conditions is met, every attempt should be made to support the patient by means other than putting him or her on a ventilator.

VENTILATION–PERFUSION MISMATCH

Ideally, the lung should match the flow of blood to those areas of the lungs that are best ventilated. In practice, there are always some parts of the lung that are poorly ventilated and receive blood, and others that are well ventilated, but do not receive much blood. This leads to a slight reduction in the level of oxygenation in the blood leaving the lung compared to what would be achieved if the ventilation and perfusion were perfectly matched (see *blood gases*). The pulmonary arteries are very responsive to *hypoxia*, thereby reducing the blood flow to areas that are underventilated. In conditions that cause destruction of the substance of the lung (*emphysema*, *pulmonary fibrosis*, etc.), blood may be shunted from the pulmonary arterial circuit directly into the pulmonary veins without passing through the gas exchange units, increasing the ventilation–perfusion mismatch. Acute administration of a *β2-agonist* causes a transient worsening of the ventilation–perfusion mismatch, and it is therefore recommended that nebulized *bronchodilators* should be given with *oxygen* when treating sick patients with *asthma*.

VERNAL KERATOCONJUNCTIVITIS

One form of *allergic keratoconjunctivitis*.

VERY LATE ANTIGEN 4 (VLA-4)

VLA-4 ($\alpha4\beta1$) is a $\beta1$ *integrin* expressed on *lymphocytes*, *monocytes*, and *eosinophils*, but not on *neutrophils*. It mediates binding to *vascular cell adhesion molecule-1* (VCAM-1), an *adhesion molecule* expressed on activated *endothelial cells* in *allergic inflammation*.

V GENE

V *genes* are genomic sequences encoding the N-terminal variable region of an *immunoglobulin* or *T cell antigen receptor* chain. The variable region shows great diversity due to the different V gene copies and the *gene recombination* process. The *genome* encodes a large number of V gene segments to ensure the *antigen receptor* repertoire of *B cells* and *T cells*.

VIP

(See *vasoactive intestinal peptide*.)

VIRAL INFECTION

A wide range of respiratory viruses can cause *asthma exacerbations*. Human *rhinoviruses* are perhaps the most common agents, especially in children. *Respiratory syncytial virus* is an important cause of bronchiolitis in children, and commonly causes *wheeze* in infants. The role of viral infections in adult *asthma* is more controversial. Many patients with *intrinsic asthma* state that their symptoms started after a viral "flu-like" infection, and they report exacerbations of their asthma with succeeding viral infections. However, most people experience three to four viral respiratory infections each year, and these may disclose incipient asthma rather than cause it. Several groups have sought evidence of persistent viral infection in asthma, but this has not been convincingly demonstrated.

VITAL CAPACITY

The amount of air that can be blown out starting from full lung capacity. This may be achieved through a *forced expiratory maneuver*, in which case it is called the *forced vital capacity*, or it may be achieved through a steady exhalation (slow vital capacity).

VLA-4

(See *very late antigen-4*.)

VNTR

(See *variable number of tandem repeats*.)

VOCAL CORD DYSFUNCTION SYNDROME

A small proportion of patients who present with *asthma*-like symptoms turn out to have incoordination of the vocal cords, which close inappropriately during inspiration, causing *stridor* and audible *wheeze*. It is often misdiagnosed as asthma (pseudoasthma). Some clues may be obtained from a *flow volume loop*, which will show extrathoracic obstruction. The condition can be visualized using a fiber optic laryngoscope or bronchoscope. Treatment is by physiotherapy. The condition should be suspected in asthmatic patients who fail to respond to standard therapy (see *asthma treatment strategies*).

W

WASP VENOM ALLERGY

A subtype of *hymenoptera allergy*.

WEED POLLEN

These *pollens* are a major source of outdoor *aeroallergens*. Weed pollens vary among different geographic regions. In the eastern U.S., the most important weed pollen is from short ragweed (Ambrosia, see *ragweed pollen*); the ragweed season runs from August through October. In Mediterranean regions, Parietaria is the major pollen source. Pollination of mugwort occurs in July and August in Europe.

WEIBEL–PALADE BODIES

Weibel–Palade bodies are intracellular structures within *endothelial cells* that carry the *adhesion molecule* P-*selectin*. Activation of endothelial cells with inflammatory *mediators*, such as *leukotrienes* (e.g., LTB$_4$), *complement factors* (e.g., *C5a*), or *histamine*, results in redistribution of P-selectin to the surface of the endothelium. Together with E-selectin, P-selectin mediates a reversible adherence to the vessel wall that is a requirement for the *recruitment of inflammatory cells*.

WESTERN BLOT

Western blotting is a method to detect specific proteins in a mixture of proteins, e.g., cellular lysates. It is used to measure the expression of specific proteins in cells. It can also be used to detect *antibodies* in serum against *allergens* (other methods would be *RAST*, *Phadiatop*, and *CAP-system*). In general, proteins are first separated on SDS-page, and then transferred to a nitrocellulose filter. These filters are then incubated with specific *antibodies* or serum, washed, and again incubated with secondary labeled antibodies to determine protein expression or the presence of allergen-specific antibodies.

WHEAL

A basic skin lesion, with an elevated, white, compressible, evanescent area produced by dermal *edema* and often surrounded by a red, axon-mediated flare.

WHEAT ALLERGEN

(See *flour allergens*.)

WHEEZE

A whistling sound made by air passing through a narrowed airway (see *airway obstruction*). Characteristically in *asthma*, there are polyphonic wheezes due to air passing through many different airways of different caliber. Wheeze can also be generated by upper airway narrowing, and can be confused with *stridor*. Monophonic wheeze is relatively less common but represents partial obstruction of a single airway, as happens in lung cancer, localized plugging, or localized bronchial stenosis.

WHO/IUIS NOMENCLATURE

(See *allergen nomenclature*.)

WISKOTT–ALDRICH SYNDROME

Wiskott-Aldrich syndrome is a rare, hereditary, X-linked recessive, congenital syndrome with the triad of thrombocytopenia, eczematous skin lesions resembling *atopic dermatitis*, and an immune defect (bacterial, viral, and fungal infections). Patients surviving to adolescence have a tendency toward malignant lymphoma. The *gene* is located on *chromosome* X p11.22-p11.23 and encodes for WASP, a protein likely to be involved in CD43 expression (see *CD antigens*).

W-LOCUS

(See *mast-cell-deficient mice*.)

WOOD DUST

Occupational asthma may be due to exposure to wood dust. Western red cedar is the most common cause. Plicatic acid is the chemical responsible for red cedar *asthma*. The pathogenic mechanisms are not known. *IgE* specific to plicatic acid can be demonstrated in only 20% of the patients. Other types of wood such as oak, mahogany, African maple, African zebra wood, Central America walnut, California redwood, Cocabolla, Iroko, and Kejaat have also been reported to cause asthma.

WOOL INTOLERANCE

The cutaneous intolerance to wool clothing, a feature typical of *atopic dermatitis*, is one of the diagnostic features from the *Hanifin–Rajka criteria*.

WOUND HEALING

Wound healing is a continuum that begins immediately after injury and may proceed for long periods of time. Different overlapping phases have been identified in tissue response to injury: *inflammation*, granulation tissue, *extracellular matrix* formation, and *remodeling*. *Mast cells* participate in all stages of this process, because of their effect on vascular permeability, angiogenesis, and *collagen* formation by *fibroblasts*. Among the various mast cell *mediators* released during *mast cell activation*, *histamine* was shown to enhance human lung fibroblast proliferation.

X, Y, Z

XANTHINE

(See *phosphodiesterase inhibitors*.)

XEROSIS

More a dermatologic lesion than a skin disease, xerosis represents an ill-defined state of dry, non-smooth skin (see *dry skin*) with an increased transepidermal water loss and a disturbance of the epidermal lipid distribution.

X-LINKED DISEASES

Diseases caused by mutations of *genes* that are located on the X *chromosome* (see *hyper-IgM-syndrome, Wiskott–Aldrich syndrome*).

X-RAY CRYSTALLOGRAPHY

Technique for determining the *three-dimensional structure* of macromolecules. A beam of X-rays is applied to a crystal of the protein of interest; electrons of the protein scatter the X-rays, and the diffracted beams are detected by film or by an electronic detector. The image of the protein is reconstructed from the intensities of the diffracted waves, or reflections, which are proportional to the number of electrons at a given position in the crystal. Initially, the reflections are mathematically manipulated by Fourier transform into an electron density map, and the structure is then interpreted from this map. X-ray crystallographic analysis has been helpful in understanding how *conformational epitopes* from *allergens* initiate *B cell antigen receptor* and *high-affinity IgE receptor* activation, and therefore *immediate hypersensitivity* reactions.

YEAST INFECTION

Oropharyngeal candidiasis has been documented as a side effect of *inhaled corticosteroids*. Large-volume *spacer devices* prevent the deposition of these drugs in the oropharynx, and therefore reduce the risk of yeast infections.

ZAFIRLUKAST

A potent *leukotriene receptor antagonist*.

ZILEUTON

A potent *5-lipoxygenase inhibitor*.